Health and Development Across the Lifespan

Health and Development Across the Lifespan

Editor: Bernard Yates

MURPHY & MOORE
www.murphy-moorepublishing.com

www.murphy-moorepublishing.com

MURPHY & MOORE

Cataloging-in-Publication Data

Health and development across the lifespan / edited by Bernard Yates.
p. cm.
Includes bibliographical references and index.
ISBN 978-1-63987-296-1
1. Health. 2. Human growth. 3. Life cycle, Human. 4. Medical care.
5. Health promotion. I. Yates, Bernard.
RA776.5 .H43 2022
613--dc23

Murphy & Moore Publishing,
1 Rockefeller Plaza,
New York City, NY 10020, USA

ISBN 978-1-63987-296-1 (Hardback)

Contents

Preface

The research on health and development across the lifespan primarily focuses on four specific age groups. These divisions are small children, older children, adults and elderly. Life course health development (LCHD) is a framework that explains how the dynamic course of health and illness develops over an individual's lifetime and how this knowledge can be used to guide new approaches to policy and research. It shows that the health of an individual is a result of multiple determinants such as biological, social, genetic, behavioral and economic circumstances that change as a person develops. LCHD also shows that development of health is an adaptive process that is governed by multiple transactions between these circumstances and bio-behavioral regulatory systems that define human functions. It offers a conceptual model for health development and an approach to understand diseases on the basis of the relationship between experience and biology. This book outlines the processes and applications of life course health development in detail. It will also provide interesting topics for research which interested readers can take up. The extensive content of this book provides the readers with a thorough understanding of the subject.

This book is a comprehensive compilation of works of different researchers from varied parts of the world. It includes valuable experiences of the researchers with the sole objective of providing the readers (learners) with a proper knowledge of the concerned field. This book will be beneficial in evoking inspiration and enhancing the knowledge of the interested readers.

In the end, I would like to extend my heartiest thanks to the authors who worked with great determination on their chapters. I also appreciate the publisher's support in the course of the book. I would also like to deeply acknowledge my family who stood by me as a source of inspiration during the project.

Editor

1

Using the Panel Study of Income Dynamics (PSID) to Conduct Life Course Health Development Analysis

Narayan Sastry, Paula Fomby, and Katherine McGonagle

1 Introduction

The Panel Study of Income Dynamics (PSID) is a nationally representative, longitudinal study of families in the USA that began in 1968—nearly 50 years ago. It is the longest-running household panel survey in the world, and has been the model for similar studies launched in a number of other countries. Data from PSID are widely used by researchers for scientific and public policy research. The study is a unique resource for answering many questions that can be answered with no other data source.

PSID data are a cornerstone of social science research in the USA. To date, approximately 3800 publications have used PSID data, including over 700 dissertations. Nine US federal agencies use the data in fulfilling their missions. Each year, nearly 25,000 data extracts are downloaded by over 2500 different users, and there are nearly five million visits to the PSID web site. As an indicator of its significance, the study's lead sponsor, the National Science Foundation (NSF), named PSID one of the 60 most important innovations that NSF played a key role in creating.

N. Sastry (✉) • P. Fomby • K. McGonagle
Survey Research Center, Institute for Social Research, University of Michigan,
426 Thompson Street, Ann Arbor, MI 48106, USA
e-mail: nsastry@umich.edu

PSID's innovative design, broad content, and long duration have been central to understanding many key research and policy issues, including income and poverty dynamics; demographic behavior such as marriage and cohabitation, teen childbearing, and migration; child health and development; cyclical behavior of wages, labor supply, and consumption; savings and wealth accumulation; disparities in health and health behaviors including obesity, exercise, and smoking; the intergenerational transmission of socioeconomic status; and the effects of neighborhoods. PSID data have shaped a new and still emerging definition of economic well-being by transforming research in this area from a static and narrow view of rich and poor to a dynamic one in which families experience episodes of poverty or affluence (e.g., Brooks-Gunn and Duncan 1997; Hirschl et al. 2003; Sandoval et al. 2009; Rank and Hirschl 2014) and shocks to wealth (e.g., Stephens 2001; Conley and Thompson 2013). The growing number of three- and four-generation families is now supporting important new analyses of multigenerational associations in socioeconomic status attainment (e.g., Sharkey and Elwert 2011; Hertel and Groh-Samberg 2014; Pfeffer 2014; Wightman and Danziger 2014).

Across these and other topics, research based on PSID data has demonstrated the importance of a life course approach, in which factors much earlier in life have lasting influences on outcomes later in life. The PSID data allow researchers unique opportunities to test specific hypotheses that emerge from the seven principles of life course health development (see Halfon and Forrest 2017). In particular, by spanning the entire life course from conception to death, the study allows researchers to focus on multiple specific life course functional phases for individuals within their social and economic context. Researchers can examine *generativity* by examining the family and socioeconomic context of mothers during the preconception and prenatal period; *acquisition of capacity*, through components of the study that focus on health and development during childhood; *maintenance of capacity*, by examining how individuals function across the prime adult years; and *managing decline*, through focused components of PSID that examine how individuals manage, adjust, and adapt to old age (see Halfon and Forrest 2017: Principle 2, health development evolves over the life course).

Beginning in the late 1990s, several developments further increased the research potential of the PSID archive for studying life course health development. Most notably, content was expanded in the areas of health, wealth, expenditures, philanthropy, development, the transition to adulthood, and time use. Two important supplements were also added to the study, focusing on child health and development and the young adult years.

In this chapter we provide a profile of PSID and its recent supplemental studies, highlighting features that support life course health development research. In the next section, we describe the origins of PSID. We then provide an overview of the design and evolution of PSID. This is followed by a description of the content of the PSID interviews and the unique features of PSID for life course health development analysis. Next, we provide an introduction to PSID supplements that focus on children and young adults—the Child Development Supplement and the Transition into Adulthood Supplement. We then provide illustrations of topics of life course health development research using PSID, highlighting prominent studies that have used the PSID data. This is followed by a description of PSID's companion international studies. Finally, we explain how to obtain data from PSID and its supplements and end the chapter with an outline of future plans for the PSID project.

2 Origins of PSID[1]

PSID started with the "War on Poverty," which President Lyndon B. Johnson launched in the 1960s. Although the Social Security Retirement, Unemployment Insurance, and the Aid to Dependent Children programs were established in the mid-1930s at the height of the Great Depression, welfare programs were greatly expanded in the mid-1960s with the establishment of the Food Stamp Program in 1964, Medicare and Medicaid in 1965, and the School Lunch and Breakfast Programs in 1966. In order to assess the effectiveness of these new programs, the US Office of Economic Opportunity directed the US Bureau of the Census to design and field a survey that was later named the Survey of Economic Opportunity (SEO). In 1966 and 1967, SEO conducted interviews with approximately 30,000 households.

There was subsequently an interest at the Office of Economic Opportunity in extending the duration of the SEO study, in order to better understand the dynamics of poverty. However, there was also a desire to avoid the bureaucratic difficulties associated with conducting the study through the Census Bureau. These circumstances led the Office of Economic Opportunity to the Survey Research Center (SRC) at the University of Michigan and to commissioning SRC to conduct a 5-year follow-up survey with approximately 2000 low-income households from SEO.

The goal of the SEO follow-up study was to understand a number of crucial and highly policy-relevant issues related to poverty dynamics. A key question was tracking the reasons for changes in household poverty over time. In particular, if

[1]This section draws on previous descriptions of the history of PSID, including publications by McGonagle et al. (2012), Brown et al. (1996), and Hill (1992).

household poverty rates were estimated at 20% each year over the 5-year study period, were the same 20% of households in poverty in each of those 5 years, or were households entering and leaving poverty during that time? In order to answer this question and other similar questions, it was essential for the study to include not just low-income households, but also to include a representative sample of nonpoor households. SRC researchers convinced the Office of Economic Opportunity to launch the study with a nationally representative sample by adding 3000 households from the SRC national sampling frame to the 2000 households from the SEO sample. The 5000 households that comprised PSID at its launch in 1968 were representative of the entire US population, while also including a large oversample of low-income households.

A second major design innovation at the launch of the study was to incorporate into the sample the family members who "split off" from study households to form their own independent households. These split-off households were largely comprised of adult children of the original sample members who were forming their own nuclear families. This design feature allowed the study to remain representative over time of all (nonimmigrant) households and, combined with the study's high wave-to-wave response rates, led to substantial growth in the study's sample size and supported research on outcomes across multiple generations of the same family.

Although the study was planned to last for just 5 years, at the end of this initial period its considerable value became clear, and there was support for its continuation. At the same time, responsibility for PSID was shifted from the Office of Economic Opportunity to the Office of the Assistant Secretary for Planning and Evaluation in the US Department of Health, Education, and Welfare. As the study continued, its prominence grew steadily as a major data source for analyzing changes in poverty over time, over the life course, and across generations, as well as for studying a wide range of additional topics. In the early 1980s, the NSF became the primary sponsor for PSID. NSF currently initiates funding for PSID and provides the majority of support for the Core PSID component, although the National Institute on Aging and the *Eunice Kennedy Shriver* National Institute of Child Health and Human Development also provide major support for the Core PSID and additional funding comes from other sponsors and agencies such as the Food and Nutrition Service of the US Department of Agriculture. Since 1982, PSID has had an NSF-sponsored Board of Overseers that provides input to the study from a national and international community of researchers and survey research experts.

3 Design and Evolution of PSID

The Core PSID survey was conducted annually from 1968 through 1997 and has been conducted biennially since 1997. As of 2015, a total of 39 waves of data have been collected over 47 years. In 1997, because of the escalation in costs driven by the doubling of the sample size during its 30-year history, PSID was forced to drop some families from the study. The cuts were made from the SEO sample. Between 1997 and 1999, an immigrant refresher added to the PSID sample a total of 441 families who had moved to the USA between 1968 and 1997. Because some of the 441 immigrant families created split-off families, by 2013 the number of post-1968 immigrant families increased to 685. In 2013, the PSID sample comprised 9063 family units with 13,693 heads and spouses and 9747 other family members, for a total of 23,440 individuals. Table 1 shows the age composition in 2013 of PSID heads and spouses and other family members. Heads and spouses are largely prime-aged adults. Other

Table 1 PSID sample members (heads and spouses and other family members), by age, 2013

	Heads and spouses		Other family members	
Age group	N	%	N	%
≤18 years	20	0.1	7485	76.8
19–39	5917	43.2	1778	18.2
40–59	5009	36.6	285	2.9
60+	2747	20.1	199	2.0
All ages	13,693	100.0	9747	100.0

family members are largely composed of children and young adults—almost all of whom are the children of the heads and spouses. The 2013 interview was about 82 min in length, which is slightly higher than the average length of the post-1997 biennial interviews but about twice as long as the pre-1997 annual interviews.

Core PSID includes a telephone interview with a single respondent in each household, using computer-assisted interview software. Interviews are conducted by SRC's Survey Research Operations group, and households receive a financial incentive for completing the interview. The PSID respondent is typically the head or the spouse of the head, but may be another adult household member. An attempt is made to interview the same family member in each wave in order to maximize the consistency of respondent reports over time; approximately 95% of families that appear in successive waves have the same respondent for both interviews. The respondent provides information on himself or herself, the spouse or partner, other household members, and characteristics of the household. Individuals in PSID households are classified as other family members if, at the time of interview, they are members of the respondents' family and either residing in an interviewed family unit or temporarily away in an institution (e.g., college, jail, hospital, or the military). Family members are individuals who are related to the head or spouse by blood, marriage, or adoption, although unrelated individuals are included in the family unit if they are permanently living together and share income and expenses. PSID's tracking rules call for following the sample members' children, who are themselves classified as sample members and are eligible for tracking as separate family units when they set up their own economically independent households. Adult sample members who move out of PSID family units are tracked to their new family units (see Hill 1992). Two strengths of the PSID sample are the large representation of African-Americans and families below the poverty line. Across all ages, approximately one-third of individuals in PSID families are African-American, and 14% reside in families below the poverty line; among children, 41% are black and over 20% are in poor families.

Consistently achieving high response rates is critical to the success of a long-term panel study such as PSID. Although most cross-sectional surveys and other telephone surveys have experienced major declines in response rates over the past several years (Curtin et al. 2005; National Research Council 2013), PSID has experienced no such decline (Schoeni et al. 2013). In fact, the study's response rates in the most recent waves have been as high as any in its nearly 50-year history. PSID has achieved reinterview response rates of 96–98% in virtually every wave. In 2003 and later, the 1997 immigrant sample's reinterview response rate increased to more than 93% on average. These high rates are attributable to a number of factors, including incentive payments, experienced interviewers matched with the same families, use of tailored techniques to address respondents' concerns, and inter-wave communications with respondents.

Despite PSID's extremely high wave-to-wave response rates, the cumulative loss to follow-up after nearly 50 years now exceeds 40%. Attrition has been higher for certain groups—in particular, for men and low-income individuals. However, PSID's weights are designed to adjust for attrition (Gouskova et al. 2009), after incorporating the original sampling probabilities (see Heeringa and Connor 1999). Weighted PSID estimates show close agreement with estimates based on corresponding samples from benchmark studies, including income to the Current Population Survey (Gouskova et al. 2010), wealth to the Survey of Consumer Finances (Bosworth and Anders 2008; Pfeffer et al. 2014), expenditures to the Consumer Expenditure Survey (Li et al. 2010; Andreski et al. 2014), health behaviors and outcomes to the National Health Interview Survey (Andreski et al. 2009), and children's demographic characteristics to the American Community Survey (Sastry and Duffy 2012). Moreover, research suggests that attrition is random within families (Wiemers et al. 2010), does not account for health-wealth relationships (Meer et al. 2003) or the substantial intergenerational correlations in income (Schoeni and Wiemers forthcoming), and does not consistently bias sibling models (Fitzgerald 2011).

4 PSID Interview Content

PSID interviews collect information on a wide range of economic, demographic, social, and health topics. However, a considerable focus is on individual and household economic status, with detailed information collected on employment, earnings, income from other sources, consumption expenditures, welfare program participation, borrowing and saving, and wealth. Table 2 summarizes the PSID instrument content in PSID's most recent wave, which was fielded in 2013. Many of these content domains, and many specific questions, have been included in the instrument since 1968.

PSID has collected an increasing amount of health content over the years. Beginning in 1968, information was collected on work and activity limitations, health insurance, smoking and alcohol use, and mortality. Data were later added on workers' compensation (1977), hospital and nursing care (1982), general health status and Social Security Disability Insurance (1984), and exercise, height, and weight (1986). A major increase in health content in the 1990s added information on activities of daily living and instrumental activities of daily living (1992) and health conditions, health expenditures, and general health status in childhood (1999).

Table 2 Core PSID instrument content in 2013

Section	Description of content
Roster	Family composition update, split-off information, location of family unit members
A	Housing, utilities, computer use
B, C, D, E	Employment
F	Housework, child care, food expenses, and food assistance
F	Transportation, education expenses, other expenditures
G	Income
G	Education updates for other family unit members
H	Health status and behavior, health insurance, health-care use and expenditures
J	Marriage, fertility, and newborn children
K and L	New head or spouse background and existing head and spouse updates, including education
M	Philanthropic giving, volunteering, religiosity, help received
P	Pensions
R	Off-year income and welfare receipt
W	Wealth and active savings; intergenerational transfers of time and money

Two Core PSID modules offer special opportunities for life course health development research. First, the childhood health calendar, which was added in 2007, asks a series of retrospective questions for the household head and spouse about health conditions that arose during their own childhood including asthma, diabetes, respiratory disorders, speech impairment, depression, drug or alcohol problems, and other emotional problems. These data appear to have high validity (Smith 2009) and allow researchers to examine the effects of health conditions on life course health development by providing markers very early in the life span. Second, beginning in 2009, new questions were added to Core PSID about mortgage distress, including foreclosure activity, falling behind in payments, mortgage modifications, and expectations about payment difficulties in the coming year. These data support research on the medium-term effects of the recent economic recession for family formation and dissolution, childbearing, and educational attainment. Researchers can examine, for instance, whether higher unemployment rates and declines in income and wealth have led young adults to postpone or avoid higher education, marriage and cohabitation, and childbearing.

5 Unique Features of PSID for Life Course Analysis

The extended time series and high response rates of PSID provide substantial analytic power to study the antecedents of a range of social, economic, and health factors as well as their effects on life course health development. PSID's design supports research based on several different analytical perspectives. First, PSID provides a nationally representative cross-sectional sample of families and of children and adults of all ages. Cross-sectional analyses based on PSID data are able to draw on a rich set of covariates that describe individual and family background characteristics, behavior, and outcomes. The vast majority of PSID respondents are themselves—or have family members who were—part of the original 1968 sample (the remainder come from the 1997 immigrant refresher samples), providing information (as of 2015) from 39 waves of data collection. Moreover, PSID now collects retrospective childhood health measures for all household heads and their partners and obtains them for new entrants (who marry into or split from a family unit) making this content available irrespective of timing of entry into the study.

Second, PSID provides prospective panel data for conducting longitudinal analyses of individuals and families. PSID follows adults over the entire life course, and hence, the number of observations for an individual is related to his or her current age and age at entry into the sample. However, individuals who were born into PSID families also have information on their childhood circumstances from their parents' reports. This combination of information on childhood circumstances and later adult behavior and outcomes represents a major analytical strength of PSID that supports a variety of different analyses. Moreover, these analytical samples are large—for instance, over 2700 children who were under 18 years of age in 1968 and were residing in the original PSID families have been followed for 43 years by the 2011 wave.

Third, PSID provides rich intergenerational and intragenerational samples. The intergenerational sample is composed of adult children of respondents who split off from their parents to form their own households and who are recruited into the study. In the 2011 wave of PSID, there were 4800 parent-child pairs in which both the parent and the adult child completed a core interview. This sample supports analyses of concurrent effects of one (or more) generations on another—for example, how current parental or grandparental circumstances affect adult children's outcomes (and vice versa). In 2011, PSID interviewed over 1200 triples that included grandparents, parents, and adult children. These data provide unique opportunities for research on the equality or inequality in opportunity and the extent to which the life prospects of youth in the USA are shaped by their parents' and grandparents' social and economic status. For many PSID families, self-reported information is currently available on up to four generations within the same family at various points in their life course. Intragenerational analyses using PSID have focused on outcome comparisons among siblings (and, to a lesser extent, among cousins) as a means to control for, or examine, unmeasured family effects. In PSID in 2011, there were 3647 pairs of siblings in which both were interviewed as a head or partner. As the size of PSID's three-generation sample increases, so too does the number of first cousins (who share a common grandmother and grandfather). In 2011, there were 4330 first-cousin pairs in PSID participating as a head or partner.

6 PSID Supplements Focusing on Children and Young Adults

From its inception, the Core PSID interview has collected information primarily about the activities and characteristics of adult household members, with the largest share of data pertaining to the head of household and his spouse or partner. As a result, PSID supports research on intragenerational and intergenerational mobility in adulthood, but has historically lacked direct, prospective measures of childhood experience to operationalize theoretically informed models of the role of early life events and circumstances in shaping adult status attainment and mobility.

6.1 Original PSID Child Development Supplement

To address this limitation, in 1997 PSID launched the Child Development Supplement (CDS) to gather longitudinal information on children in PSID families. The original CDS sample included up to two randomly selected children aged 0–12 years ($N = 3563$ at Wave I of CDS) and their primary caregivers (who were usually the children's mother). Eligible CDS participants were descended by blood or adoption from the original 1968 PSID lineage or the 1997 PSID immigrant refresher sample. In most cases, this means that the child's father or mother is the child or grandchild of an original 1968 PSID respondent. Following a longitudinal cohort design, the same children and their caregivers were reinterviewed in 2002/2003 and again in 2007/2008 with a child-based response rate of approximately 90% in each wave.

The content of CDS is shaped by the theoretical perspective that child development is determined by financial, time, and social-psychological resources. Research in this area generally views resources very broadly, defining them to include purchased resources, time, interpersonal connections, and institutions that parents, schools, and communities may use to promote the development of children (e.g., Bronfenbrenner 1979; Bronfenbrenner and Morris 2006). Access to and use of these resources shape the future health, cognitive ability, and productive social behavior of children, with development at each age building upon levels attained in previous periods (Kail 2006; Shonkoff and Phillips 2000). The design of the CDS instrument also incorporates the main pathways through which the intergenerational transmission of social, economic, and health status is theorized to operate—such as wealth, human capital, learning at home and at school, kin, local institutions, social interactions, and genetic factors.

To build a comprehensive portrait of family resources and child development, CDS collected information from multiple reporters in a variety of modes. Table 3 provides an overview of the measures collected in CDS. At each wave, primary caregivers completed a telephone interview about their own and their children's characteristics and home, school, and neighborhood environments.

Table 3 Domains and measures in the original CDS and in the new CDS

Domain	Measures
Child health status and behavior	*PCG*: Child's general health rating; chronic conditions; limitations; health-care use and expenditures *Child*: General health rating; nutrition; exercise; sleep; smoking; sexual behavior; height and weight for BMI; and weight status (underweight, normal, risk for overweight, and overweight)
Child psychological and social well-being	*PCG*: Child's internalizing and externalizing behavior problems index (BPI); positive behaviors scale; social well-being; closeness with parents, absent parent, and siblings *Child*: Relationship with parents, siblings, friends, peers, and romantic partners; depression, self-esteem, worry, social well-being; risky behaviors, thrill seeking, antisocial behaviors; drug and alcohol abuse/dependence; dating behaviors; parental psychological control; initiative; languishing and flourishing; non-cognitive skills such as self-regulation, optimism, conscientiousness, and coping
Family environment	*PCG*: Child's *home* environment; conflict with father and mother; financial training; whether child has an allowance and savings; whether child has own bank account; parental warmth; involvement in daily activities and school; household tasks; parental aggravation; disagreement in parenting
Parental monitoring	*PCG*: Caregivers' knowledge of the child's whereabouts, activities, and associations *Child*: Child disclosure of activities, family rules, and limits
Child education	*PCG*: Child's enrollment; type of school; tuition; attendance; participation in federal lunch and breakfast programs; participation in special class/school for gifted students; classified as needing special education; repeated grade; dropped out; parental expectations for future schooling *Child*: Goals and expectations for own future schooling and academic success; attitudes toward and connectedness with school; ability self-concepts for reading and math; peer bullying

(continued)

Table 3 (continued)

Domain	Measures
School environment	*NCES-CCD* and *PSS*: School type; student racial/ethnic composition; other enrollment characteristics; pupil/teacher ratio; completion rates; expenditures per child; other school resources *Child*: Perceived characteristics of school and classroom; discrimination experience by race, sex, etc.
Cognitive achievement	*Child*: Courses and grades; rewards, including awards and honors received *Assessment*: WISC-III Digit Span short-term memory; forward and backward scores
Child care	*PCG*: Child's type of care, frequency of use, and costs of arrangements
Child time use	*PCG*: Child's stylized time use on structured and unstructured extracurricular activities; costs and frequency of participation; activities with parents *Child*: Stylized time use on sport; extracurricular, community, religious, and part-time work activities; frequency of participation and peer group involvement *Time diary*: Child's type, number, duration, location of activities for 1 weekday and 1 weekend day; social context of activities describing who participated with child
Religiosity	*Child*: Comfort, importance of religious affiliation, or spirituality
Future work, family, and schooling expectations	*Child*: Negative economic expectations; achieved occupational certainty and identity; job values, career orientation, and expectations for future; ideal age at marriage and birth of children; attitudes toward marriage and childbearing out of wedlock; understanding of the implications of having a child, of leaving school
Sib relationships	*Child*: Type and frequency of cooperation with sibs, kindness, and helping behaviors toward sibs
PCG sociopsychological characteristics	*PCG*: Rosenberg self-esteem; Pearlin self-efficacy; psychological distress and well-being; social support; parenting attitudes and styles; family conflict; economic strain; work schedules; community involvement
Child expenses and savings	*PCG*: Child's expenses; savings mechanisms for child, including savings for future postsecondary education
Absent parents	*PCG*: Frequency/types of activities absent parents are involved with their children; conflict between resident and absent parent

During a home visit, children aged 8–17 years completed an interviewer-administered questionnaire, and older children (ages 12–17 years) responded to an audio computer-assisted self-interview covering more sensitive topics such as sexual behavior and drug and alcohol use. Children and primary caregivers also completed cognitive tests from the Woodcock-Johnson Revised battery that assessed reading and math skills and provided height and weight measurements during the home visit. A restricted-use data file includes school identifiers that analysts may link to administrative data to incorporate information about CDS participants' school composition and quality.

CDS is unique among national child health development studies for its inclusion of diaries of children's time use. At each wave, time diary instruments were mailed to households prior to the interviewer's home visit. Children (or caregivers acting on behalf of younger children) were assigned to complete diaries on one randomly selected weekday and weekend day. Each time diary provides a chronological report of a child's activities over a specified 24-hours period, beginning at midnight. It collected information about the flow of activities, such as what the child was doing at that time, when the activity began and ended, and what else they were doing (if they were engaged in multiple activities), as well as asking questions about who was doing the activity with the child and who else was present. These questions provide information on the extent and nature of both parent/child interactions and the more general availability of parents. These questions also provide unbiased estimates about activities that children do with their siblings, their peers, and nonfamily adults. The time diaries include specific questions about media use whenever it is mentioned, yielding information about the total time spent using media, the timing of media use during the day, the content of media used (e.g., names of television programs, movies, web sites, and electronic games), and the social context of media use (e.g., who was participating with the child).

6.2 The PSID Transition into Adulthood Supplement

In recognition that the early years of adulthood (ages 18–26 years) are critical for life span development, PSID began a new study in 2005 designed to follow the children from CDS who had turned age 18 years and had completed or left high school and had families still active in PSID, called the Transition into Adulthood Supplement (TAS). The primary scientific aim of TAS was to understand the causes and consequences of social, economic, and health transitions of young adults. To describe significant milestones in the transition to adulthood in their developmental context, TAS bridges substantive content from the CDS and the Core PSID survey instruments, in addition to introducing new age-appropriate content areas. Information is collected about educational pursuits, employment, occupational choices, education and career expectations, family responsibilities, skills and abilities, intimate relationships, and more. TAS respondents who also respond to the Core PSID interview (with eligibility based on establishing their own independent household) have a shorter TAS instrument because many of the questions of interest (e.g., employment and income) are already asked in the Core PSID interview.

Across CDS and TAS, detailed information is available about development from early and middle childhood through adolescence and into adulthood. Additional information will be collected on this cohort over its life course as these youth transition to economic independence and become Core PSID respondents. TAS data have been collected biennially for 2005–2013 and will be collected through 2015 at which time all children from CDS will have been observed at least once in the study. For 2017 and beyond, a successor study to TAS is planned. As of 2013, 2571 young adults had participated in at least one wave of TAS. The response rate for TAS was 90% in the most recent wave.

6.3 2014 Child Development Supplement

By 2013, all children in the original CDS cohort had aged into adulthood. A new round of CDS began in 2014 to collect information on the next generation of children in PSID families. The new CDS includes all children who were aged 0–17 years during the 2013 Core PSID interview and their primary caregivers (approximately 5800 children and 3300 primary caregivers). This universe represents two design changes compared to earlier rounds of CDS: first, the sample includes all eligible children in a household, rather than a limit of two children; and, second, the age range has been expanded to include all years in childhood and adolescence. In the future, CDS will adopt a steady-state model in which previously recruited children and their caregivers will be reinterviewed every 5 years until children reach adulthood and children born since the last round of the study will be added to the sample. This will produce a longitudinal data resource that is also cross-sectionally representative of children of all ages at each wave.

Primary caregivers in the new CDS participate in a computer-assisted 75-min telephone interview. Children aged 12–17 years complete a 30-min interviewer-administered questionnaire by telephone and then transition to a computerized telephone interview administered by interactive voice response (IVR) technology to answer questions on sensitive topics. The IVR approach was adopted in order to protect respondent privacy and confidentiality and to maximize data validity. To permit analysis of changes over time and across cohorts, all of the content domains from the original CDS are maintained in the new CDS caregiver and child interviews. Changes in the instrument reflect theoretical and methodological advancements in the relevant disciplines and the goal of a shorter overall instrument length. One significant addition is the expansion of questionnaire content about computer and media use. Children and primary caregivers report on the number and types of computers and other electronic devices used in the household; the types of online educational, social, and entertainment activities in which children engage; and household rules governing the use of computers and mobile devices. To date, no other nationally representative study of child development in the USA or elsewhere includes a similar level of detail about children's computer and media use. The new CDS provides a unique opportunity to study how health and social behavior correlate with children's use of digital technologies across the early life course.

The new CDS introduces two additional components of interest to health researchers. First, primary caregivers and children aged 5–17 years were asked to contribute saliva samples using an Oragene OG-500 DNA Genotek saliva kit for subsequent genetic analysis. This is the first effort to collect genetic material from two generations of family members in a large-scale nationally representative study. Second, primary caregivers were asked to complete administrative record linkage consent forms providing access to children's and caregivers' birth records and to children's school records including transcripts and state-standardized test scores for children aged 8 years and older. Birth record data provide objective, detailed information on children's health status at birth, and information from both the child and caregiver generation permit study of the intergenerational transmission of early health risk factors. State-standardized test scores obtained through school records data will provide objective measures of students' academic achievement, and school transcripts will summarize students' course taking and course performance, which are important predictors of eventual college readiness.

Finally, a randomly selected 50% of CDS 2014 households received supplemental home visits from interviewers. During these visits, children aged 3–17 years and caregivers completed the Woodcock-Johnson cognitive assessments used in previous rounds of CDS. Interviewers also reviewed and collected children's completed weekday and weekend time diaries and record home and neighborhood observations. Finally, during the in-person visits by interviewers, children aged 8–11 years complete an abbreviated version of the child questionnaire. Due to methodological constraints, these study components were not administered to families that were not selected for the supplemental home visit. Fieldwork for CDS 2014 began in October 2014 and is scheduled to end in April 2015. We expect to release final data from the study to researchers through the PSID Online Data Center in April 2016.

6.4 Life Course Health Development Analysis with CDS-TAS-PSID

With the addition of CDS and TAS to the PSID suite of studies, researchers have a comprehensive, nationally representative, prospective database of young children and their families for studying the dynamic process of child health development. Embedded in the context of PSID, CDS and TAS provide a unique framework for considering how long-range family background factors influence children's health development. As shown in Fig. 1, the value of these supplements continues to increase as sample children

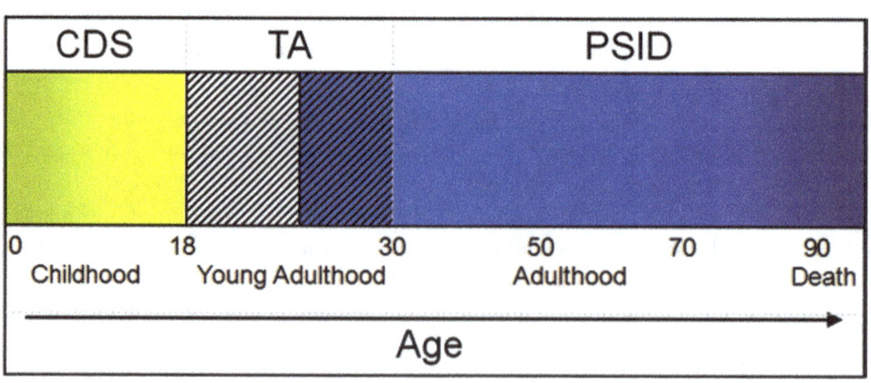

Fig. 1 Life course data from CDS-TAS-Core PSID

Table 4 Summary of key features of the original CDS, TAS, and the new CDS

	Child Development Supplement I–III (1997–2007)	Transition into Adulthood Supplement (2005–2015)	Child Development Supplement 2014
Sample eligibility	Up to two PSID children ages 0–12 years in 1997 and their primary (PCGs) and other caregivers (OCGs)	CDS children who finished or left high school and were ages 18–26 years	All PSID children ages 0–17 years in 2013 and their primary caregivers (PCGs)
Sample size	3563 children and 2394 PCGS/OCGs at Wave I	765 in 2005; 2000 in 2013	5300 children and 3000 caregivers (projected)
Response rate	Child-centered response rate of 88% at Wave I, 90% at Wave III	90% in most recent wave (2013)	Child-centered response rate of 88% (projected)
Interview mode and length	PCG: 35-min telephone or in-person Child: 20-min in-person OCG: mailback questionnaire Follow-up home visit to full sample	74-min telephone interview (for non-heads/spouses) or 51 min (for heads/spouses)	PCG: 75-min telephone Child (age 12–17 years), 30-min telephone + 15-min IVR; child (age 8–11 years, home visit sample only), 15-min in-person Follow-up home visit to half of sample
Cognitive assessments	PCG (Wave I only) and children ages 3–17 years (all waves): Woodcock-Johnson assessments of reading and math; WISC Digit Span	None	PCG and children ages 3–17 years (in-home sample): Woodcock-Johnson assessments of reading and math
Time diaries	Child: random weekday and weekend day		Child (in-home sample): random weekday and weekend day
Anthropometry	PCG and children: height and weight	Self-reported height and weight	PCG and children ages 2–17 years: height and weight
Biological samples	None	None	PCG and children (ages 5–17 years): saliva samples (Oragene OG-500 DNA Genotek saliva kit)
Administrative linkages (restricted data)	School characteristics from the National Center for Education Statistics' Common Core of Data and Private School Universe Survey Neighborhood characteristics based on residential location	Characteristics of postsecondary education institutions from the National Center for Education Statistics' Integrated Postsecondary Education Data System Neighborhood characteristics based on residential location	School characteristics from the National Center for Education Statistics' Common Core of Data and Private School Universe Survey. Future linkages to child and PCG birth records and child (age 8–17) school records Neighborhood characteristics based on residential location

age and form their own economically independent households and join the Core PSID as respondents. Table 4 summarizes the key features of the original CDS, TAS, and the new CDS.

As with Core PSID, the sample design of CDS and TAS makes it possible to analyze the data based on several different analytical perspectives. First, CDS and TAS provide nationally representative cross-sectional sample of children and young adults at each wave. Second, CDS and TAS support prospective analyses of outcomes using previously collected information on basic demographic, education, and socioeconomic outcomes, but will also provide baseline data for conducting longitudinal analyses of children and young adults. Third, CDS and TAS provide samples for conducting intergenerational and intragenerational analyses focused on childhood and the young adult years.

Almost all children in CDS and TAS have parents and grandparents who have been followed over many years in Core PSID. Approximately one-quarter of the new CDS children—a total of about 1500 children—will have a parent who participated in the original CDS and, subsequently, in the TAS study, providing extremely rich information about parent-child pairs that includes detailed developmental and behavioral data from both members of the dyad. These unique data will support innovative intergenerational analysis of key outcomes such as educational achievement, the acquisition of non-cognitive skills (e.g., self-regulation, conscientiousness, social competency, coping skills, and optimism), and behavioral problems when both individuals were children. The CDS and TAS intragenerational samples comprise of siblings and cousins. In both the original and new CDS, approximately 70% of children had a sibling in the study.

7 Topics of Life Course Research Using PSID

PSID data provide opportunities for conducting life course health development research on a variety of topics, including the dynamic process of early human capital formation; the intergenerational transmission of human capital and social capital, as well as health development assets; the historical family and contextual processes that may underlie both cohort and generational differences in children's health development; and issues related to continuity and change across generations in a wide variety of indicators of adaptive and maladaptive functioning. These data support studies of the ways in which time, social capital, and economic resources at the family, school, and neighborhood levels, as well as parenting practices and characteristics of caregivers, grandparents, extended family members, and siblings, are linked to health development over the full range of childhood, adolescence, and early adulthood. This section provides a small number of illustrations of the ways that PSID data have been used for life course health development research.

7.1 Fertility and Birth Outcomes

PSID is an important data source for understanding the causes and consequences of fertility and birth outcomes. The study has been a leading data source for understanding the causes and consequences of teen childbearing, with several articles published recently (e.g., Meadows et al. 2013; Sullivan et al. 2011; South and Crowder 2010; Wodtke 2013) that build on numerous PSID-based studies from the 1990s and early 2000s (Geronimus and Korenman 1992, 1993; Haveman et al. 1997, 2001; Corcoran and Kunz 1997; Hoffman et al. 1993; Foster and Furstenberg 1998; Foster et al. 1998). Studies of the determinants of fertility among women of all ages have examined the effects of child support (Anderson 2011), family wealth shocks (Lovenheim and Mumford 2013), and neighborhood poverty (South and Crowder 2010). PSID has become a key source of data to understand the effects of birth outcomes and health in early childhood on later health and well-being (Johnson and Schoeni 2011a, b; Johnson 2012; Johnson et al. 2012; Delaney and Smith 2012; Haas 2007; Smith 2009), reflecting the theoretical and empirical advances provided by Barker and colleagues (Barker 1998; Barker and Osmond 1986; Barker et al. 2001), by Wadsworth (1987, 1991), and by others (Kuh and Ben-Shlomo 1997; Kuh and Shlomo 2004; Hertzman and Power 2003).

7.2 Neighborhood Effects

The design of PSID and its supplements recognizes the theoretical perspective that human health development is determined by a broad set of family, social, cultural, and community resources (e.g., Bronfenbrenner 1979; Bronfenbrenner and Morris 2006). A major research focus based on this paradigm is the study of neighborhood effects on a variety of outcomes. The availability across the life course of PSID individuals' census tract of residence (and census block beginning in 2009) through a restricted-use contract permits the study of neighborhood effects. PSID has been used extensively to examine migration and the effects of neighborhoods, as evidenced by more than 400 publications on these topics with about half published in the past decade. PSID was one of the earliest data sources for studying contextual effects on socioeconomic status (Corcoran et al. 1990; Dachter 1982) and remains one of the most important and widely used sources across multiple disciplines for examining neighborhood effects on a variety of outcomes including child, adolescent, and young adult health development (Dearing et al. 2009; Jackson and Mare 2007; Timberlake 2009a, b; Wimer et al. 2008; Sharkey and Elwert 2011), health (Do and Finch 2008; Halliday 2007; Halliday and Kimmitt 2008; Johnson and Schoeni 2011b; Do et al. 2013; Wen and Shenassa 2012), education (Brooks-Gunn et al. 1993; Crowder and South 2003; Galster et al. 2007; Harding 2003; Crowder and South 2011; Galster et al. 2013; Wodtke et al. 2011), income and earnings (Islam and Tonmoy 2013; Sharkey 2008; Sharkey 2012), the intergenerational transmission of neighborhood context (Dawkins 2005a; Sharkey 2008; Sharkey and Elwert 2011; Solon et al. 2000), family migration and labor force outcomes (Blackburn 2010; Shauman 2010), and fertility behavior (South and Crowder 2010; South 1999, 2001a, b; South and Crowder 2010; Wodtke 2013). Because of its oversample of African-American families, the data have been used to examine levels and trends in racial equality in neighborhood economic status and migration (Sharkey 2008; Dawkins 2005b, 2006; Freeman 2005a, b, 2008; South and Crowder 2005; Timberlake 2007; White et al. 2005; Vartanian et al. 2007; Crowder and South 2005; Bruch 2014; Pais et al. 2012, 2014; Sharkey 2012; South et al. 2011; Wagmiller 2013).

7.3 Outcomes Across Generations of the Same Family

Because PSID follows adult children as they form their own households, it is uniquely positioned to investigate outcomes across generations of the same family. Recent studies have examined correlations across generations in health (Fitzgerald 2011; Vandewater et al. 2014; Lê-Scherban et al. 2014; Li 2015; Johnson and Schoeni 2011a), income (Bloome 2015; Chau 2012; Shore 2011), education (Roksa and Potter 2011; Torche 2011; Wightman and Danziger 2014), socioeconomic status (Eberharter 2014; Gouskova et al. 2010; Hertel and Groh-Samberg 2014), consumption expenditures (Charles et al. 2013), and cognitive ability (Sharkey and Elwert 2011). This recent research builds on the extensive work that began in the early 1990s (e.g., Corcoran et al. 1992; Solon 1992; Charles and Hurst 2003). In fact, because of the length of the panel, PSID has been used to estimate changes over time in the intergenerational transmission of economic status (Lee and Solon 2009; Mayer and Lopoo 2008). Researchers are also beginning to use the health data in conjunction with the socioeconomic data to examine the extent to which transmission of health across generations within the same family accounts for the transmission of socioeconomic status and vice versa (Johnson and Schoeni 2011b). Studies have used the CDS and TAS data in combination with the Core PSID data to examine associations across multiple generations. For example, a highly cited article in the *American Economic Review* examines the effect of parents' income on children's health to explain the intergenerational transmission of socioeconomic status (Case et al. 2002). The CDS child height and weight data were the basis of the first national study to examine the intergenerational transmission of body weight over three generations, finding an association of childhood obesity with grandparental obesity distinct from parental obesity (Davis et al. 2008).

7.4 Time Use

The CDS time diary data in particular have been the basis of a large and influential body of research examining the relationships among time spent in various activities, the family environment, and outcomes related to achievement, social and behavioral development, and health development. A frequently cited article in the *Journal of Marriage and Family* showed marked differences in child time use associated with poverty and maternal employment, with poor children spending substantially less time with fathers and more time with extended kin such as grandmothers; among poor children, those whose mothers were employed spent more time per week watching television, in daycare, and less time in sport activities (Yeung et al. 2001). Using the rich codes for television program content in CDS, an article in *JAMA Pediatrics* found that violent television programming was associated with an increased risk for antisocial behavior for boys but not for girls; neither educational nor nonviolent programming was associated with increased risk for boys or girls (Zimmerman and Christakis 2007). Several studies have used the time diary data to provide national portraits of time use among American children in various domains. A recent article in *JAMA Pediatrics* used the data to establish nationally representative sleep duration norms for US children (Williams et al. 2013). The CDS data were also featured in an article in the journal *Child Development* to document time spent by American children aged 6–12 years playing video games, using the computer, and watching TV in 1997 and 2003 and the association of early media use with academic achievement and behavior in adolescence and differences in outcomes by race (Hofferth 2010).

8 PSID's Companion International Surveys

PSID has a set of companion international studies with comparable samples and harmonized measures that allow researchers to conduct comparative international analysis of health and well-being outcomes across a range of key domains and across the life course. These companion studies are based in the UK (British Household Panel Survey/Understanding Society), Germany (Socio-Economic Panel), Canada (Survey of Labor and Income Dynamics), Australia (Household, Income and Labour Dynamics in Australia Survey), Switzerland (Swiss Household Panel), South Korea (Korea Labor and Income Panel Study), and South Africa (National Income Dynamics Study). Future studies that are planned or recently underway in China, Israel, and elsewhere will further enhance researchers' ability to conduct international comparative research that includes the USA. The Cross-National Equivalent File (CNEF) facilitates comparisons between PSID and many of these studies by providing a set of equivalently defined and constructed variables measuring income and other household attributes.

9 Obtaining Data from PSID and Its Supplements

The majority of PSID data and documentation is freely and publicly available on the Internet through the PSID Data Center (www.psidonline.org). Information is currently available on more than 70,000 variables, on approximately 75,000 individuals, and for all waves of the main PSID and its supplements. Users can create customized data extracts from any set of waves by searching or browsing for variables, obtain customized codebooks specific to their data extract, and archive data extracts for shared and later use. Data carts may be saved, allowing specific extracts to be shared with colleagues, reviewers, and students. A range of file formats is available when the user is ready to "check out," including widely used statistical software formats such as SAS, STATA, and SPSS. For researchers wishing to create genealogical samples, an application on the PSID web site called the Family Identification Mapping System (FIMS) automatically creates a customized file containing identifiers for PSID respondents' relatives (including biological and adoptive children, parents, grandparents, great-grandparents, and siblings). Online PSID courses, or webinars, are available to users on demand through the PSID web site to introduce the sample design and facilitate hands-on use of the PSID data for a variety of research purposes. PSID provides support to users through the PSID help desk, accessible by email at psidhelp@umich.edu.

PSID provides restricted data to authorized users under contract. Restricted data contain sensitive or potentially identifying information, and must be used in a secure data environment under a research plan approved by the user's institutional review board and by PSID administrators. Restricted data resources include a geocode-matched data file that provides the census tract and block codes for each dwelling occupied by PSID householders since 1968 and links PSID households to aggregated decennial census data (1970–2000) and American Community Survey data (2005 to the present). These data permit analyses of changing neighborhood context and the influence of neighborhood characteristics on health and well-being over time.

PSID has also developed links to administrative data sources in recent waves to expand opportunities for life course health development research on social context, health care, and outcomes. Since 2005, PSID has tracked known study decedents in the National Death Index (NDI). There are now nearly 6000 individuals from PSID families included in the PSID-restricted mortality files, which contain information on date of death, location of death, and International Statistical Classification of Diseases and Related Health Problems (ICD) codes for cause of death. In a separate Medicare claims file, up to 20 years of claims data (1991–2010) are available for approximately 2000 age-eligible PSID respondents and decedents. Claims data begin with a respondent's first service after Medicare entitlement, which is at age 65 or when qualification for disability insurance is met. Claims files include short-stay inpatient, skilled nursing facilities, hospital outpatient, physician/supplier, home health, and hospice services. Health plan enrollment files provide exact dates of respondent enrollment in Medicare health maintenance organizations. Although utilization information has not been reported for HMO enrollees in the past, characteristics of respondent health plans are reported. Summary files are compiled annually and by quarter.

Other external data sources provide information on housing and education. An assisted housing data file indicates whether each PSID family in every year through 2009 (except 1969, for which the addresses are not available) was living in a housing unit subsidized by the US Department of Housing and Urban Development, the Farmers Home Administration, through tax credits administered by the Department of Treasury, or state housing programs (Newman et al. 2009). PSID has also created linkable files for several data sources from the National Center for Education Statistics (NCES). Information from the Integrated Postsecondary Education Data System (IPEDS) describing the characteristics of post-secondary education institutions has been linked to the names of colleges that PSID heads and wives reported attending for all waves since 1975. Common Core of Data (CCD), Private School Universe Survey (PSS), and IPEDS data have also been linked to the CDS and TAS data and made available to users under restricted data use contract. Together, CCD and PSS provide general descriptive information on schools and school districts, data on students and staff, and fiscal data for nearly the entire universe of elementary and secondary schools attended by US students.

10 Conclusions and Future Plans

The history and evolution of PSID have resulted in a unique data set that spans 50 years, 10,000 households, and multiple generations of each family in the sample. These data have provided valuable insights into numerous topics related to life course research—most notably, the dynamics of poverty, its consequences for health development, childhood well-being, and its transmission across generations.

In this final section, we briefly discuss future plans for PSID that will likely enhance the value of the study for life course health development research. The main element of future planning for PSID is to continue the core interview every 2 years. In 2018, between the planned waves for Core PSID in 2017 and 2019, the study will mark its 50th anniversary—a major milestone for the study.

Plans for the next two waves of Core PSID include an addition to the study of a sample of post-1997 immigrants—that is, families who moved to the USA after 1997 (when PSID last added an immigrant refresher sample) and who would otherwise not be captured in the study. Screening and recruitment for this new immigrant refresher sample is planned for 2016 and 2017, with a target sample size of approximately 750 families. The proportion of the Core PSID sample these families would represent (approximately 7.5%) is similar to their representation among all US families (approximately 6.5%).

Adding a new immigrant refresher sample to PSID will provide many new research opportunities. The addition will increase the coverage of PSID's national representative sample, which is particularly salient for studying children's outcomes; expand diversity within the PSID sample, particularly by race and ethnicity; and support research that examines outcomes for new immigrant families. Hispanics are estimated to comprise 47% of the new immigrant refresher sample, Asians 26%, whites 16%, blacks 9%, and others 2%. We expect to conduct interviews with new immigrants in either English or Spanish (as is the case for Core PSID); due to cost constraints, we will likely exclude families who are unable to complete an interview in either English or Spanish. The new immigrant refresher sample will lead to virtually complete coverage by PSID of the national population of US families in 2017. The new immigrant refresher will also lead to PSID capturing the increasing diversity of the US population, especially by race and ethnicity and by immigration status. In 2017, we estimate that 12% of PSID's approximately 10,000 households will be Hispanic—a substantial increase from the current 8%. Researchers will be able to use these new data to study how the life course trajectories of individuals from recent immigrant families compare to those from nonimmigrant families and from immigrant families who arrived in earlier periods.

A second major future goal for PSID is to obtain genetic markers for all sample members. This effort has already begun, through the collection of saliva samples for children and primary caregivers in the new CDS. We expect in the future to expand the collection of saliva samples to other family members and families. Obtaining genetic markers for PSID individuals is among our top priorities because of the high scientific impact of new research on the genetic basis of social, economic, and health behavior. PSID's rich genealogical structure will allow researchers to investigate, and adjust for, the influence of gene-environment correlation by controlling for parents' and grandparents' genetic characteristics. It will allow for sharper gene-environment interaction estimates by using sibling differences—leading to better causal estimates. Among numerous topics, the data could be used to understand how genes interact with economic shocks in models that exploit both within-family and cross-time variation. Collecting genetic markers from all PSID sample members would distinguish PSID as the only national source in the USA for genetic data over multiple generations. Linking genetic information with life course data will open new opportunities to test theories that involve epigenetic and biological mechanisms (Jayasinghe 2011; Davey Smith 2012).

Future data collection activities include plans to repeat the CDS every 5 years. Future waves of CDS will collect data on all children from the previous wave who are still under age 18 years and will add all new children who were subsequently born or adopted into PSID households. We plan to field the next wave of the new CDS in 2019, on the heels of the Core PSID data collection for that year. PSID is also planning a separate initiative to directly interview all sample family members aged 18–26 years, whether they are primary respondents, spouses/partners, or other household members. This new project will build on the original TAS and will continue to focus on understanding the demographic, health, psychological, and socioeconomic development of young adults. The new CDS and the TAS successor together will offer researchers a unique opportunity to study pathways and outcomes from early and middle childhood through adolescence and into adulthood. Furthermore, the new CDS and TAS will allow researchers to study differences in early life course trajectories across cohorts, beginning with the original CDS cohort (born from 1985 to 1996) and continuing through to the most recent birth cohorts. Comparisons of life course trajectories across cohorts will provide insights into the effects of important period factors on child, adolescent, and young adult health development. For example, researchers will be able to examine the effects of the Great Recession on family behavior and outcomes and on children's health development and well-being, such as, whether parents' experience of unemployment and declines in income and wealth have led to lower investments in children (such as less schooling, a shift between private and public schools, less frequent visits to health-care providers, and changes in the time children and parents spend together and in their specific activities during this shared time).

Acknowledgment This document was supported by funding from the *Eunice Kennedy Shriver* National Institute of Child Health and Human Development (R01-HD069609; R01-HD059779; R01-HD072493; R01-HD052646).

References

Anderson, K. G. (2011). Does paying child support reduce Men's subsequent marriage and fertility? *Evolution and Human Behavior, 32*(2), 90–96.

Andreski, P., McGonagle, K. A., & Schoeni, R. F. (2009). Analysis of the quality of the health data in the panel study of income dynamics. Panel Study of Income Dynamics Technical Paper Series, #09-02.

Andreski, P., Li, G., Samancioglu, M. Z., & Schoeni, R. (2014). Estimates of annual consumption expenditures and its major components in the PSID in comparison to the CE. *The American Economic Review, 104*(5), 132–135.

Barker, D. J. P. (1998). *Mothers, babies and health in later life*. Edinburgh: Churchill Livingstone.

Barker, D. J., & Osmond, C. (1986). Infant mortality, childhood nutrition, and ischaemic heart disease in England and Wales. *Lancet, 1*(8489), 1077–1081.

Barker, D. J. P., Forsen, T., Uutela, A., Osmond, C., & Eriksson, J. G. (2001). Size at birth and resilience to effects of poor living conditions in adult life: Longitudinal study. *British Medical Journal, 323*(7324), 1273.

Blackburn, M. L. (2010). Internal migration and the earnings of married couples in the United States. *Journal of Economic Geography, 10*(1), 87–111.

Bloome, D. (2015). Income inequality and intergenerational income mobility in the United States. *Social Forces, 93*(3), 1047–1080.

Bosworth, B. B., & Anders, S. (2008). Savings and Wealth Accumulation in the PSID 1984–2005. Center for Retirement Research at Boston College Working Paper 2008–2.

Bronfenbrenner, U. (1979). *The ecology of human development*. Cambridge, MA: Harvard University Press.

Bronfenbrenner, U., & Morris, P. A. (2006). The bioecological model of human development. In R. M. Lerner & W. Damon (Eds.), *The handbook of child psychology, Vol. 1: Theoretical models of human development* (6th ed., pp. 793–828). Hoboken: Wiley.

Brooks-Gunn, J., Duncan, G. J., Klebanov, P. K., & Sealand, N. (1993). Do neighborhoods influence child and adolescent development? *American Journal of Sociology, 99*, 353–395.

Brooks-Gunn, J., & Duncan, G. J. (1997). The effects of poverty on children. *Children and Poverty, 7*(2), 55–71.

Brown, C., Duncan, G. J., & Stafford, F. P. (1996). Data watch: The panel study of income dynamics. *Journal of Economic Perspectives, 10*(2), 155–168.

Bruch, E. E. (2014). How population structure shapes neighborhood segregation. *American Journal of Sociology, 119*(5), 1221–1278.

Case, A., Lubotsky, D., & Paxson, C. (2002). Economic status and health in childhood: The origins of the gradient. *The American Economic Review, 92*, 1308–1334.

Charles, K. K., & Hurst, E. (2003). The correlation of wealth across generations. *Journal of Political Economy, 111*(6), 1155–1182.

Charles, K. K., Hurst, E., & Killewald, A. (2013). Marital sorting and parental wealth. *Demography, 50*(1), 51–70.

Chau, T. W. (2012). Intergenerational income mobility revisited: Estimation with an income dynamic model with heterogeneous age profile. *Economics Letters, 117*(3), 770–773.

Conley, D., & Thompson, J. (2013). The effects of health and wealth shocks on retirement decisions. *Federal Reserve Bank of St. Louis Review, 95*, 389–404.

Corcoran, M., & Kunz, J. P. (1997). Do unmarried births among African-American teens lead to adult poverty? *Social Service Review, 71*(2), 274–287.

Corcoran, M., Gordon, R., Laren, D., & Solon, G. (1990). Effects of family and community background on economic status. *The American Economic Review, 80*(2), 362–366.

Corcoran, M., Gordon, R., Laren, D., & Solon, G. (1992). The association between men's economic status and their family and community origins. *Journal of Human Resources, 27*(4), 575–601.

Crowder, K. D., & South, S. J. (2003). Neighborhood distress and school dropout: The variable significance of community context. *Social Science Research, 32*, 659–698.

Crowder, K. D., & South, S. J. (2005). Race, class and changing patterns of migration between poor and nonpoor neighborhoods. *American Journal of Sociology, 110*, 1715–1763.

Crowder, K. D., & South, S. J. (2011). Spatial and temporal dimensions of neighborhood effects on high school graduation. *Social Science Research, 40*(1), 87–106.

Curtin, R., Presser, S., & Singer, E. (2005). Changes in telephone survey nonresponse over the past quarter century. *Public Opinion Quarterly, 69*, 87–98.

Dachter, L. (1982). Effects of community and family background on achievement. *Review of Economics and Statistics, 64*, 32–41.

Davey Smith, G. (2012). Epigenesis for epidemiologists: Does evo-devo have implications for population health research and practice? *International Journal of Epidemiology, 41*(1), 236–247.

Davis, M., McGonagle, K., Schoeni, R., & Stafford, F. (2008). Grandparental and parental obesity influences on childhood overweight: Implications for primary care practice. *Journal of American Board of Family Medicine, 21*, 549–554.

Dawkins, C. J. (2005a). Evidence on the intergenerational persistence of residential segregation by race. *Urban Studies, 42*, 545–555.

Dawkins, C. J. (2005b). Racial gaps in the transition to first-time homeownership: The role of residential location. *Journal of Urban Economics, 58*, 537–554.

Dawkins, C. J. (2006). Are social networks the ties that bind families to neighborhoods? *Housing Studies, 21*, 867–881.

Dearing, E., Wimer, C., Simpkins, S. D., Lund, T., Bouffard, S. M., Caronongan, P., Kreider, H., & Weiss, H. (2009). Do neighborhood and home contexts help explain why low-income children miss opportunities to participate in activities outside of school? *Developmental Psychology, 45*, 1545–1562.

Delaney, L., & Smith, J. P. (2012). Childhood health: Trends and consequences over the life course. *The Future of Children, 22*(1), 43–63.

Do, D. P., & Finch, B. K. (2008). The link between neighborhood poverty and health: Context or composition? *American Journal of Epidemiology, 168*, 611–619.

Do, D. P., Wang, L., & Elliott, M. R. (2013). Investigating the relationship between neighborhood poverty and mortality risk: A marginal structural modeling approach. *Social Science and Medicine, 91*, 58–66.

Eberharter, V. V. (2014). The intergenerational dynamics of social inequality: Empirical evidence from Europe and the United States. *Global Journal of Human Social Science, 14*(1), 95–108.

Fitzgerald, J. M. (2011). Attrition in models of intergenerational links using the PSID with extensions to health and to sibling models. *The B.E. Journal of Economic Analysis and Policy, 11*(3), 3444.

Foster, E. M., & Furstenberg, F. F. (1998). Most disadvantaged children: Who are they and where do they live? *Journal of Poverty, 2*(2), 23–47.

Foster, E. M., Jones, D., & Hoffman, S. (1998). The economic impact of nonmarital childbearing: How are older, single mothers faring? *Journal of Marriage and the Family, 60*(1), 163–174.

Freeman, L. (2005a). Black homeownership: The role of temporal changes and residential segregation at the end of the 20th century. *Social Science Quarterly, 86*, 403–426.

Freeman, L. (2005b). Displacement or succession? Residential mobility in gentrifying neighborhoods. *Urban Affairs Review, 40*, 463–491.

Freeman, L. (2008). Is class becoming a more important determinant of neighborhood attainment for African-Americans? *Urban Affairs Review, 44*, 3–26.

Galster, G., Marcotte, D. E., Mandell, M., Wolman, H., & Augustine, N. (2007). The influence of neighborhood poverty during childhood on fertility, education and earnings outcomes. *Housing Studies, 22*, 723–751.

Galster, G., Marcotte, D. E., Mandell, M., Wolman, H., & Augustine, N. (2013). The influence of neighborhood poverty during childhood on fertility, education and earnings outcomes. In J. Blasius, J. Friedrichs, & G. Galster (Eds.), *Quantifying neighbourhood effects: Frontiers and perspectives* (pp. 95–123). New York: Routledge.

Geronimus, A. T., & Korenman, S. (1992). The socioeconomic consequences of teen childbearing reconsidered. *Quarterly Journal of Economics, 109*(4), 1187–1214.

Geronimus, A. T., & Korenman, S. (1993). The socioeconomic costs of teenage childbearing: Evidence and interpretation. *Demography, 30*(2), 281–290.

Gouskova, E., Heeringa, S. G., McGonagle, K. A., Schoeni, R., & Stafford, F. (2009). Construction and Evaluation of the Longitudinal Sample Weights, Panel Study of Income Dynamics, Working Paper, Institute for Social Research, University of Michigan.

Gouskova, E., Chiteji, N., & Stafford, F. (2010). Estimating the intergenerational persistence of lifetime earnings with life course matching: Evidence from the PSID. *Labor Economics, 17*, 592–597.

Haas, S. A. (2007). The long-term effects of poor childhood health: An assessment and application of retrospective reports. *Demography, 44*(1), 113–135.

Halfon, N., & Forrest, C. B. (2017). The emerging theoretical framework of life course health development. In N. Halfon, C. B. Forrest, R. M. Lerner, & E. Faustman (Eds.), *Handbook of life course health-development science*. Cham: Springer.

Halliday, T. J. (2007). Business cycles, migration and health. *Social Science and Medicine, 64*, 1420–1424.

Halliday, T. J., & Kimmitt, M. (2008). Selective migration and health in the USA, 1984–1993. *Population Studies, 62*, 321–334.

Harding, D. (2003). Counterfactual models of neighborhood effects: The effect of neighborhood poverty on high school dropout and teenage pregnancy. *American Journal of Sociology, 109*(3), 676–719.

Haveman, R., Wolfe, B., & Wilson, K. (1997). Childhood poverty and adolescent schooling and fertility outcomes: Reduced-form and structural estimates. In G. J. Duncan & J. Brooks-Gunn (Eds.), *Consequences of growing up poor* (pp. 419–460). New York: Russell Sage Foundation.

Haveman, R., Wolfe, B., & Pence, K. (2001). Intergenerational effects of nonmarital and early childbearing. In L. L. Wu & B. Wolfe (Eds.), *Out of wedlock: Causes and consequences of nonmarital fertility* (pp. 287–316). New York: Russell Sage Foundation.

Heeringa, S. G., & Connor, J. H. (1999). 1997 Panel Study of Income Dynamics Analysis Weights for Sample Families and Individuals. Panel Study of Income Dynamics, Technical Report, Institute for Social Research, University of Michigan.

Hertel, F. R., & Groh-Samberg, O. (2014). Class mobility across three generations in the U.S. and Germany. *Research in Social Stratification and Mobility, 35*, 35–52.

Hertzman, C., & Power, C. (2003). Health and human development: Understandings from life-course research. *Developmental Neuropsychology, 24*(2–3), 719–744.

Hill, M. S. (1992). *The panel study of income dynamics: A user's guide*. Newbury Park: Sage Publications.

Hirschl, T. A., Altobelli, J., & Rank, M. R. (2003). Does marriage increase the odds of affluence? Exploring the life course probabilities. *Journal of Marriage and the Family, 65*(4), 927–938.

Hofferth, S. L. (2010). Home media and children's achievement and behaviour. *Child Development, 81*, 1598–1619.

Hoffman, S., Foster, E. M., & Furstenberg, F. F. (1993). Reevaluating the costs of teenage childbearing. *Demography, 30*(1), 1–13.

Islam, T., & Tonmoy, M. (2013). Childhood neighborhood conditions and the persistence of adult income. *Regional Science and Urban Economics, 43*(4), 684–693.

Jackson, M. I., & Mare, R. D. (2007). Cross-sectional and longitudinal measurements of neighborhood experience and their effects on children. *Social Science Research, 36*, 590–610.

Jayasinghe, S. (2011). Conceptualising population health: From mechanistic thinking to complexity science. *Emerging Themes in Epidemiology, 8*(1), 2.

Johnson, R. C. (2012). Health Dynamics and the Evolution of Health Inequality over the Life Course: The Importance of Neighborhood and Family Background. *The B.E. Journal of Economic Analysis and Policy, 11*(3).

Johnson, R. C., & Schoeni, R. F. (2011a). Early-life origins of adult disease: National longitudinal population-based study of the United States. *American Journal of Public Health, 101*(12), 2317–2324.

Johnson, R. C., & Schoeni, R. F. (2011b). The influence of early-life events on human capital, health status, and labor market outcomes over the life course. *The B.E. Journal of Economic Analysis and Policy, 11*(3).

Johnson, R. C., Schoeni, R. F., & Rogowski, J. A. (2012). Health disparities in mid-to-late life: The role of earlier life family and neighborhood socioeconomic conditions. *Social Science and Medicine, 74*(4), 625–636.

Kail, R. (2006). *Children and their development*. New York: Prentice Hall.

Kuh, D., & Ben-Shlomo, Y. (1997). Introduction: A life course approach to the aetiology of adult chronic disease. In *Life course approach to chronic disease epidemiology* (pp. 3–14). Oxford: Oxford University Press.

Kuh, D., & Shlomo, Y. B. (Eds.). (2004). *A life course approach to chronic diseases epidemiology* (2nd ed.). Oxford: Oxford University Press.

Lê-Scherban, F., Diez Roux, A. V., Yun, L., & Morgenstern, H. (2014). Associations of grandparental schooling with adult grandchildren's health status, smoking, and obesity. *American Journal of Epidemiology, 180*(5), 469–481.

Lee, C. I., & Solon, G. (2009). Trends in intergenerational income mobility. *Review of Economics and Statistics, 91*, 766–772.

Li, M. (2015). Chronic exposure of grandparents to poverty and body mass index trajectories of grandchildren: A prospective intergenerational study. *American Journal of Epidemiology, 181*(3), 163–170.

Li, G., Schoeni, R. F., Danziger, S., & Charles, K. K. (2010). New expenditures in the PSID: Comparison with the CE. *Monthly Labor Review, 133*(2), 29–39.

Lovenheim, M. F., & Mumford, K. J. (2013). Do family wealth shocks affect fertility choices? Evidence from the housing market. *Review of Economics and Statistics, 95*(2), 464–475.

McGonagle, K. A., Schoeni, R. F., Sastry, N., & Freedman, V. A. (2012). The panel study of income dynamics: Overview, recent innovations, and potential for life course research. *Longitudinal and Life Course Studies, 3*(2), 268–284.

Mayer, S. E., & Lopoo, L. M. (2008). Government spending and intergenerational mobility. *Journal of Public Economics, 92*(1–2), 139–158.

Meadows, S. O., Beckett, M. K., Elliott, M. N., & Petersen, C. (2013). Maternal health status and early childbearing: A test of the weathering hypothesis. In N. Hoque, M. A. McGehee, & B. S. Bradshaw (Eds.), *Applied demography and public health*. New York: Springer.

Meer, J., Miller, D. L., & Rosen, H. S. (2003). Exploring the health-wealth nexus. *Journal of Health Economics, 22*(5), 713–730.

National Research Council. (2013). *Developing new national data on social mobility: A workshop summary*. Amy Smith, Rapporteur. Washington, DC: The National Academies Press.

Newman, S. J., Holupka, C. S., & Harkness, J. M. (2009). The long-term effects of housing assistance on work and welfare. *Journal of Policy Analysis and Management, 28*(1), 81–101.

Pais, J., Crowder, K., & Downey, L. (2014). Unequal trajectories: Racial and class differences in residential exposure to industrial hazard. *Social Forces, 92*(3), 1189–1215.

Pais, J., South, S. J., & Crowder, K. (2012). Metropolitan heterogeneity and minority neighborhood attainment: Spatial assimilation or place stratification? *Social Problems, 59*, 258–281.

Pfeffer, F. T. (2014). Multigenerational approaches to social mobility. A multifaceted research agenda. *Research in Social Stratification and Mobility, 1*(35), 1–12.

Pfeffer, F. T., Schoeni, R., Kennickell, A., & Andreski, P. (2014). Measuring wealth and wealth inequality: Comparing two U.S. surveys. PSID Technical Paper #14-03.

Rank, M. R., & Hirschl, T. A. (2014). Economic security and the American dream. In M. Crain & M. Sherraden (Eds.), *Working and living in the shadow of economic fragility* (pp. 140–156). Oxford: Oxford University Press.

Roksa, J., & Potter, D. (2011). Parenting and academic achievement: Intergenerational transmission of educational advantage. *Sociology of Education, 84*(4), 299–321.

Sandoval, D. A., Rank, M. R., & Hirschl, T. A. (2009). The increasing risk of poverty across the American life course. *Demography, 46*(4), 717–737.

Sastry, N., & Duffy, D. (2012). *An assessment of the national representativeness of children in the 2007 panel study of income dynamics* (pp. 12–01). Ann Arbor: Panel Study of Income Dynamics Technical Paper.

Schoeni, R. F., & Wiemers, E. (Forthcoming). The implication of selective attrition for estimates of intergenerational elasticity of family income. *Journal of Economic Equality.*

Schoeni, R. F., Stafford, F. P., McGonagle, K. A., & Andreski, P. (2013). Response rates in national panel surveys. *The Annals of the American Academy of Political and Social Science, 645*(1), 60–87.

Sharkey, P. (2008). The intergenerational transmission of context. *American Journal of Sociology, 113*, 931–969.

Sharkey, P. (2012). Temporary integration, resilient inequality: Race and neighborhood change in the transition to adulthood. *Demography, 49*(3), 889–912.

Sharkey, P., & Elwert, F. (2011). The legacy of disadvantage: Multigenerational neighborhood effects on cognitive ability. *American Journal of Sociology, 116*(6), 1934–1981.

Shauman, K. A. (2010). Gender asymmetry in family migration: Occupational inequality or interspousal comparative advantage? *Journal of Marriage and the Family, 72*(2), 275–392.

Shonkoff, J. P., & Phillips, D. (2000). *From neurons to neighborhoods: The science of early childhood development.* Washington, DC: National Academies Press.

Shore, S. H. (2011). The intergenerational transmission of income volatility: Is riskiness inherited? *Journal of Business and Economic Statistics, 29*(3), 372–381.

Smith, J. P. (2009). The impact of childhood health on adult labor market outcomes. *Review of Economics and Statistics, 91*(3), 478–489.

Solon, G. (1992). Intergenerational income mobility in the United States. *The American Economic Review, 82*, 93–408.

Solon, G., Page, M. E., & Duncan, G. J. (2000). Correlations between neighboring children in their subsequent educational attainment. *Review of Economics and Statistics, 82*(3), 383–392.

South, S. J. (1999). Historical changes and life course variation in the determinants of premarital childbearing. *Journal of Marriage and the Family, 61*, 752–763.

South, S. J. (2001a). The variable effects of family background on the timing of first marriage: United States, 1969–1993. *Social Science Research, 30*, 606–626.

South, S. J. (2001b). Time-dependent effects of wives' employment on marital dissolution. *American Sociological Review, 66*, 226–245.

South, S. J., & Crowder, K. D. (2005). Exiting and entering high-poverty neighborhoods: Latinos, Blacks and Anglos compared. *Social Forces, 84*, 873–900.

South, S. J., & Crowder, K. D. (2010). Neighborhood poverty and nonmarital fertility: Spatial and temporal dimensions. *Journal of Marriage and the Family, 72*(1), 89–104.

South, S. J., Crowder, K. D., & Pais, J. (2011). Metropolitan structure and neighborhood attainment: Exploring intermetropolitan variation in racial residential segregation. *Demography, 48*, 1263–1292.

Stephens, M., Jr. (2001). The long-run consumption effects of earnings shocks. *Review of Economics and Statistics, 83*(1), 28–36.

Sullivan, K., Clark, J., Castrucci, B., Samsel, R., Fonseca, V., & Garcia, I. (2011). Continuing education mitigates the negative consequences of adolescent childbearing. *Maternal and Child Health Journal, 15*(3), 360–366.

Timberlake, J. M. (2007). Racial and ethnic inequality in the duration of children's exposure to neighborhood poverty and affluence. *Social Problems, 54*, 319–342.

Timberlake, J. M. (2009a). "Scratchin' and surviving" or "movin' on up?" Two sources of change in children's neighborhood SES. *Population Research and Policy Review, 28*, 195–219.

Timberlake, J. M. (2009b). Effects of household and neighborhood characteristics on children's exposure to neighborhood poverty and affluence. *Social Science Research, 38*, 458–476.

Torche, F. (2011). Is a college degree still the great equalizer? Intergenerational mobility across levels of schooling in the United States. *American Journal of Sociology, 117*(3), 763–807.

Vandewater, E. A., Park, S. E., Carey, F. R., & Wilkinson, A. V. (2014). Intergenerational transfer of smoking across three generations and forty-five years. *Nicotine and Tobacco Research, 16*(1), 11–17.

Vartanian, T. P., Buck, P. W., & Gleason, P. (2007). Intergenerational neighborhood-type mobility: Examining differences between blacks and whites. *Housing Studies, 22*(5), 833–856.

Wadsworth, M. E. J. (1987). Follow-up of the first national birth cohort: Findings from the Medical Research Council National Survey of Health and Development. *Paediatric and Perinatal Epidemiology, 1*(1), 95–117.

Wadsworth, M. E. J. (1991). *The imprint of time: Childhood, history, and adult life.* Oxford: Oxford University Press.

Wagmiller, R. L. (2013). Blacks' and whites' experiences of neighborhood racial and ethnic diversity: Intercohort variation in neighborhood diversity and integration in early and early middle adulthood. *Urban Affairs Review, 49*(1), 32–70.

Wen, X., & Shenassa, E. (2012). Interaction between parenting and neighborhood quality on the risk of adolescent regular smoking. *Nicotine and Tobacco Research, 14*(3), 313–322.

White, K. J. C., Crowder, K. D., Tolnay, S. E., & Adelman, R. M. (2005). Race, gender, and marriage: Destination selection during the great migration. *Demography, 42*, 215–241.

Wimer, C., Simpkins, S. D., Dearing, E., Bouffard, S. M., Caronongan, P., & Weiss, H. B. (2008). Predicting youth out-of-school time participation: Multiple risks and developmental differences. *Merrill-Palmer Quarterly: Journal of Developmental Psychology, 54*, 179–207.

Wiemers, E., Schoeni, R. F., & Andreski, P. (2010). Attrition of second generation sample members in the PSID. Paper presented at the 2nd Panel Survey Methods Workshop, Mannheim Germany, July, 2010.

Wightman, P., & Danziger, S. (2014). Multi-generational income disadvantage and the educational attainment of young adults. *Research in Social Stratification and Mobility, 35*, 53–69.

Williams, J. A., Zimmerman, F. J., & Bell, J. F. (2013). Norms and trends of sleep time among US children and adolescents. *JAMA Pediatrics, 167*, 55–60.

Wodtke, G. T. (2013). Duration and timing of exposure to neighborhood poverty and the risk of adolescent parenthood. *Demography, 50*(5), 1765–1788.

Wodtke, G. T., Harding, D. J., & Elwert, F. (2011). Neighborhood effects in temporal perspective the impact of long-term exposure to concentrated disadvantage on high school graduation. *American Sociological Review, 76*(5), 713–736.

Yeung, W. J., Sandberg, J., Davis-Kean, P., & Hofferth, S. L. (2001). Children's time with fathers in intact families. *Journal of Marriage and Family, 63*, 136–154.

Zimmerman, F. J., & Christakis, D. A. (2007). Associations between content types of early media exposure and subsequent attentional problems. *JAMA Pediatrics, 120*, 986–992.

2

Pediatric Type 2 Diabetes: Prevention and Treatment Through a Life Course Health Development Framework

Pamela Salsberry, Rika Tanda, Sarah E. Anderson, and Manmohan K. Kamboj

1 Introduction

Estimates project that one in three US adults may have diabetes in 2050 (Boyle et al. 2010). The rates are even higher in some subgroups; for example, in Hispanic females it is 1 in 2 (Venkat Narayan et al. 2003). This problem is not limited to the USA. Shaw et al. 2010 estimate that 7.7% or 434 million adults will have diabetes by 2030 worldwide (Shaw et al. 2010). Until very recently, type 2 diabetes mellitus (T2DM) was a disease diagnosed in adults, but as the childhood obesity epidemic has spread in both magnitude and severity, the diagnosis of T2DM in adolescents and young adults has become more common. The prevalence of prediabetes in 12–19 years, estimated using National Health and Nutrition Examination Survey (NHANES) data, increased from 9% in 1999–2000 to 23% in 2007–2008 (May et al. 2012). Analyses using data from the SEARCH for Diabetes in Youth Study (SEARCH) indicate a 30.5% overall increase in the prevalence of T2DM in children/adolescents from 2001 to 2009 (Dabelea et al. 2014). Because of the newness of this diagnosis in children and adolescents, very little is known about the natural history of the disease, and it will likely take decades to fully understand the determinants and consequences of this new epidemic. Early indicators suggest that the disease may be more severe (Elder et al. 2012) and more difficult to manage when diagnosed in adolescents (Zeitler et al. 2012).

A recent analysis estimates that adolescents with T2DM will lose approximately 15 years of life and will experience severe and chronic complications by their 40s as a result of the disease (Rhodes et al. 2012). The mean direct cost for medical care for a man diagnosed with T2DM for less than 15 years is estimated at $2465. The economic burden of T2DM rises significantly as the

P. Salsberry, PhD, RN, FAAN (✉)
College of Public Health, Division of Health Behavior, Health Promotion, Institute for Population Health, The Ohio State University, 1841 Neil Avenue, 353 Cunz Hall, Columbus, OH 43210, USA
e-mail: Salsberry.1@osu.edu

R. Tanda, PhD, RN
College of Health Science and Professions, Ohio University, Grover Center W133B, Athens, OH 45701, USA
e-mail: tandar@ohio.edu

S.E. Anderson, PhD
The Ohio State University, College of Public Health, 336 Cunz Hall, 1841 Neil Avenue, Columbus, OH 43210, USA
e-mail: sanderson@cph.osu.edu

M.K. Kamboj, MD
The Ohio State University, College of Medicine, Endocrinology, Metabolism and Diabetes, Nationwide Children's Hospital, 700 Children's Drive (ED425), Columbus, OH 43205, USA
e-mail: Manmohan.Kamboj@Nationwidechildrens.org

years with disease increase. For those with disease 15 years or more, the costs are estimated to be 10–50% higher. This grim forecast highlights that not only will the disease burden be significant but the economic burden will be high in youth diagnosed with T2DM (Li et al. 2013). Metabolic comorbidities occur with alarming frequency (West et al. 2009). Within the SEARCH study, a significant portion of adolescents with T2DM had hypertension, high LDL cholesterol, or high triglycerides (Lawrence et al. 2009a; Mayer-Davis et al. 2009). It is clear that there is much to do to understand the epidemic, to determine effective prevention strategies, and to develop interventions for those diagnosed with the disease. It is also clear from what we are learning that preventive and treatment strategies need to begin early.

The risk for a child developing T2DM begins in utero. Individual health development trajectories emerge from this starting point and are the result of factors that accumulate across time and/or are the result of biological conditioning during sensitive periods of development. Understanding how these trajectories emerge, and which factors and events result in disease-causing pathways, is key to not only understanding the onset and variable natural history of the disease but in determining ways to prevent and treat it. There is an extensive and emergent body of literature that examines the mechanisms, pathways, and determinants of T2DM in children and adolescents. Genetic and epigenetic mechanisms are clearly a part of the story, but several studies also demonstrate the influence and importance of the social context on developing biological processes (Kempf et al. 2008). These include behaviors and psychological stressors nested within families, neighborhoods, and communities. Consistent with the principles of life course health development that are presented by Halfon and Forrest (2017), there is a growing consensus that T2DM is the result of the multilevel interaction of genetic, behavioral, social, and economic factors with the timing, sequence, and dose of exposure central to long-term outcomes.

A life course health development approach that details risks and protective factors, as well as preventive and treatment strategies, contextualized within the developmental stage of the child, is required. While one's genetic code may establish susceptibility toward T2DM development, its development is the result of a complex process of person-environment interactions that are multidimensional, multidirectional, and multilevel. A major aim of this chapter is to demonstrate that a life course health development approach to pediatric T2DM is critical to the development of a sound national strategy to prevent and treat T2DM in children. We review major factors known to influence the development of pediatric T2DM and track these across childhood. This set of factors will likely change over the next decade as our understanding of disease mechanisms deepens, but what will not change is the importance of placing these factors into context and recognizing that T2DM development is highly sensitive to the timing and social structuring of multiple environmental exposures. Research recommendations relevant to the field of maternal and child health regarding T2DM will be discussed through a life course lens. This chapter is organized around four key developmental stages: preconception and intrauterine life, infancy, childhood (early and middle), and adolescence. These health development stages unfold against the "backdrop" of each child's genetics, race/ethnicity, and family economic status.

2 The Backdrop

2.1 Genetics

Having a relative with T2DM is an established risk factor for the disease (Rosenbloom et al. 1999). Through a series of twin studies, heritability of fasting glucose levels has been estimated to range from 38% to 51% (Katoh et al. 2005; Snieder et al. 1999). Heritability is a population parameter that measures the fraction of variation, i.e., fasting glucose levels, among individuals in a population that is attributable to their genotypes (Visscher et al. 2008). At the individual level, a positive family history of T2DM has been associated with reduced insulin sensitivity at younger ages in children and adolescents when compared with children with no family history (Arslanian et al. 2005). There is a 40% increased lifetime risk for T2DM for children if one parent has T2DM; this increases to 70% if both parents have T2DM (Groop and Tuomi 1997). Studies have found that as many as 80% of youth with T2DM have a close relative with diabetes (Arslanian et al. 2005; Copeland et al. 2011).

Most of the genetic studies of T2DM have been carried out with adults; genetic studies of T2DM in children and youth are limited because of low number of subjects (Morgan 2012). An exception to this is a large meta-analysis that combined data from 6 European cohorts to test whether associations of common genetic variants identified for fasting glucose or insulin levels in nondiabetic adults were detectable in healthy children and adolescents. They found that the majority of novel fasting glucose loci identified in genome-wide associations studies (GWAS) in adults were detectable in childhood and at similar effect sizes (Barker et al. 2011). Work is progressing to examine whether associations between adult-identified susceptibility genes with T2DM hold in pediatric T2DM. For example, transcription factor 7-like 2 (TCF7L2) has been found to be associated with an increased risk of T2DM in African-American youth but not in non-Hispanic whites (Dabelea et al. 2011).

There is clear evidence that genetics plays a role in childhood susceptibility to T2DM, but significant research is needed. This research will require substantial collaboration across sites to achieve sample sizes large enough to test hypotheses. While progress is being made in elucidating underlying gene variants in adults, testing to determine if the same variants are operating in children and adolescents is required (Morgan 2012).

2.2 Prevalence and Incidence of T2DM Related to Age, Race, and Ethnicity

The prevalence of T2DM among children has risen with population increases in obesity, but compared to adolescents, T2DM in preadolescent children occurs less frequently. The highest rates are noted for adolescents aged 15–19 years, while incidence in children below 10 years in age is low. These results come from the SEARCH study, a multiethnic, population-based study designed to estimate rates of diabetes (both type 1 and type 2) based upon health-care provider assessment and in a subpopulation with further blood analyses. Data from SEARCH indicated a prevalence of diagnosed T2DM among 10–14-year-olds of 0.23 cases per 1000 children in 2009, up from 0.15 per 1000 in 2001 (Dabelea et al. 2014). Comparable prevalence estimates for adolescents (15–19 years) in 2001 and 2009 were respectively 0.54 and 0.68 per 1000 (Dabelea et al. 2014). Data from 1999 to 2010 NHANES, representative of US youth 12–19 years, indicated a total prevalence of T2DM of 0.36 per 1000 (Demmer et al. 2013). This estimate combines diagnosed and undiagnosed cases of T2DM, with approximately 1/3 of the total being undiagnosed but having a fasting glucose level of ≥126 mg/dL (Demmer et al. 2013). The prevalence of pediatric T2DM is higher for females and among minorities in the USA (Dabelea et al. 2014). SEARCH researchers modeling T2DM incidence by age and race/ethnicity report increasing incidence during the elementary school years with a peak in incidence at approximately age 14 years for all racial-ethnic groups (Imperatore et al. 2012). At any age, the incidence of T2DM for African-American, Hispanic, and Asian/Pacific Islander youth is higher than for non-Hispanic whites (Imperatore et al. 2012; Dabelea et al. 2007), and the incidence for children under 10 years old is very low (annual incidence <1 per 100,000) (Dabelea et al. 2007). However, because T2DM develops gradually, can be asymptomatic, and may be misdiagnosed as type 1 diabetes mellitus (T1DM) in children, population estimates of prevalence and incidence must be interpreted cautiously (Amed et al. 2010a).

2.3 Economic Status

Data on the relationship between economic status (of parents) and children and adolescents diagnosed with T2DM are limited, but there are indications of a positive correlation. The treatment options for T2DM in adolescents and youth study (TODAY Study) found that 41.5% of their subjects came from households with an annual income of less than $25,000, and 26.3% were in families in which the highest education level of the parent/guardian was less than a high school degree (Copeland et al. 2011). The association of economic status measured by educational level, occupation, and income with T2DM in adults has been studied extensively and likely offers clues to risk in children and adolescents. A systematic review and meta-analysis that was global in scope found associations with low levels of education (relative risk (RR) = 1.41, 95% CI: 1.28–1.51), with occupation (RR = 1.31, 95% CI: 1.09–1.57), and with low income (RR = 1.31, 95% CI: 1.09–1.57). While the data were limited from middle- and low-income countries in this study, the increased risks were independent of the income levels of countries (Agardh et al. 2011). Another systematic review examining childhood socioeconomic status (SES) as a risk for T2DM found a strong relationship; although this relationship was attenuated by adult SES, a significant relationship remained (Tamayo et al. 2010). Parental education has been found to be associated with insulin resistance in the CARDIA study participants, and the association differed by race and gender. Low parental education was associated with greater insulin resistance in African-American and white females and in African-American males, but not in white males (Tamayo et al. 2012). Smith et al. 2011 found similar results in the Framingham Offspring Study where an inverse relation between cumulative economic status and T2DM in women, but not men, was noted (Smith et al. 2011). These results highlight why untangling the pathways for risk will be difficult.

2.4 Social (Psychological) Stressors

There is strong evidence that acute or chronic stress during critical periods in early life, childhood, and/or adolescence has long-term risks for altered metabolic function including the development of T2DM (Pervanidou and Chrousos 2012). Obesity likely mediates this relation brought on by unhealthy behaviors related to eating and activity patterns as coping mechanisms for chronic stress. Furthermore, chronic stress leads to the dysregulation of the hypothalamic-pituitary-adrenal (HPA) axis, with increased cortisol, catecholamine, and elevated insulin concentrations (Pervanidou and Chrousos 2011). Key stressors in children are recognized as those related to the creation of a safe, stable, and nurturing environment, and when these are disrupted, the child's long-term health suffers (Shonkoff and Garner 2012).

2.5 Summary

These "backdrop" factors are the platform upon which health develops and emerges over time, influenced by dynamic interactions at multiple levels (biological, behavioral, social/cultural) at sensitive periods transacting simultaneously. The next sections illustrate this principle by highlighting key factors within developmental stage that have been linked to pediatric T2DM.

3 Preconception and Intrauterine Life

Over the last 20 years, a significant body of evidence from epidemiological and animal studies has established a strong link between the intrauterine environment and long-term health (Dyer and Rosenfeld 2011; Gluckman et al. 2008; McMillen and Robinson 2005; Sebert et al. 2011; Sinclair et al. 2007). The notion of biological embedding is now widely accepted, even though the mechanisms are not completely understood (Tarry-Adkins and Ozanne 2011). Maternal nutritional status, gestational diabetes, high levels of maternal stress, hypoxia/placental insufficiency, and environmental toxins have been associated with the development of T2DM in children and adolescents (Warner and Ozanne 2010; Boekelheide et al. 2012). Furthermore, the relationship of these high-risk maternal factors to intrauterine growth restriction (IUGR) and small-for-gestational-age (SGA) newborns with their predisposition for obesity, insulin resistance, and T2DM later in life has been established as well. These factors are briefly reviewed below. Several excellent papers review the underlying mechanisms of these relationships in greater depth (Dyer and Rosenfeld 2011; Armitage et al. 2004; Berends and Ozanne 2012; Martin-Gronert and Ozanne 2012; Thayer et al. 2012; Prince et al. 2014).

3.1 Maternal Nutrition: Prior to and During Pregnancy

3.1.1 Maternal Under Nutrition

A series of studies linking low birth weight, maternal undernutrition, and the development of cardiovascular disease has fueled much work on the impact of caloric restriction on the developing fetus (Hales and Barker 2001; Barker et al. 1993). Animal studies have found endocrine and metabolic abnormalities associated with food restrictions (Warner and Ozanne 2010). Data suggest that undernutrition alters the structure and/or function of the developing endocrine-metabolic axis, leading to an insulin resistance and energy conservation in light of reduced calories. An overactivation of the HPA axis leads to increased cortisol levels in growth-restricted fetuses, a situation that mimics chronic stress (Kanaka-Gantenbein 2010; Kapoor et al. 2006). The effects of the undernutrition seem to depend on the timing and extent of the deprivation. In a rodent study, a 50% caloric restriction at the end of the fetal period resulted in reduced β-cell mass (Bertin et al. 2002), and if the caloric restriction continued through early life, the reduction in β-cell mass was permanent (Garofano et al. 1998). Furthermore, the type of diet seems to be important as well. Because of the importance of amino acids in fetal development, studies on the effects of low-protein diets on fetal growth have been pursued with high interest (Fernandez-Twinn et al. 2005). Studies have shown that when dams were fed a low-protein diet, the results were growth-restricted pups, and if the maternal diets remained low protein during suckling, the growth restriction was permanent. Most importantly, these offspring then went on to develop glucose intolerance and T2DM (Hoet et al. 1992).

3.1.2 Maternal Overnutrition

Maternal obesity at the time of pregnancy is known to be associated with a greater risk for child obesity (Salsberry and Reagan 2005), placing them at increased risk for the development of T2DM. Fetal overnutrition has also been associated with insulin resistance and adult diabetes (Armitage et al. 2008). In animal studies, offspring born to obese maternal rats had higher fat-to-lean ratios at birth, and by 3 months of age, these pups were insulin resistant (Samuelsson et al. 2008). When pregnant dams are fed a high-fat content, the offspring are noted to develop a phenotype resembling the human metabolic syndrome (Armitage et al. 2008).

3.2 Maternal Stress

Increased maternal stress is associated with adverse birth outcomes, in particular low birth weight and preterm birth (Christian 2012). Studies demonstrate that maternal exposure to glucocorticoids reduces birth weight in sheep and rats (Tarry-Adkins and Ozanne 2011). Meaney et al. (2007) have suggested that these birth outcomes are mediated by effects on the HPA axis. Stressors in the environment alter maternal physiology and behavior, which then programs HPA activity in the offspring (Meaney et al. 2007). These changes have been linked to the development of T2DM and other components of the metabolic syndrome in the offspring (Brunton 2010).

3.3 Maternal Hypoxia/Placental Insufficiency

Fetal oxygenation is also an independent risk factor for fetal growth abnormalities and long-term development of T2DM. Reduction in fetal oxygenation has also been associated with IUGR, a known risk factor for metabolic syndrome.

Multiple underlying pathophysiological reasons for fetal hypoxia include placental insufficiency, uterine placental ligation, and smoking. These effects all result in IUGR (Tarry-Adkins and Ozanne 2011).

3.4 Environmental Exposures

Exposures to environmental toxins during pregnancy are under increased scrutiny as the evidence builds suggesting significant life course health affects with early-life exposures to a range of chemicals (Thayer et al. 2012). In particular, nicotine, arsenic, and endocrine disrupting chemicals (EDC) are tied to metabolic outcomes. For example, high levels of arsenic exposure have been linked to T2DM in adults, and there is some suggestion that even low doses may also confer an increased T2DM risk (Navas-Acien et al. 2008; Maull et al. 2012). The causal mechanisms include altered glucose metabolism, insulin resistance, and obesity as a result of exposure (Seki et al. 2012). Exposure to EDC, particularly bisphenol A (BPA), is thought to lead to functional changes in gene expression and increased risk for development of obesity and T2DM (Barouki et al. 2012; Liu et al. 2013). This is an area of intense activity that will likely result in significant new knowledge over the next decade.

3.5 Microbiome

There is growing recognition of the importance of the human microbiome in pediatrics (Johnson and Versalovic 2012). During pregnancy a woman's microbiome undergoes significant change from the first to third trimester, changes thought to be beneficial to the mother and the establishment of the neonatal microbiome (Prince et al. 2014; Koren et al. 2012). The infant's microbiota is influenced by the mode of delivery, with colonization in vaginally delivered newborns a function of maternal vaginal and intestinal microbiota, while cesarean delivered newborns exhibit the microbiome of the maternal skin microbiota. The infant's environment and nutrition further influence the infant's developing microbiome (Johnson and Versalovic 2012). These environmental influences on the developing microbiome are critical, as the microbiome is thought to play a role in health and disease (Cenit et al. 2014; Devaraj et al. 2013). Evidence from research in adults suggests that the microbiome plays a critical role in T2DM. Ongoing research is beginning to demonstrate implications for prevention and treatment of metabolic conditions based upon knowledge of the microbiome; extending this work to children is of high importance (Szajewska 2013; Versalovic 2013).

3.6 Gestational Diabetes (GDM)

GDM represents a form of impaired glucose tolerance that is first recognized during pregnancy. Insulin resistance normally occurs in pregnancy. This allows the metabolic needs of the fetus to be met, while an increased maternal insulin secretion compensates for the insulin resistance. But in GDM, this increased resistance is coupled with a failure of increased insulin secretion, resulting in hyperglycemia (Battista et al. 2011). GDM is harmful to the mother and to the fetus. GDM has been shown to alter pancreatic development and insulin sensitivity in the fetus (Warner and Ozanne 2010). Fetal growth is often affected, resulting in macrosomia or large-for-gestational-age infants (Dyer and Rosenfeld 2011). The Hyperglycemia and Adverse Pregnancy Outcome (HAPO) study found a strong linear relation between fasting glucose and post challenge glucose with macrosomia and neonatal adiposity (Metzger et al. 2008). Macrosomic infants born to diabetic mothers have been found to be more glucose intolerant between the ages of 10–16 years, are more likely to be obese, and are at a greater risk for T2DM (Silverman et al. 1998). Because of methodological differences in current studies, the long-term effect of GDM on child outcomes is not fully understood, but studies do suggest that increased rates of obesity, T2DM, and other cardiovascular conditions may result (Kim et al. 2011; Simeoni and Barker 2009).

Screening and Diagnosis Given the convincing evidence that diabetes and gestational diabetes are harmful to both the mother and fetus, considerable effort has been directed toward establishing consensus criteria for the diagnosis of diabetes in pregnancy. There is controversy over the "correct" diabetes threshold, that is, the level at which maternal blood glucose conveys a significant risk to the fetus. The HAPO study, a multisite and multinational study, was designed to address some of these questions. HAPO study results showed a linear relation between increasing levels of fasting and 1 and 2 hour plasma glucose levels post a 75 g oral glucose tolerance test (OGTT) on the primary study outcomes, including birth weight above 90th percentile, cord blood C-peptide level above the 90th percentile, primary cesarean delivery, and neonatal hypoglycemia (Hadar and Hod 2010). These results have led to guidelines issued in 2010 by the International Association of Diabetes and Pregnancy Study Groups (IADPSG) for the detection and diagnosis of hyperglycemic disorders in pregnancy. These guidelines include the determination of the diabetes status of the pregnant woman at the first prenatal visit. Following these guidelines is expected to increase the number of all women with diabetes during pregnancy. These guidelines, however, remain controversial (Moses 2010). There are concerns over increasing costs associated with the identification of a greater number of women with diabetes resulting in an increased number of women receiving treatment.

The American College of Obstetricians and Gynecologists and the National Diabetes Education program have joined together in a call for action, specifically recommending follow-up testing during the postpartum period in women who experienced GDM. Currently only approximately one-half of these women are tested. Recommendations include the following: If the postpartum test is normal, retest every 3 years and at the first prenatal visit for subsequent pregnancies. If prediabetes is diagnosed at the postpartum check, then the recommendation is to test annually (Gabbe et al. 2012).

Treatment Intrauterine conditions are being targeted in the HAPO study. The initial results showed that close control of glucose improved birth outcomes, leading to the new recommendations for the diagnosis and classification of hyperglycemia during pregnancy (Metzger et al. 2010). The HAPO study is also following the outcomes in children born to women with GDM; this longitudinal follow-up may yield important insights for the health of the offspring as well. Early results, however, on offspring at ages 4 and 5 show no difference in body mass index (BMI) in the treatment group (Gillman et al. 2010). Further work with longer follow-up is required to determine if there are latent effects of treatment that will potentially influence outcomes at a later age.

3.7 Summary

Intrauterine life is a sensitive period for T2DM risk development. Building upon the backdrop of genetic susceptibility and within the social and economic context of the mother, the fetus develops an underlying propensity toward T2DM development. Much of this comes through epigenetic changes influenced by maternal nutrition, life stressors, chemical exposures, and maternal behaviors. The occurrence of higher levels of risk is strongly correlated with maternal economic disadvantage and the result of molecular, physiological, behavioral, cultural, and evolutionary processes that interact across time and space. Consistent with the principles of life course health development (LCHD), development of a phenotype at high risk for T2DM development is thus the result of person-environment interactions that are multidimensional, multidirectional, and multilevel, which are highly sensitive to the timing and social structure of environmental exposures.

4 Infancy

4.1 Feeding

Multiple advantages of breastfeeding are well accepted (American Academy of Pedicatrics 2012; James and Lessen 2009), but clarifying the relationship between breastfeeding and future metabolic function is not simple and requires consideration of multiple factors that have effects over one's life course. Controlling social and environmental factors between infancy and some later age is difficult because information for such a long interval is often missing. Despite the limitations, there are several studies that have examined infant feeding type or breastfeeding duration and their relation to dietary habits or cardiometabolic risks. For example, a study that used the Hertfordshire cohort has found an independent association between exclusive breastfeeding (vs. mixed or bottle-feeding) and adherence to healthy dietary recommendations and less intake of processed meat in middle to late adulthood (Robinson et al. 2013). Socioeconomic factors were not associated with the dietary recommendation adherence. The authors speculate breast milk may have provided significant impact on dietary flavor learning during infancy.

In a recent study by Martin et al. (2014), the relationship between cardiometabolic risks and long-term exclusive breastfeeding was examined. This study was a follow-up study of a randomized control study where one group of new mothers was encouraged to undertake exclusive breastfeeding and the other nonexclusive breastfeeding. While the original intervention significantly prolonged breastfeeding duration and exclusiveness, the intervention effect did not influence cardiometabolic factors, such as blood pressure, fasting glucose, insulin, insulin resistance, and adiponectin, when children were at age 11.5 years. A previous follow-up study of this cohort also failed to show intervention effects on anthropometry (height, weight, BMI, and skinfold) and blood pressure at age 6.5 years (Kramer et al. 2009).

Investigating the effects of breastfeeding is complex as there are likely multiple biological and behavioral ways that breastfeeding may influence the infant's health development. Nutrition-focused research studies that examine the importance of the nutrients within breast milk are ongoing. But there are also suggestions that breastfeeding may impact an infant's ability to self-regulate behavior. For example, Taveras et al. (2004), using the US mixed-race cohort, have found that restrictive feeding style is associated with bottle-feeding and shorter breastfeeding duration, which could disrupt the infant's ability to self-regulate feeding behavior. Maternal restrictive feeding style was also found to be associated with increased child's weight for age at 18 months among an African-American sample (Thompson and Bentley 2013).

There has been particular interest in the effects of breastfeeding on children who are exposed to maternal diabetes in utero. The evidence is mixed regarding the effects of breastfeeding among offspring of diabetic mothers (ODM) and development of obesity and T2DM during childhood. A study from Germany found that high consumption of breastmilk during the first 7 days of life among ODM may pose deleterious effects on body weight and glucose tolerance measured at age 2 years (Plagemann et al. 2002). These authors suggest that certain substances contained in early milk of mother's with diabetes may program for metabolic dysregulation in their offspring.

In the Nurses' Health Study II (Mayer-Davis et al. 2006), researchers found that exclusive breastfeeding compared to exclusive formula feeding, or longer duration of breastfeeding (>9 months) compared to never breastfed, was associated with lower odds of being overweight at ages 9–14 years, controlling for child's age, gender, and pubertal development. However, further controlling for other maternal and child factors resulted in null association, and a separate analysis for ODM did not reach statistical significance. A case control study using the SEARCH participants found that longer duration of breastfeeding resulted in a reduction in T2DM, controlling for maternal, child's, and social factors. When the child's weight (measured using BMIz) was included in the analysis, the association was attenuated to null, suggesting that the child's BMIz may mediate the pathway to a diagnosis of T2DM (Mayer-Davis et al. 2008).

The mechanisms involved in the effects of breastfeeding on child's future weight status or risks for T2DM are unclear. However, insulin and other metabolic hormones that are present in breast milk likely play some role. Insulin is present at more than threefold concentration in early milk collected within the first weeks of the postpartum period than in mature milk collected 3 months postpartum (Ley et al. 2012). The insulin concentration in early milk does not appear to be affected by the mother's gestational diabetes status. While the insulin concentration in mature milk of nondiabetic women is not different from that of women with GDM (Ley et al. 2012), maternal prenatal metabolic indicators, such as BMI, fasting glucose, insulin resistance, insulin sensitivity, and adiponectin levels, can predict insulin concentration in mature milk (Ley et al. 2012; Whitmore et al. 2012).

Other research efforts have been focused on infant feeding practices, such as timing of solid food introduction and amount of sugar-sweetened drink during infancy and early childhood, and their effects on childhood obesity development (Gaffney et al. 2012). Another area is investigation of micro- and macronutrient constituents of breast milk. A randomized clinical trial demonstrated that health modifications made to the diets of pregnant and lactating women improved infant metabolic health (Aaltonen et al. 2011). More research is needed to investigate how infant feeding may influence metabolic health development over the life course. An excellent review article summarizes the critical next questions in lactation and neonatal nutrition, providing a road map for this necessary research (Neville et al. 2012).

4.2 Infant Growth Patterns

Several studies (Fabricius-Bjerre et al. 2011; Ekelund et al. 2007; Eriksson et al. 2006) highlight significant associations between infant/childhood growth patterns and development of T2DM and later cardiovascular disease. Because growth is orchestrated by a complex series of interactions between growth hormone, sex steroids, and insulin, tracking growth over time is an important global health measure. Understanding high-risk growth patterns may assist in earlier identification of high-risk children with the potential to begin interventions at an earlier age. The Helsinki Birth Cohort Study (HBCS) 1934–1944 has shown that a small body size at birth with thinness during the first year followed by higher BMIs later in childhood is associated with the development of T2DM (Eriksson 2006). Also, this study found that an early age at adiposity rebound was associated with a markedly increased risk of T2DM in adulthood (Eriksson 2011). An important recent finding suggests that breastfeeding may alter childhood growth even in children exposed to overnutrition during the pregnancy. In the Exploring Perinatal Outcomes among Children (EPOCH) study, breastfeeding was associated with long-term effects on childhood BMI growth extending into late childhood. Slower BMI growth velocity was seen among adequately breastfed (breastfeeding >6 months) children compared with infants who had low breastfeeding status, and these benefits lasted through age 9 years (Crume et al. 2012).

4.3 Sleep Duration

Shortened sleep duration is suggested as a risk factor for obesity, insulin resistance, and Type 2 diabetes among adults. Long-term effects of shortened sleep during infancy on metabolic function are unknown. A limited number of studies that examined the relationship between sleep duration during infancy and subsequent obesity in early childhood have produced conflicting results. For example, studies of US children (Taveras et al. 2008, 2014) have found chronic sleep curtailment from infancy to age 7 years was associated with increased BMI z-scores. Because short sleep hours were associated with longer TV viewing time, the investigators suggested the screen time as one of the potential pathways for the association. Similarly, Bell and Zimmerman (2010) using sample from the Panel Survey of Income Dynamics-Child Development Supplement, reported that shortened night time sleep (less than 9 hours) during early childhood (ages 0–59 months) but not during school age was associated with increased likelihood of being overweight or obese at follow-up at age 5–10 years. Both US studies include relatively large number of minority population (30–50%) whose nighttime sleep is on average shorter than white children. However, studies of Dutch children and Australian children have shown no such association (Hiscock et al. 2011; Klingenberg et al. 2013). The latter two studies utilized objective measures of sleep duration such as actinography, while the US studies have relied on parental report. Improvement in measurement of child's sleep duration and other behavioral markers in longitudinal studies are needed to advance the knowledge in this area.

4.4 Parenting and Postpartum Depression

The impact of maternal postpartum depression on parenting is significant during the first year of life. Mothers who suffer from postpartum depression may lack responsiveness to infant cues for hunger or satiety. However, the studies examining the association between maternal depressive symptoms and child weight status have produced mixed results. Several studies conducted in the USA have shown the association between maternal postpartum depressive symptoms and inappropriate parenting practices such as shorter or less intense breastfeeding (McLearn et al. 2006; Gaffney et al. 2014), inappropriate early feeding practices (Gaffney et al. 2014), and fewer healthy interactions with infants (McLearn et al. 2006). Exposure to chronic maternal depressive symptoms has also been associated with increased risk of childhood overweight (Wang et al. 2013). Cumulative exposure to maternal depressive symptoms in early infancy can lead to disruption of behavioral and metabolic cues for sensation of hunger and satiety. A study involving five European countries, however, has shown no relationship between maternal depressive symptoms and adiposity measures at age 24 months (Grote et al. 2010). The investigators of the latter study noted that prevalence of high depressive symptom scores differed significantly by the participating countries, and therefore, the instrument to measure depressive symptoms used in this study may not be comparably used by the participants across different study sites. More prospective cohort studies focused on the relationship between infant/child development and maternal lifestyles as well as infant's surrounding environment are needed. Cohort studies such as the Amsterdam Born Children and their Development (ABCD) study (van Eijsden et al. 2011) may provide further knowledge on this area.

4.5 Summary

Infant development occurs within a context of "backdrop" factors and as an extension of what has happened during the prior period (fetal life). Because evolutionary life-history theory suggests that development during fetal life prepares the neonate for a particular external environment, when conditions in utero match the conditions in infancy, development unfolds as an extension of pathways begun in utero. When a mismatch occurs between these environments, aspects of development may be compromised. This may be the case when undernutrition in fetal life is followed by an abundance of nutrients postnatally, a particularly risky circumstance for metabolic health. The important point is that infant health development must be seen as conditioned by the interaction of processes and conditions during intrauterine life, and that this wider lens brings into sharper focus the multiple interacting risks contributing to the development of T2DM. Our examinations of how experiences in infancy feed forward into this continuously evolving health developmental process suggest that long-term health behaviors are beginning to be set through complex transactions between maternal behaviors and preferences regarding feeding and sleep (both of which are influenced by the mother's own environment and psychological state) and the infant's developing behavioral response patterns.

5 Childhood

5.1 Childhood Overweight and Obesity

Almost all children and adolescents with T2DM are also overweight or obese, and excess adiposity, particularly visceral adiposity, is associated with insulin resistance (Dabelea et al. 2007; Haines et al. 2007; Amed et al. 2010b). Studies with US and Canadian youth have found that 75–95% of those with T2DM are obese (BMI percentile > 95th for age and sex) (Mayer-Davis et al. 2009; Amed et al. 2010b; Liu et al. 2009; Lawrence et al. 2009b; Bell et al. 2009). Another study in obese children found that 25% of obese children 4–10 years of age and 21% of 11–18 years of age were found to have an impaired glucose tolerance. Silent T2DM was identified in 4% of the obese adolescents (Sinha et al. 2002). Researchers in the UK using the International Obesity Task Force (IOTF) cut point for defining obesity (which is higher than the US reference (Rolland-Cachera 2011)) found that 83% of youth with T2DM were obese (Haines et al. 2007). These results clearly point to the importance of understanding the underlying factors that contribute to childhood obesity, and also point toward the complex path that underlies the development of T2DM. Further understanding of how multiple factors interact, with a key emphasis toward the timing of these factors in reference to the life course is needed (Ong 2010; Tounian 2011).

5.2 Impaired Glucose Tolerance and Progression to T2DM

Obese children may have deficits in glucose regulation that predict future T2DM, as well as less favorable risk factor profiles for cardiovascular disease (West et al. 2009; Burns et al. 2014). Evidence of impaired glucose tolerance, elevated fasting glucose, insulin resistance, and/or previously undiagnosed "silent" T2DM has been documented in multiple samples of obese youth (Wabitsch et al. 2004; Sinha et al. 2002; Morrison et al. 2012). Morrison et al. (2012) studied 259 overweight and obese children and adolescents (aged 5–17 years) who were seeking weight-loss treatment and found that >20% had prediabetes—impaired glucose tolerance as measured by an oral glucose tolerance test or elevated fasting glucose (Morrison et al. 2012). Among these youth with prediabetes, a majority with impaired glucose tolerance did not have elevated fasting glucose levels (Morrison et al. 2012), which is consistent with findings from an Italian study (Morandi et al. 2014). The current American Diabetes Association (ADA) guidelines (American Diabetes Association 2010) recommend that overweight children ≥10 years or pubertal with two or more additional risk factors for T2DM have their fasting glucose measured (see Table 1). ADA guidelines do not recommend screening youth with an oral glucose tolerance test. Morrison et al. found that the sensitivity and specificity of the ADA criteria to identify youth with prediabetes were respectively 39% and 70%. Furthermore, in their sample the prevalence of prediabetes in children 5–9 years old was not significantly different from that of youth ≥10 years old (Morrison et al. 2012). Some evidence indicates that elevated fasting triglycerides may help to identify obese children and adolescents who would benefit from an oral glucose tolerance test (Morrison et al. 2012; Morandi et al. 2014). More longitudinal studies of children at risk for T2DM are needed to elucidate the natural history and progression of the disorder. In a sample of 117 obese children and adolescents (4–18 years) in which two oral glucose tolerance tests were administered between 18 and 24 months apart, Weiss et al. 2005 found that of 38 youth with impaired glucose tolerance at the first time point, 8 developed T2DM, 10 still had impaired glucose tolerance, and 15 (46%) had normal glucose tolerance at the second time point (Weiss et al. 2005). Among the 84 youth with normal glucose tolerance initially, 8 had impaired glucose tolerance at the follow-up assessment (Weiss et al. 2005). Progression from prediabetes to T2DM has been studied among adults (Morris

Table 1 Summary of screening guidelines for T2DM: Childhood overweight and obesity

	Year	Recommendations	Other risk factors
Diabetes screening			
Expert Committee (Barlow 2007)	2007	BMI > 85th% and aged ≥ 10 years with ≥2 other risk factors FGT or 2 h. GTT; BMI ≥ 95th% and aged ≥ 10 years FGT every 2 years	Parental obesity Family history Current lifestyle BMI trajectory CVD risk factors (HBP, cholesterol)
ADA (Amercian Diabetes Association 2000)	2012	BMI > 85th% or weight > % of ideal for height with ≥2 other risk factors screened every 3 years beginning at age 10 years or onset of puberty, whichever is earlier. Testing done every 2 years	Family history of T2DM in first or second-degree relatives Certain race/ethnic groups[b] Signs of insulin resistance or conditions associated with insulin resistance (AN, HTN, dyslipidemia, PCOS, SGA) Maternal diabetes or GDM
ISPAD[a] (International Society for Pediatric and Adolescent Diabetes)	2011	BMI > 85th% with other risk factors. In Asian children, screen with low or high birth weight with 1 risk factor, regardless of BMI	Immediate family history of T2DM, early family history of CVD, or Signs of insulin resistance (AN, dyslipidemia, HBP, PCOS)
Overweight/Obesity screening			
USPSTF (Barton 2010)	2010	Screen at 6 year and older for obesity	
Expert Committee (Barlow 2007)	2007	Every well child visit: height and weight, calculate and plot BMI	

[a]The ISPAD guidelines are also sensitive to country resources, so that screening decisions will likely be tied directly to the health-care resources with a country

[b]Native American, African-American, Latino, Asian American, Pacific Islander

et al. 2013), and although less is currently known about how the disease develops in children and adolescents, this is an area of active investigation.

5.3 Diabetes Prevention

A number of lifestyle interventions to prevent T2DM in youth at high risk have been evaluated in randomized trials. The Yale Bright Bodies Healthy Lifestyle program is an intensive 6-month behavioral intervention for obese youth and their families that has been evaluated in multiple randomized controlled trials (Savoye et al. 2007, 2011, 2014). Among 174 ethnically diverse children and adolescents aged 8–16 years—69 assigned to the control condition—the youth in the intervention group showed reductions in adiposity at 6 months that were maintained at 1 year as well as reductions in fasting insulin levels, which were seen at 6 months and also maintained for 1 year (Savoye et al. 2007). These youth were also assessed 24 months after the start of the trial and the favorable changes in body composition and insulin sensitivity seen at 6 and 12 months were sustained at similar levels at 24 months (Savoye et al. 2011). A subsequent trial among 10–16-year-olds with prediabetes ($n = 38$ receiving the Bright Bodies intervention and $n = 37$ standard clinical care) also demonstrated improvements in glucose metabolism and insulin sensitivity as well as reductions in adiposity and improved fitness (Savoye et al. 2014). Such results are encouraging, and although the intervention is intensive, it uses a standardized curriculum and is likely to be cost-effective long term (Savoye et al. 2014).

The HEALTHY Study was a national 3-year middle-school intervention program designed to reduce risk factors for type 2 diabetes. It used a randomized trial designed to determine whether changes to the school environment of middle-school students over a 3-year period could impact their risk for T2DM (Foster et al. 2010; Hirst et al. 2009). Prevention of T2DM in youth involves encouraging changes in eating and activity behaviors that should also reduce risk for obesity. Although many large and well-conducted randomized trials of school-based interventions to prevent obesity have had limited impact on obesity prevalence (Luepker et al. 1996; Caballero et al. 2003; Brown and Summerbell 2009), such interventions may improve glucose homeostasis and other risk factors for T2DM (Trevino et al. 2004; Rosenbaum et al. 2007). The Healthy Study was a group randomized trial conducted in 42 middle schools (21 intervention, 21 control) in 7 areas of the USA between fall 2006 and spring 2009 (Hirst et al. 2009). Students were in 6th grade when enrolled and in 8th grade when outcomes were assessed. The interventions in the Healthy Study included changes to the school environment with regard to nutrition (Gillis et al. 2009), physical activity (McMurray et al. 2009), and health messaging (Venditti et al. 2009). The primary outcome was prevalence of BMI ≥85th percentile (overweight and obesity), and at baseline about 50% of students in intervention and control schools were overweight or obese (Kaufman et al. 2009). Over the course of the study, this prevalence decreased in intervention schools to 45.8% and in control schools to 45.2%, and thus there was not an effect of the intervention on the prevalence of overweight and obesity (Foster et al. 2010). However, the intervention did have a modest and statistically impact on the secondary outcomes of obesity, mean BMI z-score, high waist circumference, and fasting insulin levels (Foster et al. 2010). These results suggest that changes to the school environment regarding nutrition, physical activity, and health messaging may reduce the risk of childhood onset of T2DM (Foster et al. 2010)

Some evidence suggests that interventions targeting physical fitness may be as effective in reducing risk for T2DM in youth as multicomponent interventions. Among obese 7–11-year-old children, a program of 40 min of aerobic exercise 5 days per week for 4 months reduced adiposity and insulin levels, but these effects were not sustained in the absence of the program (Ferguson et al. 1999). A dose-response effect for the benefit of time spent in exercise on fitness and cardiometabolic measures of T2DM risk was demonstrated in a subsequent study of overweight and obese 7–11-year-olds randomized to a 10–15-week program of 20 or 40 min per school day of aerobic activity or to a control group (Davis et al. 2012). Similar findings were noted in a pilot randomized study in which physical activity was added to a family-based weight control treatment. The exercise group had lower visceral abdominal fat posttreatment, a result that may be key in future work to reduce diabetes risk (Saelens et al. 2011). In a YMCA-based program targeted to prevent the development of T2DM in high-risk inner-city African-American children (TAT: Taking Action Together), initial results were encouraging with improvement in glucoregulation in boys (but not girls) and a decrease in BMI z-scores in the treatment group (Ritchie et al. 2010; Raman et al. 2010).

5.4 Obesity Prevention

Because of the strong association between obesity and T2DM, much of the literature that discusses prevention of T2DM focuses on weight reduction or healthy weight maintenance throughout childhood. In a systematic review of the effectiveness of weight management interventions in children, the US Preventative Services Task Force (USPSTF) results support at least in the short term benefits of comprehensive medium-to-high intensity behavioral interventions in children 6 years and older (Whitlock et al. 2010). The outcomes studied in the USPSTF review were limited to childhood weight and not the progression to T2DM (see Table 1).

Recent evidence points to the importance and benefit of intervening early in children's lives to reduce obesity (Knowlden and Sharma 2012), and a number of randomized controlled treatment trials in preschool-aged children have demonstrated success. An intensive 16-week multidisciplinary program for overweight or obese Dutch children aged 3–5 years and their parent was compared to a "usual-maintained care" control, and results showed reductions in BMI and waist circumference that were for 12 months (Bocca et al. 2012a). Among 33 obese preschool-aged (2–5 years) children in the Midwest USA, a pilot randomized trial compared two 6-month multidisciplinary treatment programs (one in which all sessions were held at a clinic and another program that alternated between clinic sessions and individual home-based visits by a pediatric psychology fellow); both interventions were consistent with Expert Committee (Barlow 2007) stage 3 recommendations and were compared to a control condition of pediatrician counseling as recommended by the Expert Committee as stage 1 treatment (Stark et al. 2014). Compared to pediatrician counseling, children in the intervention with home visits group had greater reductions in BMI z-score at 6 months (end of intervention) and at 12 months than did children in the clinic only intervention (Stark et al. 2014). These results suggest that parents of obese preschool-aged children may benefit from in-home guidance regarding implementation and maintenance of parenting behaviors related to weight reduction. In an observational study of children aged 6–16 years seeking treatment for obesity in Sweden, researchers evaluated whether age and severity of obesity impacted the likelihood of treatment success over a 3-year period (Danielsson et al. 2012). They found that younger children (6–9 years) were more likely to have clinically meaningful reductions in weight status than older children and adolescents, and that treatment success was rare for adolescents particularly if they were severely obese (Danielsson et al. 2012). The difficulties associated with treating obesity once it is established underscore the need to prevent excess weight gain in young children before they become obese.

It is well established that parents play a key role in obesity treatment efforts directed at youth (Kitzmann et al. 2010), and for obvious reasons parents are the main audience for obesity prevention efforts in early childhood (Skouteris et al. 2011, 2012; Hesketh and Campbell 2010). Interventions directed at parents of infants have shown promise in reducing children's risk for obesity (Campbell et al. 2013; Wen et al. 2012), and parents of infants may be receptive to messaging aimed at increasing adoption of healthy eating and activity behaviors. Emerging evidence also suggests that interventions to promote positive parenting in general may help to reduce risk for childhood obesity (Harvey-Berino and Rourke 2003; Brotman et al. 2012). Maternal warmth and sensitivity are associated in prospective cohort studies with lower risk for obesity (Anderson et al. 2012, 2014). An explanatory mechanism may involve the impact of responsive parenting on the child's developing stress response system and regulatory pathways in the limbic areas of the brain (McEwen 2008; Schore 2005). In a national sample of preschool-aged children, the household routines of having family meals, ensuring that children get adequate sleep, and limiting time spent watching television were associated with lower prevalence of obesity (Anderson and Whitaker 2010). A randomized trial of a 6-month home-based intervention to promote these household routines in a sample of low-income families of 2–5-year-old children reduced children's BMI (Haines et al. 2013).

Recent evidence points to the importance of intervening early. In a randomized clinical trial targeting 3–5-year-old overweight or obese children, a multidisciplinary program reduced BMI, BMI z-scores, waist circumference, and waist circumference z-scores compared to a usual treatment control group. The treatment results were still present 12 months after the start of the intervention (Bocca et al. 2012b). A 6-month intensive home-based behavioral intervention program aimed at obese preschoolers (ages 2–5 years) has also shown promise in reducing BMI z-scores, both during the treatment period and at 12 months follow-up (Saelens et al. 2011). In an observational study of obese children ages 6–16 years, all were exposed to a behavioral treatment; changes in BMIs across a 3-year treatment window showed that younger aged children (6–9 compared with 14–16 years) were more successful in improving outcomes (Danielsson et al. 2012).

5.5 Screening Guidelines

Given what we know about factors associated with diabetes, screening for T2DM in children and adolescents is linked to weight status of the child, age of the child, and pubertal status. Several groups have published guidelines for T2DM screening in children. These guidelines are summarized in Table 1.

5.5.1 Growth in Childhood

Birth weight and growth trajectories have both been recognized as factors that are associated with the life course risk of T2DM. Given this, it seems key that individuals from the start understand their risk and that primary-care providers collect these data for all children. Surprisingly few guidelines currently recommend including birth weight as a component of a child's risk assessment for T2DM. An exception to this is the ISPAD screening guidelines that include birth size in their guidelines for Asian children. No recommendations were found that considered the actual growth of the child with respect to possible high-risk trajectories. Including birth size and growth as screeners for high-risk children has yet to be fully examined. A better understanding of the growth trajectory may be useful in identifying high-risk children earlier, but further work is needed in this area.

5.6 Summary

Childhood is the period where health behaviors are formed. While there is evidence that these behaviors are influenced by experience in the prior developmental periods, there is also evidence that significant change is still possible, especially in children under 5 years. Increasing evidence from both observational and intervention studies suggests that behavioral change is possible early on, but by middle childhood it becomes increasingly more difficult to affect real behavior change. These findings are pushing the research community to design studies that include young children, and the evidence is accumulating that interventions at the youngest ages achieve the best outcomes. During this period the child's world widens as he/she transitions into preschool and kindergarten, raising further the need to widen the focus of intervention beyond the family.

6 Adolescence

6.1 Transition into Adolescence

Puberty is an important phase in the life course that needs to be considered in studying the risks for T2DM. During puberty there is a known physiological insulin resistance and hyperinsulinemia that is thought to facilitate pubertal weight gain and growth (Burt Solorzano and McCartney 2010). The timing of the start of this insulin resistance has been reported to begin in mid-childhood, some years before puberty (Jeffery et al. 2012). Understanding this insulin resistance as it relates to the pubertal process is of high importance, as the rates of childhood diabetes continue to rise. Obesity exaggerates this pubertal insulin resistance, especially in girls, and may partially explain advanced maturation in obese females (Burt Solorzano and McCartney 2010).

6.2 Diagnosis of T2DM

The rising prevalence of both type 1 and type 2 among children and adolescents, in conjunction with increasing obesity throughout the population, has complicated the diagnosis of diabetes type. Past reliance on phenotype to distinguish and diagnose type of diabetes is not reliable (Amed et al. 2010a; Rosenbloom et al. 2008). In obese adolescents who present with new-onset diabetes, measurement of pancreatic autoantibodies is recommended as necessary to differentiate the type of diabetes (Zeitler 2010).

6.3 Treatment

Overall, there are few published evidence-based treatment studies for pediatric T2DM. The ADA and the ISPAD have published treatment recommendations, but these are primarily consensus based and built on current guidelines for adult T2DM (Amed et al. 2010a; Herbst et al. 2014). There are a handful of studies that have either been conducted or are ongoing specifically to address pediatric T2DM, studies which address both questions of prevention and treatment.

Treatment for T2DM has been addressed in a large multicenter randomized clinical trial, the Treatment Options for T2DM in Adolescents and Youth (known as the TODAY Study) (Copeland et al. 2011). Subjects were between the ages of 10 and 17, diagnosed with T2DM for less than 2 years, and had a BMI percentile at or above the 85th percentile for age and sex. Subjects were randomized into one of 3 comparison groups: metformin monotherapy, metformin plus rosiglitazone, or metformin plus an intensive family lifestyle program. Rates of failure (defined as poor glycemic control) were 52% in metformin alone, 39% in metformin plus rosiglitazone, and 47% in metformin plus the lifestyle program. Greatest weight loss was seen in the metformin plus the lifestyle program (Zeitler et al. 2012). These results highlight the difficulty that the majority of adolescents have in maintaining good glycemic control and suggest that many will require insulin within a few years of diagnosis. Ongoing research is needed to determine optimal management strategies in adolescents with T2DM.

The goal of therapy is to achieve euglycemia. The blood glucose levels should be monitored based on individual needs. Self- monitored blood glucose testing may be done at premeal times, or limited to before breakfast and before dinner only. Postprandial blood glucose levels, obtained 2 h after dinner, also offer helpful data for dose titration. The hemoglobin A1c is monitored at the time of clinic follow-up every 3 months. This reflects the average blood glucose over the past 3-month period. The aim of treatment is to achieve a hemoglobin A1c of less than 6.5% and the target blood glucose range = 70–120 mg/dl.

The first intervention for treatment of T2DM remains healthy lifestyle modifications including dietary modifications (including decreasing caloric intake) and increasing physical activity and exercise regimens to achieve weight stabilization and ultimately weight loss. Data from a recent study suggests that regular exercise was associated with lowering of the hemoglobin A1c (Herbst et al. 2014). Initiating changes in portion control as well as food choices and implementing modest amounts of exercise often prove difficult. Often adolescents have long-standing overweight and obesity concerns. Lifestyle changes tend to be more successful if initiated by the whole family instead of the particular individual being targeted.

If the diagnostic parameters are consistent with T2DM, pharmacologic treatment will need to be initiated. The particular therapeutic regimen initiated is determined by the initial presentation of T2 DM. If the adolescent presents in diabetic ketoacidosis, insulin therapy is instituted, initially intravenously, with subsequent transition to subcutaneous insulin therapy after the resolution of the acute diabetes ketoacidosis phase. Oral medication, specifically metformin, is initiated as well once the ketosis has resolved. If the presentation of T2DM is less acute, with the diagnosis being made on routine office testing, and hemoglobin A1c is less than 9%, medication therapy may be initiated first with metformin. In patients with symptomatology in between these 2 scenarios, where hemoglobin A1c is more than 9% in the presence of typical symptomatology, but no diabetes ketoacidosis, therapy may be initiated with metformin along with basal insulin (Zeitler et al. 2014). Other medications used for treatment of T2DM in adults are not approved for adolescents below 16 years of age.

Adherence to therapeutic interventions is key for achieving adequate diabetes control and is strongly emphasized. Modifications to regimen are based on hemoglobin A1c and review of blood glucose data. Adolescents who are on metformin therapy as well as basal insulin may need additional rapid acting insulin to cover their meals. Adolescents who were initiated on insulin and metformin, and achieve goal A1c, are feasible to gradually decrease the insulin dose, after they are on maximal metformin dosing. If adolescents are able to modify lifestyle factors as well as manage medication therapy adequately, it may be feasible to discontinue insulin altogether, while continuing on metformin therapy, albeit done very gradually with close monitoring.

6.3.1 Bariatric Surgery

Bariatric surgery for weight loss or uncontrolled T2DM is not commonly undertaken in the adolescent population. Results obtained in studies with adults that report weight loss and improvement in T2DM after bariatric surgery procedures (Courcoulas et al. 2014) has caused increased interest in its use in adolescents with morbid obesity. When bariatric surgery has been used as a treatment strategy for extreme obesity in adolescents, it has been found to be effective in improving or reversing abnormal glucose metabolism, but long-term outcome data in this age group is not yet available. This treatment option is limited to a very specific population because of potential complications (Brandt et al. 2010).

6.4 Surveillance

Comorbidities associated with T2DM should be investigated and treated as needed based on individual clinical presentation. The ADA and the ISPAD have published guidelines for comorbidity screening in youth diagnosed with T2DM. These guidelines are summarized in Table 2.

In a study examining adherence to ADA recommendations for lipid levels, blood pressure, hemoglobin A1c, microalbuminuria, and eye examinations, 95% of the participants reported having their blood pressure checked at all or most visits, 88% had lipid levels measured, 83% had kidney function tested, 68% underwent HbA1c testing, and 66% underwent an eye examination (Waitzfelder et al. 2011). Participants aged 18 years or older, particularly those with T2DM, tended to have fewer tests of all kinds performed. Age and family income emerged as important correlates of overall quality of care in multivariate models: older age and lower income were associated with not meeting the guidelines. Overall, while there was good compliance with the ADA-recommended guidelines, efforts to improve HbA1c testing and eye examinations were needed, especially among older adolescents and young adults (Waitzfelder et al. 2011).

6.5 Comorbidities

The TODAY study has demonstrated that a significant portion of adolescents with T2DM develop comorbidities. Careful attention to these

Table 2 Summary of surveillance guidelines for comorbidities

	Year	Recommendations
ADA (Amercian Diabetes Association 2000)	2012	Blood pressure measurement annually Fasting lipid profile Microalbuminuria assessment Dilated eye examination performed at the time of diagnosis Evaluation of polycystic ovarian disease and other comorbidities such as sleep apnea, hepatic steatosis, orthopedic complications, and psychosocial concerns
ISPAD (ISPAD 2011)	2011	Blood pressure measured at least annually Initial eye examination within 3 months of diagnosis and then annually from 11 years on after 2 years of diabetes duration Annual screening for microalbuminuria from age 11 and after 2 years of diabetes duration Fasting blood lipids after initial diagnosis and stabilization of diabetes ≥12 years; if family history of hypercholesterolemia, early CVD, or family history is unknown, screening should start at 2 years Peripheral and autonomic neuropathy assessed by history and physical exam from age 11 years with 2 years of diabetes duration

must be part of any management plan for these youths. Common comorbidities include hypertension and other metabolic conditions. Table 2 summarizes guidelines for monitoring the development of comorbidities in children/adolescents with T2DM.

6.6 Care Transition into Adult Practice

The emerging adult period (ages 18–30 years) is a high-risk time for youth with T2DM. These transitions from the pediatric to adult care setting often result in loss to follow-up at a time when the emergence of complications is occurring and the youth are engaging in high-risk health behaviors (Peters and Laffel 2011). In the majority of health-care institutions, there are no well-structured, seamless processes in place to ensure smooth transitions of care for any chronic care condition. Furthermore, there is little evidence-based research to guide practice on the management of this care transition in youth with T2DM. In the absence of evidenced-based programs and because of concerns about this transition, many programs are in the process of designing and/or implementing transition of care initiatives (Lee 2013). In 2011, a consensus-based document outlining recommendations for transition from pediatric and to adult diabetes care systems was published. Part of this document specifically highlighted the need for research to determine the best strategies for transition to diabetic adult care to assure optimal outcomes for the youth (Peters and Laffel 2011).

6.7 Summary

Because T2DM is most likely diagnosed during or shortly after puberty, the emphasis in adolescence is focused on understanding the components of care for the disease, including the surveillance for and management of comorbidities. In adolescence the consequences of the child's early environments are becoming clear and the window for prevention has narrowed.

7 Summary and Recommendations

7.1 Summary

- Pediatric T2DM is a life course problem—this chapter demonstrates that no one factor and no one time period provides the explanation; prevention and treatment is not simple. To optimize childhood metabolic health, we must begin prior to conception and at every age seize the opportunities to shape the child's environment to enhance metabolic health development.
- Significant progress has been made in describing the growing pediatric T2DM epidemic and in identifying individual risk factors that contribute to its development. Work is ongoing to understand the underlying mechanisms of pediatric T2DM. This knowledge base will likely grow rapidly over the next decade.
- A major limitation of much of this work is that the studies tend to be singularly focused on exploring and understanding a particular risk, and are completed using a specific disciplinary approach. What is missing from most of this literature is the recognition that these risks exist within a dynamic developmental context with implications from micro- to macrosystems. The next generation of studies needs to consider how risks play out differently depending upon prior or current exposures and environments. What are the risk modifiers and mediators?
- Accounting for the influence of time-specific exposures during sensitive developmental periods in conjunction with exposures across time is limited in the current research, and must be addressed more thoroughly in future studies.
- Another major task facing pediatric T2DM researchers is to understand the developmental similarities and differences in T2DM between children and adults. When T2DM "threatens" or occurs in children/adolescents, the challenges of understanding and intervening are different from those in the adult population, both biologically and behaviorally.

- Pediatric T2DM must be understood within the dynamic context of the child's overall health development. Research on the factors and developmental processes occurring early in life has shown how the emergence of T2DM children and adolescents is conditioned by prior experiences, exposures, and response patterns earlier in the life course.
- Translating the current knowledge into practice-relevant evidence is lagging and must be accelerated.

7.2 Recommendations

7.2.1 Recommendation 1: To Continue to Elucidate Mechanisms that Contributes to Pediatric T2DM by Focusing the Research in Key Areas

There are several parts to this recommendation including the identification of substantive research areas to guide further work, as well as recommendations about the process for doing the work. Life course health development research will require transdisciplinary teams of scientists that examine phenomenon across different levels (genetic, cellular, biological systems, families, neighborhoods, and large and complex macro-systems) at different developmental stage of the child. No one individual, and no one discipline, can achieve this knowledge by working in a disciplinary silo.

There are several areas that will require further investigation, and in particular we need to increase our understanding of factors that may mitigate the effects of adverse early-life programming. Childhood adversity, including the type of adversity (e.g., resource lack compared with family chaos), and chronic stress are noted as likely to be involved in the biological programming of several chronic health conditions including pediatric T2DM, but this is poorly accounted for in most of the current studies. Inclusion of poverty and family stress get at some of these factors, but better conceptual and empirical models are needed. Furthermore, the timing of the exposure for these risks is also not well documented, and their time-specific impacts are not well understood (i.e., is it poverty during pregnancy, during early childhood, or both?). On the positive side, there is a small but growing literature on the importance of parenting style, particularly nurturing behaviors, as possibly ways of mitigating the negative effects of various types of adverse environmental contexts.

Research priorities include:

- Understanding the health capital and health development capacity that mothers (and fathers) bring to conception and determine which of these factors are most important for child health development
- Determining how adult-recognized T2DM genetic susceptibility applies in pediatric T2DM
- Increased work to identify the epigenetic changes that occur in response to risk exposures (e.g., environmental toxins, stressors)
- Nutrition research, at every stage of childhood
- Understanding how health behaviors develop across time

But none of these are factors will provide a satisfactory explanation in isolation; each must be conditioned on prior and co-occurring factors. A life course health development perspective suggests that research must be embedded within the life stage of the child, taking into account the child's full developmental history, including the intrauterine period. Exploring contemporaneous factors, e.g., physical activity, and their association with T2DM should be done conditional on prior life course exposures, not simply on current factors; for example, knowing that the child was exposed to diabetes in utero and the birth size of the infant may be key markers for understanding differential effects of contemporaneous factors. Figure 1 integrates these ideas to display the life stages along the horizontal axis and prevention, screening, and treatment/surveillance along the y axis. Embedded within this figure but not displayed because of the complexity is that at each point multiple factors from multiple levels are transacting simultaneously to bring about an outcome.

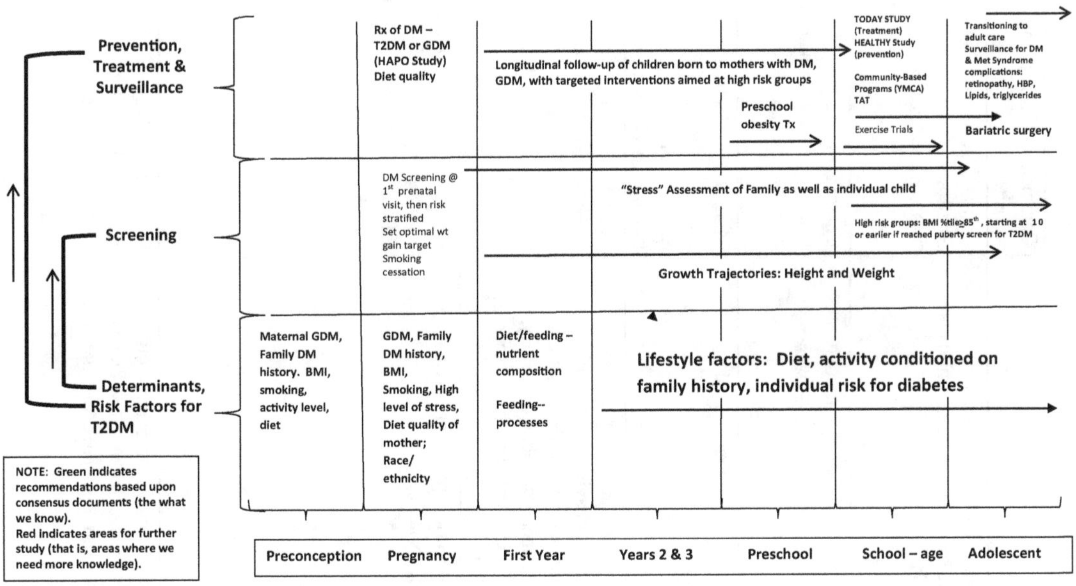

Fig. 1 A life course approach for understanding the risks, prevention and treatment of type 2 diabetes

7.2.2 Recommendation 2: To Strengthen Data and Methods Used to Address Identified Research Priorities and Explore the Feasibility of an International Effort to Harmonize Ongoing Birth Cohorts for the Purpose of Developing a Better Understanding of the Timing, Dose, and Interaction of Factors that Contribute to Pediatric T2DM Worldwide

Few data sets used to study the onset and impacts of T2DM include significant information on the broader context of the family, school, or neighborhood. In studies with good social data, biological data are often not included. A wider (micro to macro contexts) and longer (birth through adolescence) lens is needed to study T2DM. The need for longitudinal studies that can provide this lens is widely noted in the research literature, but because of the costs and subject burden, these long-term studies are difficult to carry out. However, there are a large number of longitudinal birth cohort studies ongoing worldwide that may have the potential for improving the understanding of pediatric T2DM. The recommendation here is to explore the feasibility of an international effort to harmonize ongoing birth cohorts to develop a better understanding of the timing, dose, and interactions of factors that contribute to T2DM worldwide. An added benefit of the development of such a data set is that it would provide the data to generate and test hypotheses, not just about T2DM but data directly relevant to the testing of the life course health development theoretical framework.

Table 3 presents an overview of international birth cohort studies. Of these studies, one dates to the 1950s, one to the 1960s, two during the 1970s, and another two in the 1980s. Twelve of the birth cohorts began data collection in the 1990s and 21 began data collection between 2000 and 2011. From this list, there are a handful of studies with data elements (birth data, multiple data collection points throughout childhood, including adolescent health and height and weight) pertinent to informing a life course picture of key pathways in this epidemic. Six birth cohorts were identified as having collected data beyond 1995 and included at least one data collection point in adolescence (defined as data

Table 3 Birth cohort longitudinal studies

Cohort/country	Years	Ages/data collection points	Sample characteristics	Measures	Comments: PI/Managing entity// website
Early Childhood Longitudinal Study—Birth cohort/US (ECLS)	Births in 2001	Birth through kindergarten entry: 9 months, 2 years, 4 years, and kindergarten	14,000 diverse nationally rep. sample; oversampling of API, AI, and Alaskan natives, twins, LBW	Cognitive, social, emotional, physical development—assessments, parents, child care settings, and KGT	National Center for Education Statistics http://nces.ed.gov/ecls
National Child Development Study (NCDS): UK 1958 Cohort	Births in 1958	1958, 7, 11, 16, 23, 33, 42, 46, 50; in 2003 @45, 9000 in biomedical screens	17,000 born during 1 week in 1958 in England, Scotland, Wales	Physical, educational, economic, employment, family life, health behaviors, well-being, social participation, attitudes	Centre for Longitudinal Studies, Institute of Education: Jane Elliot, PI http://www.cls.ioe.ac.uk/
1970 British Cohort Study	Births in 1970	1970, 5, 10, 16, 30, 34, and 42 (in 2012)	17,000 people born in England, Scotland, Wales in single week in 1970	Health, physical educational and social development, economic circumstances	Managed by Centre for Longitudinal Studies, Institute of Education; Alice Sullivan, PI http://www.cls.ioe.ac.uk/
Millennium Cohort Study	Births in 2000–2001	9 months, 3, 5, 7, 11 (in 2012) plus health visitor survey report and fertility survey report	19,000 people in the UK	Sibling and parent info; parenting, childcare, school choice, child behavior and cognitive development, child and parent health, parent's employment and education, income, poverty, neighborhood, and residential mobility; social capital and ethnicity	Managed by Centre for Longitudinal Studies, Institute of Education Lucinda Platt, PI http://www.cls.ioe.ac.uk/
Growing up in Scotland (GUS)	Births in Scotland: 2003/2004 birth cohort 1 and 2010/2011 birth cohort 2	Data collection yearly on the early cohorts; for the 2010 cohorts—only at key transitions	8000 children were enrolled into the study in 2005–20065000 were babies (~10 months) born between 6/ 2004 and 5/ 20053000 were toddlers (~34 months) born between 6/2002 and 5/ 2003. 6000 children born between 3/2010 and 2/ 2011 will be enrolled during 2010–2011; data collection at 10 months old.	Education, social work/support for parents, health, childcare, social inclusion	*Centre for Research onFamilies and Relationships*—University of Edinburghhttp://growingupinscotland.org.uk/
Growing up in Ireland	Births in 1999/2000 for older cohort; 2007/2008 for infant cohort	Two rounds of data collections with each group	8500 9-year-olds and 11,000 9-month-olds interviewed during September 2008 to April 2009. Second round data collection took place between January and August 2011.	The main aim of the study is to paint a full picture of children in Ireland and how they are developing in the current social, economic, and cultural environment	PI: Professor James Williams at Trinity College Dublin. http://www.growingup.ie/

(continued)

Table 3 (continued)

Cohort/country	Years	Ages/data collection points	Sample characteristics	Measures	Comments: PI/Managing entity// website
NLSY: Children of the '79	US	The NLSY child sample is comprised of all children born to the NLSY79 mothers; mothers have been interviewed biennially; data on child begins at birth through adulthood	More than 11,000 children have been identified; birth years range from 1979 through 2010	Cognitive, behavioral, health status, home environment, psychosocial, parental involvement, economic conditions of the family, risky behaviors	Access to in data available at Bureau of Labor Statistics web site www.bls.gov/nls/nlsy79.htm
Panel study of income dynamics (PSID)	US Birth 1968 and ongoing	Birth through adulthood. Annually from 1968 to 1997, biennially 1998. Child development supplement 1n 1997 from birth –12 and 2002/2003 for 5–18 years. 2007/2008 at 10–18 years. 18 years transition to adulthood at '05,'07, '09, '11	70,000 individuals over four decades. Includes initial participants from 1968 and their biological/adopted descendants. 1997 and 1999 included 511 immigrants to the USA	Cognitive, behavioral and health status. Afterschool physical activities, home environment, psychosocial, parental involvement, schooling and school environment	http://psidonline.isr.umich.edu/Guide/default.aspx
National Longitudinal Survey of Children and Youth	Canada 1994 and ongoing	Birth to early adulthood—eight cycles with varying age ranges (0–25 years)	Cycle 8: 35,795 children	Child health, family psychosocial, emotional, development, teenage risk behaviors	http://www.statcan.gc.ca/start-debut-eng.html

Danish Longitudinal Survey of Children	Denmark 1995 and 2003	Birth to adulthood: Birth 1995, 1996, 1999, 2003, 2007 (11 years old)	6011 children (born Sept 15-Oct 31, 1995 and mothers are Danish citizens); 611 children (born April 1-Dec 31, 1995 and mothers had been residing in Demark for 3 years); 6000 children born in 1995 who were placed in group homes/foster care—data collection began in 2003	Effect of differences in the socioeconomic situation, way of life, ethnicity, upbringing, and organization of home life within the family and its effects on childhood development. Consequences of the institutionalized childhood. Effectiveness of societal support of families and children. Effect of leave-of-absence schemes on the parents' perception of the father/mother role, or their perception of the role of the family/"the public sector." Effect of parents' mutual relations (conflict/harmony) on their children's daily life. Effect of parental education, way of life, cultural background and working conditions of the parents on the way they prioritize family life. Conditions in childhood/adolescence that effect social integrate. What social mechanisms influence child resiliency	http://www.sfi.dk/the_danish_longitudinal_survey_of_children-3214.aspx
Growing up in France (ELFE)	France 2011 (children born on specific days of year 2009 [4 days in each of the four different quarters])	Birth to adulthood: birth, 2 months, 3, 6, 11	1000 children (goal is 20,000)	To study the various factors interacting all over the life course up to adulthood (family structure, social and physical environment, schooling, health, and nutritional behavior) and to clarify the impact of the experience lived during infancy on the individual's physical, psychological, social, and professional development. Measure the cumulative exposures to specific environmental conditions or behaviors year after year and to analyze their consequences on social and health inequalities	http://www.cls.ioe.ac.uk/page.aspx?&sitesectionid=326&sitesectiontitle=ELFE+%28Growin%20g+up+in+France

(continued)

Table 3 (continued)

Cohort/country	Years	Ages/data collection points	Sample characteristics	Measures	Comments: PI/Managing entity// website
European Longitudinal Study of Pregnancy and Childhood (ELSPAC)	Europe born 1991 to 1995: Great Britain, Isle of Man, Czech Republic, Slovakia, Russia, Ukraine, Croatia and Estonia; recently added: Spain and Greece.	Pregnancy, birth to 19 years: 6 and 18 months; 3, 5, 7, 11, 15, 18 and 19 years	7589 children	Detect biological, psychological, and social factors as well as factors of external environment associated with survival and health of the fetus, infant and a child. Biopsychosocial determinants of the child's development from conception until the end of school age, while taking into consideration a lifestyle of the family, environment, care, or relationships among family members as well as personalities of the mother and the father. Furthermore, we are aiming to find the links between biopsychosocial determinants as well as origin and development of health disorders of a fetus, newborn, and a child. Medical issues during pregnancy—bleeding, eclampsia, infections, adolescent mothers. Specific termination of pregnancy—preterm delivery, intrauterine growth retardation of the fetus, abortions, child of diabetic mother. Growth— weight; height; length of long bones; circumference of head, waist, and arm; skin folders; and other anthropometric data. Development—developmental landmarks, motoric coordination, intellectual abilities	Research Institute of Preventive and Social Paediatrics at the Faculty of Medicine, Masaryk University Brno, Czech Republic: Lubomír Kukla, PI; Website: http://www.aloe-app.com/index-en.php
Growing up in Australia	Australia 2004	Two cohorts—families with 4–5-year-old children (4–19 years) and families with 0–1-year-old infants (birth to 16 years) Interviewed biennially	10,000 children – infant cohort (Dabelea et al. 2014; Grote et al. 2010) and child cohort (4991)	Children's social, economic, and cultural environments to their adjustment and well-being	Daryl Higgins, PI Website: http://www.aifs.gov.au/growingup/index.html

Birth to twenty	South Africa 1990	Birth through adulthood Birth to 14 years annually and 14 through adulthood biennially; multigenerational	3273 children (1594 recruited antenatal); 3273 women (singleton births)	Lifecycle approach and attempts to integrate historical, personal, social, and economic information with data collected during all major developmental stages. In the early years, the emphasis was on physical growth, health and health service usage; in the preschool years attention turned to social behavior, and home and center support for learning; during primary school, data has been collected on educational progress; in the teen years the study is concentrating on precursors to adult health and adjustment, including sexual behavior, school achievement, substance use, diet, activity, and conflict with the law. Regularly assessments are made of children's residential circumstances, household composition, and socioeconomic conditions. Growth measurements are taken and blood and urine samples subjected to a number of biochemical tests. Body composition, blood pressure and physical activity are also assessed	Child Youth Family and Social Development, Human Sciences Research Council: Linda Richter, PI http://www.wits.ac.za/academic/health/research/birthto20/10274/home.html
The Avon Longitudinal Study of Parents and Children 1992 (ALSPAC)—Children of the '90s study	UK	Birth to early adulthood	14,000 mothers in the former county of Avon enrolled during pregnancy in 1991 and 1992. The health and development of their children has been followed in great detail ever since	During pregnancy: medical history and physical health of mother and grandparents, exposure to environmental pollutants, sleeping patterns, diet, caffeine and alcohol consumption, smoking, illegal drug taking, psychological well-being of parents, their expectations and attitudes, social support networks. Early childhood: health, lifestyle, and development. At focus clinics, physical measurements and psychological tests, regular biological samples, DNA extraction, school performance on SATS and GCSEs. ALSPAC links to additional sources of data on participants include national pupil database and school census data, and information on death and cancer	http://www.bristol.ac.uk/alspac/

(continued)

Table 3 (continued)

Cohort/country	Years	Ages/data collection points	Sample characteristics	Measures	Comments: PI/Managing entity// website
Childhood Obesity – Early Programming by Infant Nutrition (CHOPIN)	Germany: 2002 to 2004 enrollment	Follow through to age 11; data collection yearly through 8 and then again at 11	1678 infants in Belgium, Germany, Italy, Poland, Spain	Birth outcomes (wt, length, gestational age, Apgar, sex); child exposures infancy through age 11; development; child health, biological samples. Also included a 1 year multicenter intervention trial on newborn infants, to test whether feeding infant formulae (differing in protein content), can influence growth trajectories during the first year of life	PI: Berthold Koletzko, Div. Metabolic and Nutritional Medicine, Dr. von Hauner Children's Hospital, Ludwig-Maximilians-University of Munich Medical http://www.ist-world.org/ProjectDetails.aspx?ProjectId=c63efc2bdd954069bed34a6d65d33dd4&SourceDatabaseId=e4fcfde0182a45898e8741a1abae3984
All Babies in Southeast Sweden	Sweden: Oct 1st 1997 to Oct 1st 1999	Multiple—beginning during fetal life, including bio-samples during pregnancy through age 14 years	17,000 infants	Main exposure: nutrition, physical activity, sleep pattern, infections, psychosocial factors, child care, stress, drugs, vaccinations, genetics, Outcomes: autoimmunity (Type 1 DM, celiac disease, RA), allergy, obesity, Type 2 DM	PI Johnny Ludvigsson; Dept of Clin Exp Medicine, Linköping university, Sweden http://www.researchweb.org/is/lio/ansokan/56531
Aarhus Birth Cohort	Births beginning in 1990 Denmark	Pre-pregnancy, second and third trimester	100,000 children and 100,000 mothers who gave birth at the Dept of Obst and Gyn, Aarhus Univ Hospital, Skejby	Fetal programming hypothesis and on various aspects of pregnancy, birth, and neonatal care. Birth outcomes (wt, lt, GA at birth, Apgar, congenital malformations, stillbirth, sex)	Dept. of Pediatrics and Perinatal Epidemiology Research Unit, Aarhus University Hospital, Skejby, Denmark:Tine Brink Henriksen, PI http://fetotox.au.dk/the-fetotox-birth-cohorts/aarhus-birth-cohort-biobank-abcb/
Amsterdam Born Children and their Development (ABCD study)	2003–2004	Pre-pregnancy, pregnancy (1st, 2nd, 3rd trimester), birth, 5 and 6 years to adulthood	6161 infants and 8266 mothers	Association between lifestyle, psychosocial conditions and nutritional status during pregnancy, and the child's health at birth (birth weight, pregnancy duration, perinatal mortality) and in later life (growth, physical development, behavior and cognitive functioning)	Academic Medical Centre/ University of Amsterdam: Manon van Eijsden; Tanja G.M. Vrijkotte, PI http://www.abcd-study.nl/
Babies After SCOPE: Evaluating the Longitudinal Impact using Neurological and Nutritional Endpoints	Ireland: Aug 1st 2008 to Oct 31 2011	Birth to 5 years, birth to 1, 2, and 5 years	2185 children born in Ireland	Maternal health, fetal growth, and childhood nutrition, growth and development in the first 2 years of life. Birth outcomes (wt, lt, GA at birth, sex)	University College Cork: PI Deirdre Murray, PI http://www.nationalchildrensresearchcentre.ie/research/baseline-study-babies-after-scope-evaluating-longitundinal-impact-using-neurological-and-nutritional-endpoints/

Bologna Birth Cohort	Italy 2004–2005	Birth to adulthood: birth, 1, 2, 3, and 7 years	654 children, 651 mothers, 593 fathers delivering at the University Hospital of Bolonga	Exposure: passive smoking, breastfeeding, nutrition, allergens, indoor pollution, motor vehicles pollution Outcome: wheezing, asthma, eczema, atopic dermatitis, sleep, cognitive development. Birth outcomes (wt, lt, GA at birth, Apgar, stillbirth, sex)	Maria Pia Fantini, PI
Born in Bradford	UK Jan 1st 2007 to Dec 24th 2010	Birth to adulthood: 1, 2, and 3 years	14,000 children, 14,000 mothers, and 3000 fathers	Describe health and ill-health within a largely bi-ethnic population; identify modifiable causal pathways that promote well-being, or contribute to ill-health; develop, design and evaluate interventions to promote health and well-being; Develop a model for integrating operational, epidemiological, and evaluative research into practice within the NHS and other health-related systems; build and strengthen the local research capacity	Bradford Institute for Health Research: John Wright, PI http://www.borninbradford.nhs.uk/
Copenhagen Child Cohort 2000 (CCC2000)	Denmark Births in 2000	Pregnancy, birth to adulthood: birth, 1, 6, and 11 years	6090 children, 6090 mothers	Developmental trajectories of psychopathology and mental disorders from birth in a general population birth cohort and to determine at risk states of mental illness in childhood and adolescence. Birth outcomes (wt, lt, GA at birth, Apgar, congenital malformations, stillbirth, sex)	Child and Adolescent psychiatric Centre, University Hospital of Copenhagen: Anne Mette Skovgaard, PI
Danish National Birth Cohort (DNBC)	Denmark Births 1996–2002	Pregnancy, birth to adulthood: birth—7 years, 11 years	95,000 children, 100,418 mothers	Pregnancy complications and diseases in offspring as a function of factors operating in pregnancy/fetal and early life. Fetal growth as an outcome and as a determinant of later health. Main exposures: infection, alcohol, tobacco, environments, medication, psychosocial factors. Nutrition in pregnancy, in general but with focus upon fish intake Outcome measures: life-long follow-up of children—mortality and morbidity. Birth outcomes (wt, lt, GA at birth, Apgar, congenital malformations, stillbirth, sex)	Statens Serum Institut, Copenhagen: Jørn Olsen, PI http://www.ssi.dk/English/RandD/Research%20areas/Epidemiology/DNBC/
Dortmund Nutritional and Anthropometric Longitudinally Designed Study (DONALD)	Germany Births from 1985 and ongoing	Infants 3–6 months old to adulthood: birth—18 years	1300 each children, mothers, and fathers; open cohort study. Annual recruitment of 30–40 infants	Environmental exposure is not the main focus of the birth outcomes (wt, lt, GA at birth, apgar, sex). Child exposures: child care, second hand smoke, smoking, alcohol, breastfeeding, diet, PA, medications, head circumference, sexual maturation, allergies, infections, cardiac, cancer, DM, BP, sleep, urine samples	Research Insitute of Child Nutrition: Anette Buyken, Thomas Remer, Ute Alexy, Mathilde Kersting – Pis

(continued)

Table 3 (continued)

Cohort/country	Years	Ages/data collection points	Sample characteristics	Measures	Comments: PI/Managing entity//website
Gateshead Millennium Study	UK births from June 1st 1999 to May 31st 2000	Birth to adulthood: birth, 1, 7, 9, and 12 years	1029 children and 1011 mothers	Feeding, weaning, and growth, including characteristics of maternal feeding style, eating attitudes, and depression. Childhood aspects of developmental psychopathology, behavioral and emotional development, and repetitive behaviors. Origins of childhood obesity, with particular reference to food intake, physical activity and sedentary behavior. Original purpose was investigation of weight faltering	Newcastle University: Ashley Adamson, PI http://www.cls.ioe.ac.uk/page.aspx?&sitesectionid=332&sitesectiontitle=Gateshead+Millennium+Study
GECKO Drenthe cohort	Netherlands born April 1st 2006 to April 1st 2007	Pregnancy, birth to adulthood: birth—5 years	2997 children born in Drenthe, Netherlands. Pregnant mothers recruited in the third trimester	The overall aim of the GECKO Drenthe cohort is to study the prevalence and early risk factors for the development of childhood overweight and fat distribution at very young age. Within this birth cohort the growth of the children is closely followed, starting at birth until adulthood. The children are followed using questionnaires that the parents have to answer and the regular visits to the Well Baby Clinics, where length, weight, head circumference, and hip and waist circumference are measured. Furthermore, physical activity is measured using accelerometers. At birth, cord blood was sampled and stored for (epi)genetic analysis and biomarkers. During the first 9 months of life, the children were measured every month (incl. questionnaire); thereafter this frequency decreased until once every 2 years from 3 years onward. The children are now 5 years old	University Medical Center Groningen: E. Corpeleijn, PI
Generation R	Netherlands birth Jan 21st 2002 to Feb 1st 2006	Pregnancy, birth to adulthood: birth—5, 7, and 9 years	10,000 children, 97,780 mothers, and 6500 fathers	Identification of early critical periods and causal pathways for growth, development, and health. Birth outcomes (wt, length, GA at birth, Apgar, congenital malformation, still birth, sex)	Erasmus Medical Center Rotterdam: Vincent Jaddoe, PI http://research.lunenfeld.ca/eagle/?page=841

Genetic and Environment: Prospective Study on Infancy in Italy (GASPII)	Italy June 1st 2003 to Oct 31st 2004	Birth to 20 years: birth, 1, 3, and 8 years	708 children, 693 mothers (>18 years), and 63 fathers	Environmental exposures, diet, air pollution asthma and allergies, accidents and injuries, obesity, minor birth defects, neurodevelopment. Birth outcomes (wt, length, GA at birth, Apgar, congenital malformation, still birth, sex)	Department of Epidemiology Regional Health Service lazio Region: Daniela Porta, PI
German Infant Study on the influence of Nutrition Intervention (GINIplus)	Germany births Jan 1st 1995 to Jan 1st 1998	Birth to adulthood: birth—4, 6, 10, and15 years	5991 children, maternal pregnancy outcomes	Intervention substudy; double -blinded randomized trial for hypoallergenic formulae, observational substudy: natural course of atopic diseases and metabolic disorders; mental health, nutrition, body weight and physical activity; Birth outcomes (wt, lt, GA at birth)	HelmholtzZentrum München: D. Berdel; A.v. Berg; C.P. Bauer; U. Krämer; S. Koletzko; J. Heinrich – PIs
Healthy Habits for two (HHf2)	Denmark births April 1st 1984 to April 1st 1987	Pregnancy, birth annually through 18 to 20 years	11,144 children of live birth singleton pregnancy, 11,980 mothers who attended 2 midwife in Aalborg or Odense during week 35 to 38 of pregnancy	Birth outcomes (wt, lt, GA at birth, Apgar, congenital malformations, sex). Converted from a trial to a birth cohort	The Danish Epidemiology Science Centre: Jørn Olsen, PI
KOALA Birth Cohort Study (KOALA)	Netherlands Birth Jan 1st 2000 to Oct 1st 2002	Pregnancy, Birth to adulthood: birth—2, 5–9 years	2843 children, 2900 mothers >14 weeks in a pregnancy pelvic pain or from an alternate lifestyle practices, 2900 fathers	Main outcomes: 1. allergy and asthma development, 2. growth and overweight development (inflammatory, immunological, metabolic, cardiorespiratory and cardiovascular aspects) Main exposures: microbial (infections, gut microbiota), breastfeeding and breast milk composition, nutrition, physical activity, parenting practices and parenting styles; home, neighborhood, and childcare environment. Birth outcomes (wt, lt, GA at birth, Apgar, congenital malformations, sex)	Maastricht University: Carel Thijs, PI http://www.koala-study.nl/
Lifeways Cross-Generation Cohort Study	Ireland 2001 to 2003	Pregnancy, birth: birth—3, 5, and 10 years	1074 children, 1061 mothers, 325 fathers	Physical and psychological health status, socioeconomic circumstances, birth, childhood, early adulthood and early middle age. Birth outcomes (wt, GA at birth, Apgar, congenital malformations, stillbirth, sex)	University College Dublin: Cecily Kelleher, PI http://www.ucd.ie/phpps/research/clinicalepidemiologygroup/lifewayscross-generationcohortstudy/

(continued)

Table 3 (continued)

Cohort/country	Years	Ages/data collection points	Sample characteristics	Measures	Comments: PI/Managing entity// website
Mother Child Cohort in Crete (RHEA)	Greece Feb 1st 2007 to Feb 29th 2008	Pregnancy, birth to 16 years: birth—4 years	1590 children; 1610 mothers >16 years and 9–13 wks gestation; 37 fathers	1. The evaluation of nutritional, environmental, biological, and psychosocial exposures in the prenatal period and in early childhood. 2. The evaluation of the association of these exposures with the development of the fetus and the child, reproductive outcomes, endocrine-related outcomes, neurodevelopment, obesity, and the occurrence of chronic diseases including asthma and allergies, metabolic syndrome, and endocrine disorders that appear first in childhood but that may perpetuate to adulthood. 3. The evaluation of mother's health during and after pregnancy. 4. The evaluation of genetic susceptibility and the interactions between genetic and environmental factors affecting child health. Birth outcomes (wt, lt, GA at birth, Apgar, stillbirth, sex)	Dept of Social Medicine, Medical School, Heraklion, University of Crete, Greece and CREAL, Barcelona, Spain: Manolis Kogevinas and Leda Chatzi – PIs
Norwegian Human Milk Study (HUMIS)	Norway 2003 to 2009	Birth to adulthood: Birth –2 years, 8 years	2500 children breastfeeding at 2 wks of age, 2500 mothers, 2400 fathers	Exposures: environmental toxicants, gut microbiota, pops, Pfos, organotins, gut microbiota, *Bifidobacterium*, *Lactobacillus*, early nutrition, human milk composition, duration of breastfeeding. Main outcomes: child health, reproductive health, asthma and allergy, ADHD, neuropsychological development, depression, overweight. Birth outcomes (wt, lt, GA at birth, Apgar, congenital malformations, sex)	Norwegian Institute of Public Health: Merete Eggesbø, PI
Norwegian Mother and Child Cohort Study (MoBa)	Norway Jan 1st 1999 to Dec 31 2008	Pregnancy, birth to adulthood: birth, 1, 3, 5, 7, 8 years	10,500 children, 90,700 mothers 17–20 wks pregnant, 72,100 fathers	Causes of diseases. Additional aims are to detect early signs of disease and to describe the development of diseases. Birth outcomes (wt, lt, GA at birth, apgar, congenital malformations, stillbirth)	Norwegian Institute of Public Health: Per Magnus, PI http://www.fhi.no/eway/default.aspx?pid=240&trg=Main_6664&Main_6664=6894:0:25,7372:1:0:0:::0:0&MainContent_6898=6671:0:25,7899:1:0:0:::0:0&List_6673=6674:0:25,7905:1:0:0:::0:0

Odense Child Cohort	Denmark Births beginning in 2010	Infants 0–5 months to 18 years	1650 children, 2249 mothers, 2102 fathers—living in Odense, Denmark	Interaction between the fetus/infant/child during pregnancy, birth, and childhood and the social and environmental determinants for health and disease. Birth outcomes (wt, lt, GA at birth, Apgar, stillbirth, sex)	Odense University Hospital, Hans Christian Andersen Children's Hospital, Paediatric Research Unit: Steffen Husby, PI http://www.sdu.dk/en/Om_SDU/Institutter_centre/Klinisk_institut/Forskning/Forskningsenheder/Paediatri/Odense+Børnekohorte
Study on the pre- and early postnatal determinants of child health and development (EDEN – France)	France Births 2003 to 2005	Pregnancy, birth to 8 years: birth to 5 years and 8 years	1900 children, 2000 mothers >18 years and <24 wks pregnant, 1800 fathers	Pre- and postnatal determinant of the child's development and health. Birth outcomes (wt, lt, GA at birth, Apgar, congenital malformations, stillbirth, sex)	CESP INSERM: Heude Barbara, PI

The cohorts outlined here met the following criteria: Enrollment of the mother/child into the cohort was either prior to the pregnancy, during the pregnancy, or at birth; there was data collected with some frequency in childhood; the studies were not single/narrow focused)

Key source is http://www.birthcohorts.net; this site is an inventory of birth cohort longitudinal studies maintained by Department of Public Health, University of Copenhagen, Professor Anne-Marie Nybo Andersen collection at 15 years or beyond). These cohorts also gathered data for childhood weight, height, health assessment, and various social parameters. The cohorts were the Canadian National Longitudinal Survey of Children and Youth (NLSCY, data collected at various age points from birth through age 25 over the course of 8 cycles), the European Longitudinal Study of Pregnancy and Childhood (ELSPAC, data collected at nine points from birth through 19 years and includes the countries of Great Britain, Isle of Man, Czech Republic, Slovakia, Russia, Ukraine, Croatia, Estonia, Spain and Greece), the Growing Up in Australia survey (data collected through two separate cohorts with one beginning at birth to 1 year and the second at 4/5 years with follow-up to age 19 years), the South Africa's Birth to 20 longitudinal study (data collected through two separate cohorts that followed children ages birth to 14 years and age 14 years through adulthood), the UK's Avon Longitudinal Study of Parents and Children (ALSPAC) (data collected on children born between 1990 and 1992 from birth through adulthood), and finally, the German Infant Study on the Influence of Nutrition Intervention (GINIplus), collected data on children born between 1995 and 1998 annually from birth through 4 years and then at 6, 10, and 15 years of age.

In addition to the data limitations currently facing the pediatric T2DM research community, there are also methodological/analytical challenges. To make progress in all of these research priorities, large amounts of data will be needed. These data will be diverse ranging from genetic and other biologicals to social structure factors. Management and analyses of such diverse data will require new methods and collaborations that will include basic scientists, mathematicians, data engineers, practitioners, and translational scientists. Researchers will need to employ big data analytics and a complex system perspective that can address multiple causes and outcomes. The challenges are significant, but the opportunities vast to make a real difference to the health development of all children

7.2.3 Recommendation 3: To Translate the Growing Body of Knowledge into Evidenced-Based Prevention and Treatment Strategies

There are clear needs for both prevention and treatment trials in children and adolescents. There is a dearth of evidence-based studies and guidelines available to pediatric practitioners and pediatric endocrinologist to address the multiple management issues faced when treating patients with T2DM. Areas of clear need include prevention strategies for children born at high risk. For example, low birth weight newborns, offspring of diabetic mothers, could be placed in programs to test interventions to modify risk. This is a very important area of pediatric and diabetes research with implications on health status and care for large number of children into adulthood and should be of high priority for funding agencies.

Prevention trials are needed that can identify strategies to reduce the risk for developing T2DM, and as recent work demonstrates, understanding the age at intervention is key. Prevention strategies may be gleaned from longitudinal data collected for other reasons. While not a prospective trial, the primary data elements could be supplemented either through new data collection efforts (e.g., during adolescence collecting insulin, glucose, etc.), or by combining the primary data with other administrative data—child electronic health records of heights and weights throughout childhood—or both. With home address information, child contexts could be tracked over time and neighborhoods accounted for in the analyses.

Finally, there is much work to be done to translate the knowledge into policy at every level. Pediatric practitioners need up-to-date guidelines to identify children at high risk for T2DM at young ages. Families must be given the information about the possible long-term consequences of decisions made in early life. Local, state, and national governments also need policies in place that enhance child health development throughout childhood. Only then will we be able to achieve the goal of optimal health development for every child.

References

Aaltonen, J., Ojala, T., Laitinen, K., Poussa, T., Ozanne, S., & Isolauri, E. (2011). Impact of maternal diet during pregnancy and breastfeeding on infant metabolic programming: A prospective randomized controlled study. *European Journal of Clinical Nutrition, 65*(1), 10–19.

Agardh, E., Allebeck, P., Hallqvist, J., Moradi, T., & Sidorchuk, A. (2011). Type 2 diabetes incidence and socio-economic position: A systematic review and meta-analysis. *International Journal of Epidemiology, 40*(3), 804–818.

Amed, S., Daneman, D., Mahmud, F. H., & Hamilton, J. (2010a). Type 2 diabetes in children and adolescents. *Expert Review of Cardiovascular Therapy, 8*(3), 393–406.

Amed, S., Dean, H. J., Panagiotopoulos, C., Sellers, E. A., Hadjiyannakis, S., Laubscher, T. A., et al. (2010b). Type 2 diabetes, medication-induced diabetes, and monogenic diabetes in Canadian children: A prospective national surveillance study. *Diabetes Care, 33*(4), 786–791.

Amercian Diabetes Association. (2000). Type 2 diabetes in children and adolescents. *Pediatrics, 105*(3 Pt 1), 671–680.

American Academy of Pedicatrics. (2012). Breastfeeding and the use of human milk. *Pediatrics, 129*(3), e827–e841.

American Diabetes Association. (2010). Diagnosis and classification of diabetes mellitus. *Diabetes Care, 33*(Suppl 1), S62–S69.

Anderson, S. E., & Whitaker, R. C. (2010). Household routines and obesity in US preschool-aged children. *Pediatrics, 125*(1), 420–428.

Anderson, S. E., Gooze, R. A., Lemeshow, S., & Whitaker, R. C. (2012). Quality of early maternal-child relationship and risk of adolescent obesity. *Pediatrics, 129*(1), 132–140.

Anderson, S. E., Lemeshow, S., & Whitaker, R. C. (2014). Maternal-infant relationship quality and risk of obesity at age 5.5 years in a national US cohort. *BMC Pediatrics, 14*(1), 54.

Armitage, J. A., Khan, I. Y., Taylor, P. D., Nathanielsz, P. W., & Poston, L. (2004). Developmental programming of the metabolic syndrome by maternal nutritional imbalance: How strong is the evidence from experimental models in mammals? *The Journal of Physiology, 561*(Pt 2), 355–377.

Armitage, J. A., Poston, L., Taylor, P., & D. (2008). Developmental origins of obesity and the metabolic syndrome: The role of maternal obesity. *Frontiers of Hormone Research, 36*, 73–84.

Arslanian, S. A., Bacha, F., Saad, R., & Gungor, N. (2005). Family history of type 2 diabetes is associated with decreased insulin sensitivity and an impaired balance between insulin sensitivity and insulin secretion in white youth. *Diabetes Care, 28910*, 115–119.

Barker, D. J., Hales, C. N., Fall, C. H., Osmond, C., Phipps, K., & Clark, P. M. (1993). Type 2 (non-insulin-dependent) diabetes mellitus, hypertension and hyperlipidaemia (syndrome X): Relation to reduced fetal growth. *Diabetologia, 36*(1), 62–67.

Barker, A., Sharp, S. J., Timpson, N. J., Bouatia-Naji, N., Warrington, N. M., Kanoni, S., et al. (2011). Association of genetic loci with glucose levels in childhood and adolescence: A meta-analysis of over 6,000 children. *Diabetes, 60*(6), 1805–1812.

Barlow, S. E. (2007). Expert committee recommendations regarding the prevention, assessment, and treatment of child and adolescent overweight and obesity: Summary report. *Pediatrics, 120*(Suppl 4), S164–S192.

Barouki, R., Gluckman, P. D., Grandjean, P., Hanson, M., & Heindel, J. J. (2012). Developmental origins of non-communicable disease: Implications for research and public health. *Environmental Health : A Global Access Science Source, 11*, 42.

Barton, M. (2010). Screening for obesity in children and adolescents: US preventive services task Force recommendation statement. *Pediatrics, 125*(2), 361–367.

Battista, M. C., Hivert, M. F., Duval, K., & Baillargeon, J. P. (2011). Intergenerational cycle of obesity and diabetes: How can we reduce the burdens of these conditions on the health of future generations? *Experimental Diabetes Research, 2011*, 596060. doi:10.1155/2011/596060.

Bell, J. F., & Zimmerman, F. J. (2010). Shortened nighttime sleep duration in early life and subsequent childhood obesity. *Archives of Pediatrics & Adolescent Medicine, 164*(9), 840–845.

Bell, R. A., Mayer-Davis, E. J., Beyer, J. W., D'Agostino, R. B., Jr., Lawrence, J. M., Linder, B., et al. (2009). Diabetes in non-Hispanic white youth: Prevalence, incidence, and clinical characteristics: The SEARCH for diabetes in youth study. *Diabetes Care, 32*(Suppl 2), S102–S111.

Berends, L. M., & Ozanne, S. E. (2012). Early determinants of type-2 diabetes. *Best Practice & Research. Clinical Endocrinology & Metabolism, 26*(5), 569–580.

Bertin, E., Gangnerau, M. N., Bellon, G., Bailbe, D., Arbelot De Vacqueur, A., & Portha, B. (2002). Development of beta-cell mass in fetuses of rats deprived of protein and/or energy in last trimester of pregnancy. *American Journal of Physiology. Regulatory, Integrative and Comparative Physiology, 283*(3), R623–R630.

Bocca, G., Corpeleijn, E., Stolk, R. P., & Sauer, P. J. J. (2012a). Results of a multidisciplinary treatment program in 3-year-old to 5-year-old overweight or obese children: A randomized controlled clinical trial. *Archives of Pediatrics & Adolescent Medicine, 166*(12), 1109–1115.

Bocca, G., Corpeleijn, E., Stolk, R. P., & Sauer, P. J. (2012b). Results of a multidisciplinary treatment program in 3-year-old to 5-year-old overweight or obese children: A randomized controlled clinical trial. *Archives of Pediatrics & Adolescent Medicine, 166*(12), 1109–1115.

Boekelheide, K., Blumberg, B., Chapin, R. E., Cote, I., Graziano, J. H., Janesick, A., et al. (2012). Predicting later-life outcomes of early-life exposures. *Environmental Health Perspectives, 120*(10), 1353–1361.

Boyle, J. P., Thompson, T. J., Gregg, E. W., Barker, L. E., & Williamson, D. F. (2010). Projection of the year 2050 burden of diabetes in the US adult population: Dynamic modeling of incidence, mortality, and prediabetes prevalence. *Population Health Metrics, 8*, 29. doi:10.1186/1478-7954-8-29.

Brandt, M. L., Harmon, C. M., Helmrath, M. A., Inge, T. H., McKay, S. V., & Michalsky, M. P. (2010). Morbid obesity in pediatric diabetes mellitus: Surgical options and outcomes. *Nature reviews. Endocrinology, 6*(11), 637–645.

Brotman, L. M., Dawson-McClure, S., Huang, K. Y., Theise, R., Kamboukos, D., Wang, J., et al. (2012). Early childhood family intervention and long-term obesity prevention among high-risk minority youth. *Pediatrics, 129*(3), e621–e628.

Brown, T., & Summerbell, C. (2009). Systematic review of school-based interventions that focus on changing dietary intake and physical activity levels to prevent childhood obesity: An update to the obesity guidance produced by the National Institute for health and clinical excellence. *Obesity Reviews, 10*(1), 110–141.

Brunton, P. J. (2010). Resetting the dynamic range of hypothalamic-pituitary-adrenal axis stress responses through pregnancy. *Journal of Neuroendocrinology, 22*(11), 1198–1213.

Burns, S. F., Lee, S., Bacha, F., Tfayli, H., Hannon, T. S., & Arslanian, S. A. (2014). Pre-diabetes in overweight youth and early atherogenic risk. *Metabolism, 63*(12), 1528–1235.

Burt Solorzano, C. M., & McCartney, C. R. (2010). Obesity and the pubertal transition in girls and boys. *Reproduction, 140*(3), 399–410.

Caballero, B., Clay, T., Davis, S. M., Ethelbah, B., Rock, B. H., Lohman, T., et al. (2003). Pathways: A school-based, randomized controlled trial for the prevention of obesity in American Indian schoolchildren. *American Journal of Clinical Nutrition, 78*(5), 1030–1038.

Campbell, K. J., Lioret, S., McNaughton, S. A., Crawford, D. A., Salmon, J., Ball, K., et al. (2013). A parent-focused intervention to reduce infant obesity risk behaviors: A randomized trial. *Pediatrics, 131*(4), 652–660. doi:10.1542/peds.2012-2576.

Cenit, M. C., Matzaraki, V., Tigchelaar, E. F., & Zhernakova, A. (2014). Rapidly expanding knowledge on the role of the gut microbiome in health and disease. *Biochimica et Biophysica Acta, 1842*(10), 1981–1992.

Christian, L. M. (2012). Physiological reactivity to psychological stress in human pregnancy: Current knowledge and future directions. *Progress in Neurobiology, 99*(2), 106–116. doi:10.1016/j.pneurobio.2012.07.003.

Copeland, K. C., Zeitler, P., Geffner, M., Guandalini, C., Higgins, J., Hirst, K., et al. (2011). Characteristics of adolescents and youth with recent-onset type 2 diabetes: The TODAY cohort at baseline. *Journal of Clinical Endocrinology and Metabolism, 96*(1), 159–167.

Courcoulas, A., Goodpaster, B., Eagleton, J., Belle, S., Kalarchian, M., Lang, W., et al. (2014). Surgical vs medical treatments for type 2 diabetes mellitus: A randomized clinical trial. *JAMA Surgery, 7*(149), 707–715.

Crume, T. L., Ogden, L. G., Mayer-Davis, E. J., Hamman, R. F., Norris, J. M., Bischoff, K. J., et al. (2012). The impact of neonatal breast-feeding on growth trajectories of youth exposed and unexposed to diabetes in utero: The EPOCH study. *International Journal of Obesity, 36*(4), 529–534.

Dabelea, D., Bell, R. A., D'Agostino, R. B., Jr., Imperatore, G., Johansen, J. M., Linder, B., et al. (2007). Incidence of diabetes in youth in the United States. *JAMA, 297*(24), 2716–2724.

Dabelea, D., Dolan, L. M., D'Agostino, R., Jr., Hernandez, A. M., McAteer, J. B., Hammon, R. F., et al. (2011). Association testing of TCF7L2 polymorphisms with type 2 diabetes in multi-ethnic youth. *Diabetologia, 54*(3), 535–539.

Dabelea, D., Mayer-Davis, E. J., Saydah, S., Imperatore, G., Linder, B., et al. (2014). Prevalence of type 1 and type 2 diabetes among children and adolescents from 2001 to 2009. *JAMA, 311*(17), 1778–1786.

Danielsson, P., Kowalski, J., Ekblom, O., & Marcus, C. (2012a). Response of severely obese children and adolescents to behavioral treatment. *Archives of Pediatrics & Adolescent Medicine, 166*(12), 1103–1108.

Danielsson, P., Kowalski, J., Ekblom, O., & Marcus, C. (2012b). Response of severely obese children and adolescents to behavioral treatment. *Archives of Pediatrics & Adolescent Medicine, 166*(12), 1103–1108.

Davis, C. L., Pollock, N. K., Waller, J. L., Allison, J. D., Dennis, B. A., Bassali, R., et al. (2012). Exercise dose and diabetes risk in overweight and obese children: A randomized controlled trial. *JAMA, 308*(11), 1103–1112.

Demmer, R. T., Zuk, A. M., Rosenbaum, M., & Desvarieux, M. (2013). Prevalence of diagnosed and undiagnosed type 2 diabetes mellitus among US adolescents: Results from the continuous NHANES, 1999-2010. *American Journal of Epidemiology, 178*(7), 1106–1113.

Devaraj, S., Hemarajata, P., & Versalovic, J. (2013). The human gut microbiome and body metabolism: Implications for obesity and diabetes. *Clinical Chemistry, 59*(4), 617–628.

Dyer, J. S., & Rosenfeld, C. R. (2011). Metabolic imprinting by prenatal, perinatal, and postnatal overnutrition: A review. *Seminars in Reproductive Medicine, 29*(3), 266–276.

van Eijsden, M., Vrijkotte, T. G., Gemke, R. J., & van der Wal, M. F. (2011). Cohort profile: The Amsterdam born children and their development (ABCD) study. *International Journal of Epidemiology, 40*(5), 1176–1186.

Ekelund, U., Ong, K. K., Linne, Y., Neovius, M., Brage, S., Dunger, D. B., et al. (2007). Association of weight gain in infancy and early childhood with metabolic risk in young adults. *The Journal of Clinical Endocrinology and Metabolism, 92*(1), 98–103.

Elder, D. A., Herbers, P. M., Weis, T., Standiford, D., Woo, J. G., & D'Alessio, D. A. (2012). Beta-cell dysfunction in adolescents and adults with newly diagnosed type 2 diabetes mellitus. *Journal of Pediatrics, 160*(6), 904–910.

Eriksson, J. G. (2006). Early growth, and coronary heart disease and type 2 diabetes: Experiences from the Helsinki birth cohort studies. *International Journal of Obesity, 30*(Suppl 4), S18–S22.

Eriksson, J. G. (2011). Early growth and coronary heart disease and type 2 diabetes: Findings from the Helsinki birth cohort study (HBCS). *The American Journal of Clinical Nutrition, 94*(6 Supplement), 1799S–1802S.

Eriksson, J. G., Osmond, C., Kajantie, E., Forsen, T. J., & Barker, D. J. (2006). Patterns of growth among children who later develop type 2 diabetes or its risk factors. *Diabetologia, 49*(12), 2853–2858.

Fabricius-Bjerre, S., Jensen, R. B., Faerch, K., Larsen, T., Molgaard, C., Michaelsen, K. F., et al. (2011). Impact of birth weight and early infant weight gain on insulin resistance and associated cardiovascular risk factors in adolescence. *PloS One, 6*(6), e20595. doi:10.1371/journal.pone.0020595.

Ferguson, M. A., Gutin, B., Le, N. A., Karp, W., Litaker, M., Humphries, M., et al. (1999). Effects of exercise training and its cessation on components of the insulin resistance syndrome in obese children. *International Journal of Obesity and Related Metabolic Disorders, 23*(8), 889–895.

Fernandez-Twinn, D. S., Wayman, A., Ekizoglou, S., Martin, M. S., Hales, C. N., & Ozanne, S. E. (2005). Maternal protein restriction leads to hyperinsulinemia and reduced insulin-signaling protein expression in 21-mo-old female rat offspring. *American Journal of Physiology. Regulatory, Integrative and Comparative Physiology, 288*(2), R368–R373.

Foster, G. D., Linder, B., Baranowski, T., Cooper, D. M., Goldberg, L., Harrell, J. S., et al. (2010). A school-based intervention for diabetes risk reduction. *New England Journal of Medicine, 363*(5), 443–453.

Gabbe, S. G., Landon, M. B., Warren-Boulton, E., & Fradkin, J. (2012). Promoting health after gestational diabetes: A National Diabetes Education Program call to action. *Obstetrics and Gynecology, 119*(1), 171–176.

Gaffney, K. F., Kitsantas, P., & Cheema, J. (2012). Clinical practice guidelines for feeding behaviors and weight-for-age at 12 months: A secondary analysis of the infant feeding practices study II. *Worldviews on Evidence- Based Nursing, 9*(4), 234–242.

Gaffney, K. F., Kitsantas, P., Brito, A., & Swamidoss, C. S. (2014). Postpartum depression, infant feeding practices, and infant weight gain at six months of age. *Journal of Pediatric Health Care, 28*(1), 43–50.

Garofano, A., Czernichow, P., & Breant, B. (1998). Beta-cell mass and proliferation following late fetal and early postnatal malnutrition in the rat. *Diabetologia, 41*(9), 1114–1120.

Gillis, B., Mobley, C., Stadler, D. D., Hartstein, J., Virus, A., Volpe, S. L., et al. (2009). Rationale, design and methods of the HEALTHY study nutrition intervention component. *International Journal of Obesity, 33*(Suppl 4), S29–S36.

Gillman, M. W., Oakey, H., Baghurst, P. A., Volkmer, R. E., Robinson, J. S., & Crowther, C. A. (2010). Effect of treatment of gestational diabetes mellitus on obesity in the next generation. *Diabetes Care, 33*(5), 964–968.

Gluckman, P. D., Hanson, M. A., Cooper, C., & Thornburg, K. L. (2008). Effect of in utero and early-life conditions on adult health and disease. *New England Journal of Medicine, 359*(1), 61–73.

Groop, L. C., & Tuomi, T. (1997). Non-insulin-dependent diabetes mellitus–a collision between thrifty genes and an affluent society. *Annals of Medicine, 29*, 37–53.

Grote, V., Vik, T., von Kries, R., Luque, V., Socha, J., Verducci, E., et al. (2010). Maternal postnatal depression and child growth: A European cohort study. *BMC Pediatrics, 10*, 14. doi:10.1186/1471-2431-10-14.

Hadar, E., & Hod, M. (2010). Establishing consensus criteria for the diagnosis of diabetes in pregnancy following the HAPO study. *Annals of the New York Academy of Sciences, 1205*, 88–93.

Haines, L., Wan, K. C., Lynn, R., Barrett, T. G., & Shield, J. P. (2007). Rising incidence of type 2 diabetes in children in the U.K. *Diabetes Care, 30*(5), 1097–1101.

Haines, J., McDonald, J., O'Brien, A., Sherry, B., Bottino, C. J., Schmidt, M. E., et al. (2013). Healthy habits, happy homes: Randomized trial to improve household routines for obesity prevention among preschool aged children. *JAMA Pediatrics, 167*(11), 1072–1079.

Hales, C. N., & Barker, D. J. (2001). The thrifty phenotype hypothesis. *British Medical Bulletin, 60*, 5–20.

Halfon, N., & Forrest, C. B. (2017). The emerging theoretical framework of life course health development. In N. Halfon, C. B. Forrest, R. M. Lerner, & E. Faustman (Eds.), *Handbook of life course health-development science*. Cham: Springer.

Harvey-Berino, J., & Rourke, J. (2003). Obesity prevention in preschool native-American children: A pilot study using home visiting. *Obesity Research, 11*(5), 606–611.

Herbst, A., Kapellen, T., Schober, E., Graf, C., Meissner, T., & Holl, R. (2014). Impact of regular physical activity on blood glucose control and cardiovascular risk factors in adolescents with type 2 diabetes mellitus – a multicenter study of 578 patients from 225 centres. *Pediatric Diabetes, 16*(3), 204–210.

Hesketh, K. D., & Campbell, K. J. (2010). Interventions to prevent obesity in 0-5 year olds: An updated systematic review of the literature. *Obesity, 18*(Supple 1), S27–S35.

Hirst, K., Baranowski, T., DeBar, L., Foster, G. D., Kaufman, F., Kennel, P., et al. (2009). HEALTHY study rationale, design and methods: Moderating risk of type 2 diabetes in multi-ethnic middle school students. *International Journal of Obesity, 33*(Suppl 4), S4–20.

Hiscock, H., Scalzo, K., Canterford, L., & Wake, M. (2011). Sleep duration and body mass index in 0-7-year olds. *Archives of Disease in Childhood, 96*(8), 735–739.

Hoet, J. J., Dahri, S., Snoeck, A., Reusens-Billen, B., & Remacle, C. (1992). Importance of diets and their effect on fetal development: Function and structure of the endocrine pancreas following protein deficiency during intrauterine life. *Bulletin et Mémoires de l'Académie Royale de Médecine de Belgique, 147* (3–5), 174–181. discussion 81–83.

Imperatore, G., Boyle, J. P., Thompson, T. J., Case, D., Dabelea, D., Hamman, R. F., et al. (2012). Projections of type 1 and type 2 diabetes burden in the U.S. population aged <20 years through 2050: Dynamic modeling of incidence, mortality, and population growth. *Diabetes Care, 35*(12), 2515–2520.

ISPAD. (2011). *Global IDF/ISPAD guideline for childhood and Pediatric diabetes*. Brussels, Belgium: International Diabetes Foundation.

James, D. C., & Lessen, R. (2009). Position of the American dietetic association: Promoting and supporting breastfeeding. *Journal of the American Dietetic Association, 109*(11), 1926–1942.

Jeffery, A. N., Metcalf, B. S., Hosking, J., Streeter, A. J., Voss, L. D., & Wilkin, T. J. (2012). Age before stage: Insulin resistance rises before the onset of puberty: A 9-year longitudinal study (EarlyBird 26). *Diabetes Care, 35*(3), 536–541.

Johnson, C. L., & Versalovic, J. (2012). The human microbiome and its potential importance to pediatrics. *Pediatrics, 129*(5), 950–960.

Kanaka-Gantenbein, C. (2010). Fetal origins of adult diabetes. *Annals of the New York Academy of Sciences, 1205*, 99–105.

Kapoor, A., Dunn, E., Kostaki, A., Andrews, M. H., & Matthews, S. G. (2006). Fetal programming of hypothalamo-pituitary-adrenal function: Prenatal stress and glucocorticoids. *The Journal of Physiology, 572*(Pt 2), 31–44.

Katoh, S., Lehtovirta, M., Kaprio, J., Harjutsalo, V., Koskenvuo, M., Eriksson, J., et al. (2005). Genetic and environmental effects on fasting and postchallenge plasma glucose and serum insulin values in Finnish twins. *Journal of Clinical Endocrinology and Metabolism, 90*(5), 2642–2647.

Kaufman, F. R., Hirst, K., Linder, B., Baranowski, T., Cooper, D. M., Foster, G. D., et al. (2009). Risk factors for type 2 diabetes in a sixth-grade multiracial cohort: The HEALTHY study. *Diabetes Care, 32*(5), 953–955.

Kempf, K., Rathmann, W., & Herder, C. (2008). Impaired glucose regulation and type 2 diabetes in children and adolescents. *Diabetes/Metabolism Research and Reviews, 24*, 427–437.

Kim, S. Y., England, J. L., Sharma, J. A., & Njoroge, T. (2011). Gestational diabetes mellitus and risk of childhood overweight and obesity in offspring: A systematic review. *Experimental Diabetes Research, 2011*, 541308.

Kitzmann, K. M., Dalton, W. T., 3rd, Stanley, C. M., Beech, B. M., Reeves, T. P., et al. (2010). Lifestyle interventions for youth who are overweight: A meta-analytic review. *Health Psychology, 29*(1), 91–101.

Klingenberg, L., Christensen, L. B., Hjorth, M. F., Zangenberg, S., Chaput, J. P., Sjodin, A., et al. (2013). No relation between sleep duration and adiposity indicators in 9-36 months old children: The SKOT cohort. *Pediatric Obesity, 8*(1), e14–e18.

Knowlden, A. P., & Sharma, M. (2012). Systematic review of family and home-based interventions targeting paediatric overweight and obesity. *Obesity Reviews, 13*(6), 499–508.

Koren, O., Goodrich, J. K., Cullender, T. C., Spor, A., Laitinen, K., Backhed, H. K., et al. (2012). Host remodeling of the gut microbiome and metabolic changes during pregnancy. *Cell, 150*(3), 470–480.

Kramer, M. S., Matush, L., Vanilovich, I., Platt, R. W., Bogdanovich, N., Sevkovskaya, Z., et al. (2009). A randomized breast-feeding promotion intervention did not reduce child obesity in Belarus. *The Journal of Nutrition, 139*(2), 417S–421S.

Lawrence, J., Mayer-Davis, E., Ryeynolds, K., Beyer, J., Pettitt, D., D'Agostino, R. B., et al. (2009a). Diabetes in Hispanic American youths. *Diabetes Care, 32*(Supplement 2), S123–S132.

Lawrence, J. M., Mayer-Davis, E. J., Reynolds, K., Beyer, J., Pettitt, D. J., D'Agostino, R. B., et al. (2009b). Diabetes in Hispanic American youth: Prevalence, incidence, demographics, and clinical characteristics: The SEARCH for diabetes in youth study. *Diabetes Care, 32*(Suppl 2), S123–S132.

Lee, Y. (2013). Diabetes care for emerging adults: Transition from pediatric to adult diabetes care systems. *Annals of Pediatric Endocrinology & Metabolism, 18*, 106–110.

Ley, S. H., Hanley, A. J., Sermer, M., Zinman, B., & O'Connor, D. L. (2012). Associations of prenatal metabolic abnormalities with insulin and adiponectin concentrations in human milk. *The American Journal of Clinical Nutrition, 95*(4), 867–874.

Li, R., Bilik, D., Brown, M. B., Zhang, P., Ettner, S. L., Ackerman, R. T., et al. (2013). Medical costs associated with type 2 diabetes complications and comorbidities. *The American Journal of Managed Care, 19*(5), 421–430.

Liu, L. L., Yi, J. P., Beyer, J., Mayer-Davis, E. J., Dolan, L. M., Dabelea, D. M., et al. (2009). Type 1 and type 2 diabetes in Asian and Pacific Islander U.S. youth: The SEARCH for diabetes in youth study. *Diabetes Care, 32*(Suppl 2), S133–S140.

Liu, J., Yu, P., Qian, W., Li, Y., Zhao, J., Huan, F., et al. (2013). Perinatal bisphenol a exposure and adult glucose homeostasis: Identifying critical windows of exposure. *PloS One, 8*(5), e64143.

Luepker, R. V., Perry, C. L., McKinlay, S. M., Nader, P. R., Parcel, G. S., Stone, E. J., et al. (1996). Outcomes of a field trial to improve children's dietary patterns and physical activity. The child and adolescent trial for cardiovascular health. CATCH collaborative group. *The Journal of the American Medical Association, 275*(10), 768–776.

Martin, R. M., Patel, R., Kramer, M. S., Vilchuck, K., Bogdanovich, N., Sergeichick, N., et al. (2014). Effects of promoting longer-term and exclusive breastfeeding on cardiometabolic risk factors at age 11.5 years: A cluster-randomized, controlled trial. *Circulation, 129*(3), 321–329.

Martin-Gronert, M. S., & Ozanne, S. E. (2012). Mechanisms underlying the developmental origins of disease. *Reviews in Endocrine & Metabolic Disorders, 13*(2), 85–92.

Maull, E. A., Ahsan, H., Edwards, J., Longnecker, M. P., Navas-Acien, A., Pi, J., et al. (2012). Evaluation of the association between arsenic and diabetes: A National Toxicology Program workshop review. *Environmental Health Perspectives, 120*(12), 1658–1670.

May, A. L., Kuklina, E. V., & Yoon, P. W. (2012). Prevalence of cardiovascular disease risk factors among US adolescents, 1999–2008. *Pediatrics, 129*(6), 1035–1041.

Mayer-Davis, E. J., Rifas-Shiman, S. L., Zhou, L., Hu, F. B., Colditz, G. A., & Gillman, M. W. (2006). Breastfeeding and risk for childhood obesity: Does maternal diabetes or obesity status matter? *Diabetes Care, 29*(10), 2231–2237.

Mayer-Davis, E. J., Dabelea, D., Lamichhane, A. P., D'Agostino, R. B., Jr., Liese, A. D., et al. (2008). Breast-feeding and type 2 diabetes in the youth of three ethnic groups: The SEARCh for diabetes in youth case-control study. *Diabetes Care, 31*(3), 470–475.

Mayer-Davis, E. J., Beyer, J., Bell, R. A., Dabelea, D., D'Agostino, R., Jr., Imperatorek, G., et al. (2009). Diabetes in African American youth: Prevalence, incidence, and clinical characteristics: The SEARCH for diabetes in youth study. *Diabetes Care, 32*(Supplement 2), S112–S122.

McEwen, B. S. (2008). Understanding the potency of stressful early life experiences on brain and body function. *Metabolism Clinical and Experimental, 57*(Suppl 2), S11–S15.

McLearn, K. T., Minkovitz, C. S., Strobino, D. M., Marks, E., & Hou, W. (2006). Maternal depressive symptoms at 2 to 4 months post partum and early parenting practices. *Archives of Pediatrics & Adolescent Medicine, 160*(3), 279–284.

McMillen, I. C., & Robinson, J. S. (2005). Developmental origins of the metabolic syndrome: Prediction, plasticity, and programming. *Physiological Reviews, 85*(2), 571–633.

McMurray, R. G., Bassin, S., Jago, R., Bruecker, S., Moe, E. L., Murray, T., et al. (2009). Rationale, design and methods of the HEALTHY study physical education intervention component. *International Journal of Obesity, 33*(Suppl 4), S37–S43.

Meaney, M. J., Szyf, M., & Seckl, J. R. (2007). Epigenetic mechanisms of perinatal programming of hypothalamic-pituitary-adrenal function and health. *Trends in Molecular Medicine, 13*(7), 269–277.

Metzger, B. E., Lowe, L. P., Dyer, A. R., Trimble, E. R., Chaovarindr, U., Coustan, D. R., et al. (2008). Hyperglycemia and adverse pregnancy outcomes. *The New England Journal of Medicine, 358*(19), 1991–2002.

Metzger, B. E., Gabbe, S. G., Persson, B., Buchanan, T. A., Catalano, P. A., Damm, P., et al. (2010). International association of diabetes and pregnancy study groups recommendations on the diagnosis and classification of hyperglycemia in pregnancy. *Diabetes Care, 33*(3), 676–682.

Morandi, A., Maschio, M., Marigliano, M., Miraglia Del Giudice, E., Moro, B., Peverelli, P., et al. (2014). Screening for impaired glucose tolerance in obese children and adolescents: A validation and implementation study. *Pediatric Obesity, 9*(1), 17–25.

Morgan, A. R. (2012). Determining genetic risk factors for pediatric type 2 diabetes. *Current Diabetes Reports, 12*(1), 88–92.

Morris, D. H., Khunti, K., Achana, F., Srinivasan, B., Gray, L. J., Davies, M. J., et al. (2013). Progression rates from HbA(1c) 6.0-6.4% and other prediabetes definitions to type 2 diabetes: A meta-analysis. *Diabetologia, 56*(7), 1489–1493.

Morrison, K. M., Xu, L., Tarnopolsky, M., Yusuf, Z., Atkinson, S. A., & Yusuf, S. (2012). Screening for dysglycemia in overweight youth presenting for weight management. *Diabetes Care, 35*(4), 711–716.

Moses, R. G. (2010). New consensus criteria for GDM: Problem solved or a pandora's box? *Diabetes Care, 33*(3), 690–691.

Navas-Acien, A., Silbergeld, E. K., Pastor-Barriuso, R., & Guallar, E. (2008). Arsenic exposure and prevalence of type 2 diabetes in US adults. *JAMA, 300*(7), 814–822.

Neville, M. C., Anderson, S. M., McManaman, J. L., Badger, T. M., Bunik, M., Contractor, N., et al. (2012). Lactation and neonatal nutrition: Defining and refining the critical questions. *Journal of Mammary Gland Biology and Neoplasia, 17*(2), 167–188. doi:10.1007/s10911-012-9261-5.

Ong, K. K. (2010). Early determinants of obesity. *Endocrine Development, 19*, 53–61.

Pervanidou, P., & Chrousos, G. P. (2011). Stress and obesity/metabolic syndrome in childhood and adolescence. *International Journal of Pediatric Obesity, 6*(Supplement 1), 21–28.

Pervanidou, P., & Chrousos, G. P. (2012). Metabolic consequences of stress during childhood and adolescence. *Metabolism, 61*(5), 611–619.

Peters, A., & Laffel, L. (2011). Diabetes care for emerging adults: Recommendations for transition from pediatric to adult diabetes care systems: A position statement of the American Diabetes Association. *Diabetes Care, 34*(11), 2477–2485.

Plagemann, A., Harder, T., Franke, K., & Kohlhoff, R. (2002). Long-term impact of neonatal breast-feeding on body weight and glucose tolerance in children of diabetic mothers. *Diabetes Care, 25*(1), 16–22.

Prince, A. L., Antony, K. M., Ma, J., & Aagaard, K. M. (2014). The microbiome and development: A mother's perspective. *Seminars in Reproductive Medicine, 32*(1), 14–22.

Raman, A., Ritchie, L. D., Lustig, R. H., Fitch, M. D., Hudes, M. L., & Fleming, S. E. (2010). Insulin resistance is improved in overweight African American boys but not in girls following a one-year multidisciplinary community intervention program. *Journal of Pediatric Endocrinology & Metabolism, 23*(1–2), 109–120.

Rhodes, E. T., Prosser, L. A., Hoerger, T. J., Lieu, T., Ludwig, D. S., & Laffel, L. M. (2012). Estimated morbidity and mortality in adolescents and young adults diagnosed with type 2 diabetes mellitus. *Diabetic Medicine, 29*(4), 453–463.

Ritchie, L. D., Sharma, S., Ikeda, J. P., Mitchell, R. A., Raman, A., Green, B. S., et al. (2010). Taking action together: A YMCA-based protocol to prevent type-2 diabetes in high-BMI inner-city African American children. *Trials, 11*, 60.

Robinson, S., Ntani, G., Simmonds, S., Syddall, H., Dennison, E., Sayer, A. A., et al. (2013). Type of milk feeding in infancy and health behaviours in adult life: Findings from the Hertfordshire cohort study. *The British Journal of Nutrition, 109*(6), 1114–1122.

Rolland-Cachera, M. F. (2011). Childhood obesity: Current definitions and recommendations for their use. *International Journal of Pediatric Obesity, 6*(5–6), 325–331.

Rosenbaum, M., Nonas, C., Weil, R., Horlick, M., Fennoy, I., Vargas, I., et al. (2007). School-based intervention acutely improves insulin sensitivity and decreases inflammatory markers and body fatness in junior high school students. *The Journal of Clinical Endocrinology and Metabolism, 92*(2), 504–508.

Rosenbloom, A. L., Joe, J. R., Young, R. S., & Winter, W. E. (1999). Emerging epidemic of type 2 diabetes in youth. *Diabetes Care, 22*(2), 345–354.

Rosenbloom, A. L., Silverstein, J. H., Amemiya, S., Zeitler, P., & Klingensmith, G. J. (2008). ISPAD clinical practice consensus guidelines 2006-2007. Type 2 diabetes mellitus in the child and adolescent. *Pediatric Diabetes, 9*(5), 512–526.

Saelens, B. E., Grow, H. M., Stark, L. J., Seeley, R. J., & Roehrig, H. (2011). Efficacy of increasing physical activity to reduce children's visceral fat: A pilot randomized controlled trial. *International Journal of Pediatric Obesity, 6*(2), 102–112.

Salsberry, P. J., & Reagan, P. B. (2005). Dynamics of early childhood overweight. *Pediatrics, 116*(6), 1329–1338.

Samuelsson, A. M., Matthews, P. A., Argenton, M., Christie, M. R., McConnell, J. M., et al. (2008). Diet-induced obesity in female mice leads to offspring hyperphagia, adiposity, hypertension, and insulin resistance: A novel murine model of developmental programming. *Hypertension, 51*(2), 383–392.

Savoye, M., Shaw, M., Dziura, J., Tamborlane, W. V., Rose, P., Guandalini, C., et al. (2007). Effects of a weight management program on body composition and metabolic parameters in overweight children: A randomized controlled trial. *JAMA, 297*(24), 2697–2704.

Savoye, M., Nowicka, P., Shaw, M., Yu, S., Dziura, J., Chavent, G., et al. (2011). Long-term results of an obesity program in an ethnically diverse pediatric population. *Pediatrics, 127*(3), 402–410.

Savoye, M., Caprio, S., Dziura, J., Camp, A., Germain, G., Summers, C., et al. (2014). Reversal of early abnormalities in glucose metabolism in obese youth: Results of an intensive lifestyle randomized controlled trial. *Diabetes Care, 37*(2), 317–324.

Schore, A. N. (2005). Back to basics: Attachment, affect regulation, and the developing right brain: Linking developmental neuroscience to pediatrics. *Pediatrics in Review, 26*(6), 204–217.

Sebert, S., Sharkey, D., Budge, H., & Symonds, M. E. (2011). The early programming of metabolic health: Is epigenetic setting the missing link? *The American Journal of Clinical Nutrition, 94*(6 Supplement), 1953S–1958S.

Seki, Y., Williams, L., Vuguin, P. M., & Charron, M. J. (2012). Minireview: Epigenetic programming of diabetes and obesity: Animal models. *Endocrinology, 153*(3), 1031–1038.

Shaw, J. E., Socree, R. A., & Zimmet, P. Z. (2010). Global estimates of the prevalence of diabetes for 2010 and 2030. *Diabetes Research and Clinical Practice, 87*, 4–14.

Shonkoff, J. P., & Garner, A. S. (2012). The lifelong effects of early childhood adversity and toxic stress. *Pediatrics, 129*(1), e232–e246.

Silverman, B. L., Rizzo, T. A., Cho, N. H., & Metzger, B. E. (1998). Long-term effects of the intrauterine environment. The Northwestern University diabetes in pregnancy Center. *Diabetes Care, 21*(Suppl 2), B142–B149.

Simeoni, U., & Barker, D. J. (2009). Offspring of diabetic pregnancy: Long-term outcomes. *Seminars in Fetal & Neonatal Medicine, 14*(2), 119–124.

Sinclair, K. D., Lea, R. G., Rees, W. D., & Young, L. E. (2007). The developmental origins of health and disease: Current theories and epigenetic mechanisms. *Society of Reproduction and Fertility Supplement, 64*, 425–443.

Sinha, R., Fisch, G., Teague, B., Tamborlane, W. V., Banyas, B., Allen, K., et al. (2002). Prevalence of impaired glucose tolerance among children and adolescents with marked obesity. *The New England Journal of Medicine, 346*(11), 802–810.

Skouteris, H., McCabe, M., Swinburn, B., Newgreen, V., Sacher, P., & Chadwick, P. (2011). Parental influence and obesity prevention in pre-schoolers: A systematic review of interventions. *Obesity Reviews, 12*(5), 315–328.

Skouteris, H., McCabe, M., Ricciardelli, L., Milgrom, J., Baur, L., Aksan, N., et al. (2012). Parent–child interactions and obesity prevention: A systematic review of the literature. *Early Child Development and Care, 182*(2), 153–174.

Smith, B. T., Lynch, J. W., Fox, C. S., Harper, S., Abrahamowicz, M., Almeida, N. D., et al. (2011). Life-course socioeconomic position and type 2 diabetes mellitus: The Framingham offspring study. *American Journal of Epidemiology, 173*(4), 438–447.

Snieder, H., Boomsma, D. I., van Doornen, L. J., & Neale, M. C. (1999). Bivariate genetic analysis of fasting insulin and glucose levels. *Genetic Epidemiology, 16*(4), 426–446.

Stark, L. J., Clifford, L. M., Towner, E. K., Filigno, S. S., Zion, C., Bolling, C., et al. (2014). A pilot randomized controlled trial of a behavioral family-based intervention with and without home visits to decrease obesity in preschoolers. *Journal of Pediatric Psychology, 39*(9), 1001–1012. doi:10.1093/jpepsy/jsu059.

Szajewska, H. (2013). Microbiota modulation: Can probiotics prevent/treat disease in pediatrics? *Nestle Nutrition Institute Workshop Series, 77*, 99–110.

Tamayo, T., Christian, H., & Rathmann, W. (2010). Impact of early psychosocial factors (childhood socioeconomic factors and adversities) on future risk of type 2 diabetes, metabolic disturbances and obesity: A systematic review. *BMC Public Health, 10*, 525. doi:10.1186/1471-2458-10-525.

Tamayo, T., Jacobs, D. R., Jr., Strassburger, K., Giani, G., Seeman, T. E., Matthews, K., et al. (2012). Race- and sex-specific associations of parental education with insulin resistance in middle-aged participants: The CARDIA study. *European Journal of Epidemiology, 27*(5), 349–355.

Tarry-Adkins, J. L., & Ozanne, S. E. (2011). Mechanisms of early life programming: Current knowledge and future directions. *The American Journal of Clinical Nutrition, 94*(6 Supplement), 1765S–1771S.

Taveras, E. M., Scanlon, K. S., Birch, L., Rifas-Shiman, S. L., Rich-Edwards, J. W., & Gillman, M. W. (2004). Association of breastfeeding with maternal control of infant feeding at age 1 year. *Pediatrics, 114*(5), e577–e583.

Taveras, E. M., Rifas-Shiman, S. L., Oken, E., Gunderson, E. P., & Gillman, M. W. (2008). Short sleep duration in infancy and risk of childhood overweight. *Archives of Pediatrics & Adolescent Medicine, 162*(4), 305–311.

Taveras, E. M., Gillman, M. W., Pena, M. M., Redline, S., & Rifas-Shiman, S. L. (2014). Chronic sleep curtailment and adiposity. *Pediatrics, 133*(6), 1013–1022.

Thayer, K. A., Heindel, J. J., Bucher, J. R., & Gallo, M. A. (2012). Role of environmental chemicals in diabetes and obesity: A National Toxicology Program workshop review. *Environmental Health Perspectives, 120*(6), 779–789.

Thompson, A. L., & Bentley, M. E. (2013). The critical period of infant feeding for the development of early disparities in obesity. *Social Science & Medicine, 97*, 288–296.

Tounian, P. (2011). Programming towards childhood obesity. *Annals of Nutrition & Metabolism, 58*(Suppl 2), 30–41.

Trevino, R. P., Yin, Z., Hernandez, A., Hale, D. E., Garcia, O. A., & Mobley, C. (2004). Impact of the Bienestar school-based diabetes mellitus prevention program on fasting capillary glucose levels: A randomized controlled trial. *Archives of Pediatrics & Adolescent Medicine, 158*(9), 911–917.

Venditti, E. M., Elliot, D. L., Faith, M. S., Firrell, L. S., Giles, C. M., Goldberg, L., et al. (2009). Rationale, design and methods of the HEALTHY study behavior intervention component. *International Journal of Obesity, 33*(Suppl 4), S44–S51.

Venkat Narayan, K. M., Boyle, J. P., Thompson, T. J., Sorensen, S. W., & Willimason, D. F. (2003). Lifetime risk for riabetes mellitus in the United States. *JAMA, 290*(14), 1884–1889.

Versalovic, J. (2013). The human microbiome and probiotics: Implications for pediatrics. *Annals of Nutrition & Metabolism, 63*(Suppl 2), 42–52.

Visscher, P. M., Hill, W. G., & Wray, N. R. (2008). Heritability in the genomics era–concepts and misconceptions. *Nat Rev Genet, 9*(4), 255–266.

Wabitsch, M., Hauner, H., Hertrampf, M., Muche, R., Hay, B., Mayer, H., et al. (2004). Type II diabetes mellitus and impaired glucose regulation in Caucasian children and adolescents with obesity living in Germany. *International Journal of Obesity and Related Metabolic Disorders, 28*(2), 307–313.

Waitzfelder, B., Pihoker, C., Klingensmith, G., Case, D., Anderson, A., Bell, R. A., et al. (2011). Adherence to guidelines for youths with diabetes mellitus. *Pediatrics, 128*(3), 531–538.

Wang, L., Anderson, J. L., Dalton, W. T., Wu, T., Liu, X., & Zheng, S. (2013). Maternal depressive symptoms and the risk of overweight in their children. *Maternal and Child Health Journal, 17*(5), 940–948.

Warner, M. J., & Ozanne, S. E. (2010). Mechanisms involved in the developmental programming of adulthood disease. *The Biochemical Journal, 427*(3), 333–347.

Weiss, R., Taksali, S. E., Tamborlane, W. V., Burgert, T. S., Savoye, M., & Caprio, S. (2005). Predictors of changes in glucose tolerance status in obese youth. *Diabetes Care, 28*(4), 902–909.

Wen, L. M., Baur, L. A., Simpson, J. M., Rissel, C., Wardle, K., & Flood, V. M. (2012). Effectiveness of home based early intervention on children's BMI at age 2: Randomised controlled trial. *BMJ, 344*, e3732. doi:10.1136/bmj.e3732.

West, N. A., Hamman, R. F., Mayer-Davis, E. J., D'Agostino, R. B., Jr., Marcovina, S. M., Liese, A. S., et al. (2009). Cardiovascular risk factors among youth with and without type 2 diabetes: Differences and possible mechanisms. *Diabetes Care, 32*(1), 175–180.

Whitlock, E. P., O'Connor, E. A., Williams, S. B., Beil, T. L., & Lutz, K. W. (2010). Effectiveness of weight management interventions in children: A targeted systematic review for the US preventive service task Force. *Pediatrics, 125*(2), e396–e418.

Whitmore, T. J., Trengove, N. J., Graham, D. F., & Hartmann, P. E. (2012). Analysis of insulin in human breast milk in mothers with type 1 and type 2 diabetes mellitus. *International Journal of Endocrinology, 2012*, 296368. doi:10.1155/2012/296368.

Zeitler, P. (2010). Approach to the obese adolescent with new-onset diabetes. *The Journal of Clinical Endocrinology and Metabolism, 95*(12), 5163–5170.

Zeitler, P., Hirst, K., Pyle, L., Linder, B., Copeland, K., Arslanian, S., et al. (2012). A clinical trial to maintain glycemic control in youth with type 2 diabetes. *New England Journal of Medicine, 366*(24), 2247–2256.

Zeitler, P., Tandon, N., Nadeau, K., Urakami, T., Barrett, T., & Maahs, D. (2014). Type 2 diabetes in the child and adolescent. *Pediatric Diabetes, 20*(Supplement), 20–26.

3

Core Principles of Life Course Health Development Methodology and Analytics

Todd D. Little

The success of life course health development research is tied intimately to the measures and methods used. In this paper, I highlight a number of measurement, design, and analysis issues that researchers must consider in order to execute the highest-quality research possible. Many of the ideas presented here reflect the significant advances in statistical techniques, software functionality, and computational power, all of which afford researchers today with more options and more generalizable procedures than was possible even a decade or so ago.

The face of life course health development research in general is changing at a rapid pace. Because of the advances, teams of researchers with at least one dedicated methodology and analytics expert are needed to manage and integrate the theoretical with the methodological. The advanced techniques, improved estimation algorithms, and user-accessible software/hardware developments signal what I see as a paradigm shift in how life science research will be conducted now and in the future. Although techniques such as structural equation modeling (SEM), multilevel modeling (MLM), and mixture distribution modeling have permeated the research agenda in many fields, the capability of these tools has hardly been fully utilized. In this chapter, I intend to highlight (meaning space won't allow me the luxury of detail) many of the issues that life course health development researchers should be aware of. For more details and examples, I will refer to various sources along the way. More attention and examples to this material can also be found in Little (2013 and in Little et al. 2006a).

1 Measurement Issues

Manifest variable analytics remain popular despite their many flaws and unmet assumptions (e.g., measures are assumed to be without error, measurement invariance is assumed, indirect effects are not possible, items are supposed to be tau-equivalent and locally independent, and so on; McDonald 1999). As a result, scientific progress is mired in these untenable characteristics of classical methods. In order to progress with

Partial support for this project was provided by grant NSF 1053160 (Todd D. Little & Wei Wu, co-PIs) and by the Institute for Measurement, Methodology, Analysis, and Policy (Todd D. Little, director) and Todd Little's Stats Camp (statscamp.org). Correspondence concerning this work should be addressed to Todd D. Little, Institute for Measurement, Methodology, Analysis, and Policy, Texas Tech University, Lubbock, TX 79409. E-mail: yhat@statscamp.org. Web: immap.educ.ttu.edu and statscamp.org. Todd D. Little owns and receives remuneration from Yhat Enterprises (yhatenterprises.com), which runs educational workshops such as Stats Camp (statscamp.org), and processes his royalties and his fees for consulting on statistics and methods with life science researchers.

T.D. Little (✉)
Texas Tech University, Lubbock, TX, USA
e-mail: Todd.D.Little@ttu.edu; yhat@statscamp.org

prudent alacrity, life course health development researchers must embrace and leverage the power and sophisticated elegance of latent variable approaches. Structural equation modeling (SEM) is an overarching and general methodology that I will emphasize in this discussion; SEM is predicated on a measurement model that defines and represents latent variables (see Brown 2014, for details of the confirmatory factor analysis measurement model that underlies SEM models).

In this regard, latent variables are represented as the reliable information in a set of indicators – that is, measurement error is removed along with its attenuating and biasing effects. Removing measurement error is desirable because, when not removed, it decreases correlations and effect size estimates (e.g., Cohen's *d*) and inflates measures of dispersion, which biases any statistical tests when tested using classical procedures. When measurement error is removed, the reliable construct-related information about a set of indicators can be tested for measurement (factorial) invariance across age cohorts, measurement occasions, and life contexts. In addition to these positive features of the measurement model, SEM also affords levels of complexity that can be tied directly to theoretical models. For example, models of mediation, moderation, additive effects, and nested dependencies can be specified and easily estimated (see Little 2013, for details, and see below). Before addressing these modeling features of SEM, I turn first to a couple key issues in the measurement model of an SEM: refining measurement, modeling latent variables, factorial invariance and DIF (differential item functioning) testing, and the use of item parcels.

1.1 Refining Measurement

The constructs of life course health development are, for the most part, continuous because they reflect the continuous change across the life span. Unfortunately, researchers seem to disregard this idea when they construct response scales to measure the continuous scaled constructs. The most common scale used in behavioral science research is the Likert scale which was developed over 80 years ago (Likert 1932). It was developed to make measurement of continuous constructs easy to accomplish during the era of paper and pencil administration and laborious data entry. Other methods of measuring constructs are much more efficient and, in fact, can be more intuitive than Likert scaling. Continuous number lines using endpoint anchors (visual analog scales), for example, are easy to understand and typically provide greater information regarding the nature of the construct. Such measures are interval, not ordinal, in nature (Funke and Reips 2012; Reips and Funke 2008; Reips 2006). Such scales have also been around for a long time, but the burden of coding and the error-prone tendency of data entry made Likert scaling more appealing – that is, until now. With computer technology developed to the level that it has become, the use of rich electronically captured responses should become the norm. In this regard, methods for modeling responses, such as item response theory (IRT), will be less useful than continuous variable approaches such as SEM.

A future direction of life course health development is in the area of measurement development. Measures and scales that have been developed in the life sciences are often not designed to optimally measure change processes. The standards of measurement development to establish and model life course trajectories must be modified to include more emphasis on being sensitive to change. Because many scales of constructs such as self-efficacy, self-esteem, well-being, attitudes, and beliefs rely on Likert scales, such scales measure relative levels against an unspecified and unknowable standard. This lack of clarity can easily corrode the foundations of a measure when applied longitudinally.

For example, take a question like "in the past 2 weeks how much have you felt glad?" If I reply 7 on a 1–7 scale, the basis of my rating is unclear. It could be relative to my usual self, relative to my friends, or relative to the particular circumstances of the past 2 weeks. Also, the variability of my happiness in the past 2 weeks is not clear. Am I trending upward, trending downward, or about the same as usual? Such ambiguities of measurement make analyzing life course trajectories for constructs measured in such a way (i.e., with ambiguous referenced Likert scaling) as dubious at best and a fool's errand at worse. New tools for measuring change in such constructs must become a focal point of researchers in the area of life course health development. Modifying existing tools and adapting them to the circumstances of a given study should be encouraged rather than sanctioned.

For objective health measures, the standards for measurement are well established, and changes in them are easily tracked (CO^2, cotinine, cortisol, cholesterol, etc.). For some of these biological gold standards, however, the cost of assessment can be precipitous. Below I will highlight some techniques to reduce cost and yet still yield valid measurements of such constructs. As I intimated above, some of these new techniques for measurement are only possible with the latent variable approaches that I emphasize herein.

1.2 Modeling Latent Variables

A construct is a latent variable. A latent variable cannot be observed directly, but instead its scores are inferred by triangulating across multiple measures that we can directly observe (e.g., responses to a questionnaire scale, reaction time trials, numerous behavioral observations, and so on). When a construct's indicators are measured with four or fewer categories or the items are yes/no or right/wrong in nature, item response theory (IRT) analysis is used to examine the nature of the latent variable. When the construct's indicators are measured with five or more ordinal intervals, IRT analyses are not necessarily needed. Instead, SEM can be used to assess the nature of the latent variable (Rhemtulla et al. 2012). When variables are measured with five or more ordinal intervals, the precision of each item is generalizable across the full range of the latent variable. When four or few ordinal intervals are involved, IRT allows one to adjust and identify the precision of items for where along the latent variable they are most useful to measure the latent variable score well.

As modern measurement tools, both SEM and IRT can be used for advanced statistical features such as test equating, linking scores of the same construct that uses different indicators of it, and the like. The details of how to perform linking are beyond the scope of my discussion here (see Little 2013; McDonald 1999); instead, I simply wish to emphasize that IRT is fundamentally a special case of SEM and that both statistical approaches rely on the idea that latent variables are the level of analysis, that is, the critical level. Multiple measured indicators are the means by which a construct can be assessed. The advantage of SEM over IRT is the ability to measure multiple constructs simultaneously to allow for the idea that health is an integrated set of capacities and an emergent property of humans. IRT and SEM, however, have melded considerably recently. Software programs such as Mplus can now easily allow both categorical and continuous indicators. In this context, DIF testing explicitly becomes testing for factorial invariance.

1.3 Linking Constructs

Figure 1 displays graphically two methods for linking measures of the same construct over time to allow modeling of the growth, change, and trajectory of a construct over time. Note that the model in panel B allows estimation of a bias correction factor for one of the measures of the construct by utilizing a bifactor decomposition (see Little 2013). This model assumes that the measure B in this example is unbiased. Determining whether one measure is biased while the other is not requires strong theory and empirical support. For this example, my main point is that linking construct scores is a relatively straightforward modeling enterprise in the SEM world as well as the IRT world. Linking allows life course health development researchers to be consistent with many of the principles of life course health development by maintaining measurement continuity while allowing for items that are developmentally appropriate.

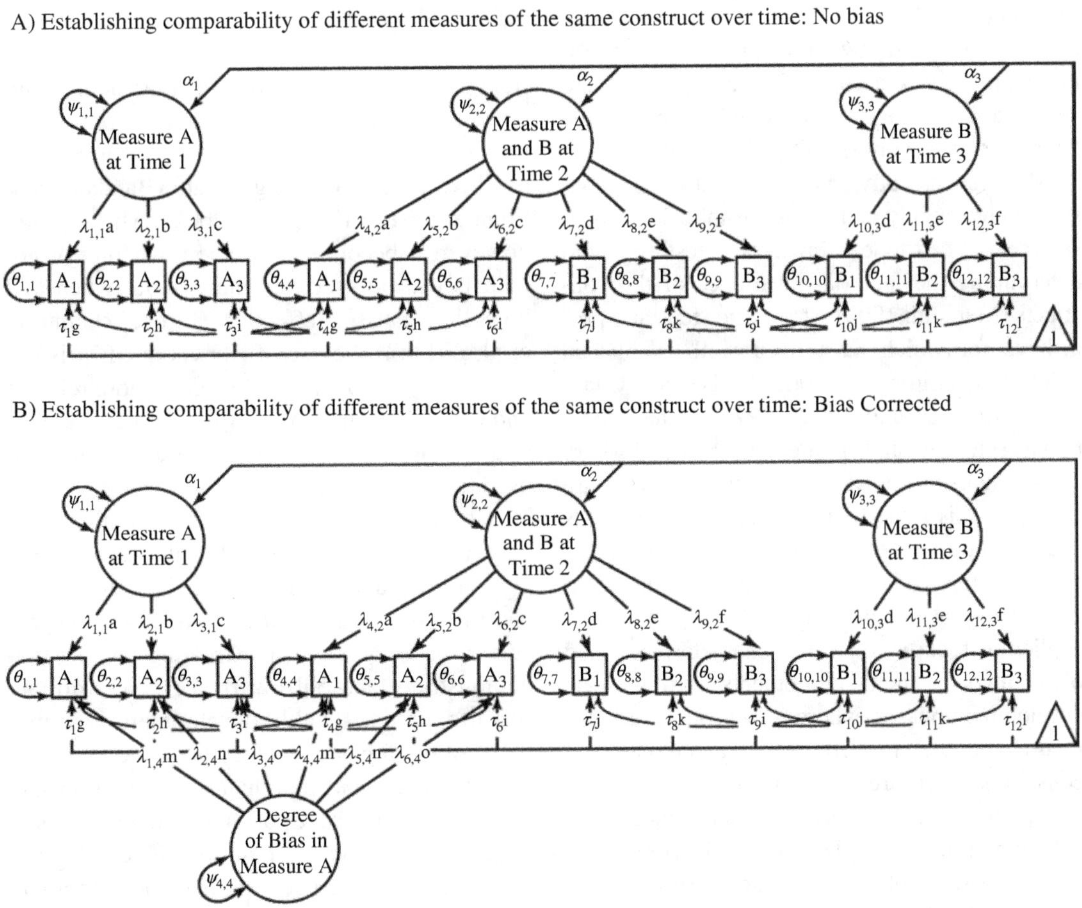

Fig. 1 Two models for establishing comparability of different measures of the same construct over time, with and without a "bias correction" factor. (**a**) Establishing comparability of different measures of the same construct over time: No bias. (**b**) Establishing comparability of different measures of the same construct over time: Bias corrected. (*Note.* The corresponding loadings and intercepts that are equated across time are designated by a superscripted letter (a-o). The residual variances among the corresponding indicators are allowed to associate over time (From Little 2013 and copyright, Todd D. Little. Reproduced with permission))

1.4 Factorial Invariance and Differential Item Functioning

One key assumption of life course health development, which is readily tested in SEM and IRT, is that the core properties of the measurement characteristics for a given construct are invariant across ages, measurement occasions, and contexts. When the measurement "DNA" of a given construct is supported by establishing strong factorial invariance, the certitude of construct comparisons is established. When factorial invariance is established, the interpretation of the observed differences in the constructs is unconfounded by any changes in the underlying psychometric characteristics of the measurement process. Measurement certainty is critical for valid life course research because observed differences across ages or contexts may be due to changes in the measurement of the construct and not changes in the construct itself. In the worlds of SEM and IRT analysis, testing for factorial invariance and differential item function (DIF) is the same thing. They both assess the certitude by which an item is psychometrically valid across different groups and across different ages when conditioned on the latent variable score (McDonald 1999).

More specifically, when indicators of constructs are roughly continuous, establishing measurement certitude involves testing and determining the factorial invariance of the constructs (Meredith 1993) – the basic steps and procedures for which have been well established (Little 1997; Little et al. 2007; Millsap and Cham 2012; Widaman and Reise 1997). In the educational sciences and related literatures, where dichotomous or polytomous item batteries are common, this issue of measurement certainty is addressed through the techniques of DIF testing – the basic steps and procedures for which have also been well established (de Ayala 2007). DIF testing explicitly focuses on item characteristics and often involves item refinements during scale development phases, whereas factorial invariance focuses on the measurement characteristics of constructs to ensure that construct comparisons are veridical during the hypothesis testing phases. A failure of invariance, however, is the continuous variable parallel of finding evidence of DIF. Life course health development research must emphasize measurement certitude for comparing constructs by testing for factorial invariance when the measures are continuous or testing for DIF when the measures or dichotomous or polytomous.

As long as partial strong factorial invariance holds (i.e., where a majority of the loadings and intercepts are proportionally equivalent), then the construct comparisons can proceed with sufficient certainty of comparison. Factorial invariance and DIF are both matters of degree. Within the SEM world, partial invariance is a simple way to allow items with evidence of DIF to not bias the construct's representation. A failure of invariance, if it involves many items however, becomes an exploratory study to determine what may have undermined the ability of the measures to reflect accurately the construct of interest across different ages or groups. Carefully planning and thoughtful measure construction can avoid the disappointment of a lack of invariance or evidence of DIF.

1.5 Parcels

Item parcels, as a measurement approach, are an essential tool for life course health development researchers. The items vs. parcels controversy has been a long-standing debate (Bandalos and Finney 2001; Little et al. 2002). This debate, however, is becoming less about whether or not parcels can be used and more about when and how they can be effective (Little, Rhemtulla et al. 2013a). The use of parcels in SEM is the process of creating a smaller set of more reliable and equally (or more) valid indicators of a construct from the larger pool of items that were used to measure the construct.

Little, Rhemtulla et al. (2013a) detail the covariance algebra of parcels and describe how knowing intimately the item-level information is critical to creating and successfully using parcels in an SEM analysis. Creating parcels that demonstrate factorial invariance is appropriate for life course health development research because the focus of inquiry is on the nature of the constructs and the change relations in and among the constructs of study. Because most longitudinal models that examine changes across the life course can become extremely large, using parcels is a matter of need rather than opinion.

2 Longitudinal Design Issues in Life Course Health Development Research

A number of design concerns arise when best practices in life course health development research are considered. Among these concerns are the timing of measurements, the model of change, and the moderating effect of lag differences. Each of these design issues is consistent with a number of the life course health development principles, particularly continuous change over time and the environmental influences that will impact health development across the life course. I will selectively address each of these issues in turn, even though other issues are certainly germane to this discussion.

2.1 Indexing Change

Life span research generally favors age-related changes, while life course research favors changes related to milestones and contextual influences. To model change well requires that the timing of measurements and the pace of change must by in sync regardless of the change emphasis. Rarely, however, is this synchronization of change with measurement achieved in actual research practice. Researchers need to carefully consider what changes and how fast it changes. In terms of the pace of change, to model change processes adequately requires that the occasions of measurement must be as fast as the fastest-changing process under scrutiny. Note that not all constructs need to be measured at the same pace or at the same occasions because imbalanced measurement intervals are easily handled in modern latent variable analytics.

To model what changes requires a reconsideration of the unit of change that should be used as the index of change. The measurement occasion is a very common index of change, and yet it confounds many factors such as cohort, age, and time of measurement. Sometimes age in years is used as the index of change. As Little (2013) emphasizes, change is a function of time, not necessarily or exclusively age or measurement occasion. Determining the right index of time to capture change is critical to accurately represent life course developmental processes.

2.2 Lag as Moderator

When measurement intervals are not precisely the same for all individuals, the difference in the elapsed interval can impact estimates of a given model. When measurements vary for individuals, this information can be used to represent the unique change processes associated with the varying measurement occasions. One model for representing the varying time lags is the recently introduced lag as moderator (LAM) model (Selig et al. 2012).

The LAM model explicitly incorporates the lag differences at a given measurement occasion to examine the influence that the differences in lag may have on the estimated model parameters. In the empirical data example reported in Selig et al., the influence of early home environment on later cognitive development showed a steeply declined effect as a function of time. When the lag in the measurement occasions was short (3 months), the influence of a rich home environment on intellective functioning was very high ($B = 2.5$), but when the lag was much longer than the intended 10-month interval (17 months), the effect had dropped to essentially zero (see Selig et al., for details of the model and of the empirical example).

One important implication of the LAM model is that lag can be used as a new design feature, with the interval of measurement becoming an element of the design that researchers can control and, with random assignment, allow a much broader universe of generalizability than the traditional longitudinal designs. Variable intervals can also be included in complex growth curve models by using some of the advance features of modern software. For example, Mplus has time scores that allow each person's time of measurement to vary, and OpenMX has definition variables that can accomplish the same goal.

3 Planned Missing Data Designs

Planned missing data designs are, in my estimation, the most underutilized weapon in a modern researcher's arsenal. Because latent variable models and modern approaches to treating missing data are able to provide efficient and unbiased estimates of parameters of interest in a quick and easy manner, not using planned missing data designs is rather difficult to justify. The family of possible planned missing procedures that can be used all provides information that is more valid than traditional ways of collecting data. They are also tremendously cost-effective. The validity component comes into play because planned missing data designs reduce the burden and fatigue on respondents. In life course health development research, the likelihood of selective attrition and other sources of unplanned missingness is also reduced because of the easy nature of responding (Little, Jorgenson et al. 2013b; Little and Rhemtulla 2013; Rhemtulla and Little 2012).

The Missing Data Mechanisms To understand unplanned missing data designs, I need to mention a few words about the mechanisms of missing data and how modern missing data treatments handle them (see Little and Rubin 2002; Enders 2010; van Buuren 2012). Three mechanisms can cause missing data: First, missing completely at random (MCAR) is, as the name indicates, a mechanism whereby their missing scores and their values are unrelated to anything that would impact the validity of inference. MCAR is the preferred mechanism for missing data because the only issue of statistical concern is the loss in power that occurs when data are missing. All missing data produce a loss in power. Only some missing data is unrelated to the observed data or any unobserved process (i.e., MCAR in origin). The second mechanism is termed missing at random (MAR). MAR occurs when the missing data are associated with a linear combination of one or more variables that are contained on the dataset. When MAR is at play, the variables that are observed on the dataset are predictive of the missing data, and, when this information is utilized in a modern treatment procedure, the information that was lost is readily retrieved.

The third mechanism is termed missing not at random (MNAR) and occurs when missing values are associated with one or more variables that are not observed. Large-scale life course research projects can reduce or eliminate the MNAR mechanism from its biasing influence by carefully and systematically including all variables that are known to associate or may likely be associated with missingness into the data collection protocol. If direct measures of these variables are not available, then proxy variables can be included. The goal here is to convert what would have been a MNAR missing data process into a MAR missing data process. The reason for this goal is that MNAR produces biased data that cannot be made unbiased, whereas MAR missing data is a process from which unbiased parameter estimates can be recovered.

The Modern Treatments The two most widely used modern approaches are full information maximum likelihood (FIML) estimation and multiple imputation (MI), which typically will utilize the expectation/maximization algorithm and/or the Markov chain Monte Carlo algorithm. FIML and MI are perfectly suited to handle MCAR missingness, and, unlike classical approaches, they provide an added benefit of restoring most of the power that was lost due to the missing data. FIML and MI are also perfectly well suited to handle data that are MAR and can also handle MNAR missingness when a study is designed to include predictors of missingness or their proxies.

FIML is an estimation procedure whose effectiveness depends on the variables that are included in the analysis model or in the auxiliary data block. If the combination of the variables associated with missingness is included in the analysis model either as a focal variable or as an auxiliary variable, FIML will produce unbiased estimates of all model parameters. MI will give the same answer as FIML when a large number of imputations are conducted (minimum $m = 20$, while 100 is generally recommended; see Enders 2010). The advantage of MI over FIML is that all variables on a dataset are involved in the imputation process. Then the variables associated with missingness are on the dataset, this information will be included in the imputation process, and the missing values will be recovered.

All things being equal, a model fit to imputed data will give the same answer as the FIML estimated model. These two modern approaches to handling missing data are state of the science in the statistical literature (see Enders 2010; van Buuren 2012) and should usurp the biased and ill-informed practices of some fields and disciplines. Techniques such as last or baseline observation carried forward or imputing and then setting the dependent variable as missing again after imputation were deemed effective treatments at one time. These treatments are biased and not recommended anymore (van Buuren 2012). If one of the two modern approaches is used, and when they take full advantage of including variables that are associated with MAR missing, then regardless of the research question, the analytic technique used, or the stakes involved, the best, most generalizable answer will emerge.

Planned Missing Protocols Two of the most effective planned missing protocols are the multiform design and the two-method design (Graham et al. 2001, 2006; Mistler and Enders 2012). The multiform design derives its name from the fact that multiple questionnaire protocols are created. These different forms can be thought of as short forms of the larger data collection protocol. Table 1 displays a layout of the simplest multiform design, the three-form design. The key to the three-form design is assigning items to be in four different blocks of items. The X block is the common block of items that all participants fill out. This block contains demographic variables, marker variables, and other essential elements that logically or theoretically are best collected on all participants. Variables that would be associated with unplanned missing data patterns and that constructs that don't have the multiple indicators of them are good candidates to include in the X block. The A, B, and C blocks each contain the remaining items evenly distributed among them. To enhance the power of this design, creating blocks of items that have high between block correlations is preferred. For longitudinal studies, using a random assignment of form to participant at each measurement occasion also enhances the power of this design. For a detailed simulation studies on the use of the three-form design for longitudinal research, see Jorgensen et al. (2014) and Jia et al. (2014).

The multiform design works so elegantly because the mechanism that produces the missingness for the unassigned items is controlled by the investigator making it an MCAR missing data mechanism. Of course, respondents will also refuse to answer some of the administered items. In such situations, the mixture of MCAR and MAR missingness is simultaneously addressed when FIML or MI is used. There modern treatments make no distinction between these two mechanisms when recovering both the information and the power that is lost due to missing data. Planned missing data designs increase validity by minimizing the fatigue and burden as well as reactivity (Harel et al. 2011). In addition to these validity gains, planned missing data designs reduce the unplanned missing data that occurs (Harel et al. 2011).

As with any design issue, sample size plays a role. As I mentioned at the outset, my focus is on latent variable approaches to modeling life course changes in health development, and as such sample sizes will be larger than many traditional studies of health in this context. Along with the validity gains by reducing respondent burden, fatigue, and reactivity, planned missing protocols allow researchers to redistribute resources to increase the number of participants by reducing the costs associated with each participant. The cost savings may be relatively small for the three-form design because the cost of 45 min vs. 1 h of a participant's reimbursement time may not translate directly into a 25% savings. The cost savings and power enhancement associated with the two-method design, on the other hand, can be dramatic.

The two-method design is based on the fact that many constructs have multiple methods by which they can be assessed. For some of these

Table 1 The general layout of a three-form planned missing data design

Form	Common variables	Variable set A	Variable set B	Variable set C
1	1/4 of Variables	1/4 of Variables	1/4 of Variables	None
2	1/4 of Variables	1/4 of Variables	None	1/4 of Variables
3	1/4 of Variables	None	1/4 of Variables	1/4 of Variables

Note: The distribution and proportions of variables across the different sets do not have to be uniform (From Little (in press))

constructs, one of the methods is considered a gold standard of assessment. Gold standard assessments are usually expensive to collect because they involve highly skilled assessors, copyrighted material, laboratory work, or time on very expensive machinery. Most studies that rely on gold standard assessments often are forced to conduct low-powered research because the costs are prohibitive. These cost barriers to using gold standard assessments, on the other hand, have lead researchers to develop and use less-expensive and easily obtained measures of the same constructs. These less-expensive measures are not as accurate as the gold standard version, but they typically are a reasonable proxy of the construct. Herein lies the beauty and elegance of the two-method design.

Using both the biased proxy measure and the gold standard measure, a given study can increase its sample size three- or more fold! Such increases in sample sizes easily move a given study into the sample size requirements of SEM. In fact, this design can only work when the appropriate SEM measurement model is employed to model the two methods of assessing the same construct. Figure 1 depicts a couple of possible variations of the two-method design. Two notable features of the measurement models shown here are that multiple indicators for each of the methods are included as indicators of the focal construct. In addition, a bifactor method factor is fit to the indicators of the biased proxy measurement tool. This bias factor or method factor extracts all the variance in the biased proxy that is unrelated to the information carried by the gold standard indicators. The indicators from the gold standard measure anchor the construct so that the resulting focal construct is an unbiased measure reflecting the construct centroid defined by the gold standard measurement tool.

This two-method design is ideally suited for researchers in the health sciences. What are the barriers to adopting this design and the associated advantages of SEM models? Lack of understanding on how planned missing designs work and lack of appreciation of the advantages of SEM appear to be the culprits. The statistical theory and the body of research evidence clearly support their use. As I mentioned earlier, research networks must coordinate and include experts in life course analytics (either instead of or in addition to the traditional biostatistics support). If they do, then the research conducted will benefit fully from the advantages and merits of all the techniques that I have outlined in this article.

Wave Missing Designs The simplest wave missing data design is the pre-post design where testing effects and retest effect are of concern. This simple design involves randomly assigning some participants to the pretest only, some to the posttest only, and some to both pre- and posttest. Unlike the flawed ANOVA framework to test the effects using such a design, a simple multiple-group longitudinal SEM with a modern treatment of the missing data provides a powerful way to analyze such data. For longitudinal studies of longer duration, participants can be randomly assigned to participate in different assessment occasions. As with the multiform design, these wave missing designs can be used even when MAR missingness is present. Clearly some participants will drop out of a study and some participants will come and go. These MAR patterns on top of the MCAR patterns are readily handled with modern missing data treatments. In addition, as mentioned, unplanned missing data are often reduced when planned missing is included (Harel et al. 2011s).

The Sequential Designs and the Accelerated Longitudinal Designs Given that MCAR and MAR are readily recoverable missing data mechanisms and MNAR can be minimized by imbuing a dataset with potential predictors of the missingness, using hybrid missing data models is easy and powerful to do. An underutilized model of this nature is the accelerated longitudinal design. To understand the accelerated longitudinal design, I display a graphical rendition of the three sequential longitudinal designs in Fig. 2. The three sequential designs are intended to unconfound two of the three factors that are confounded in a traditional longitudinal model. In a traditional longitudinal design, time of measurement is confounded with the age of the person which is also confounded with the cohort from which the sample is drawn.

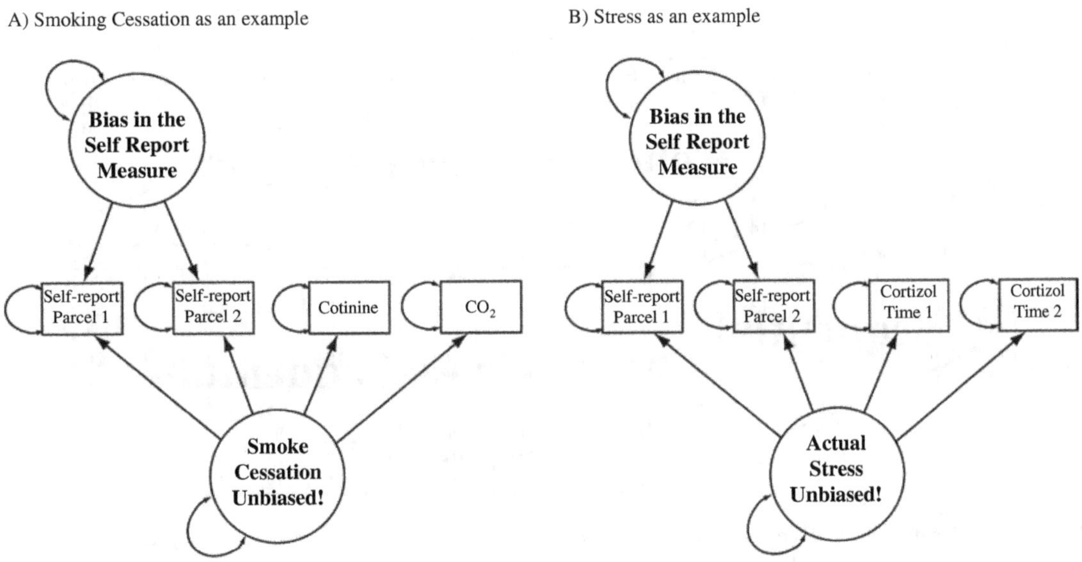

Fig. 2 Two examples of the two-method planned missing data design. (**a**) Smoking cessation as an example (**b**) Stress as an example (*Note*. From Little (2013) and copyright Todd d. Little. Reproduced with permission)

Of the sequential designs, the cross-sequential design is the most popular design. The cross-sequential design (which is commonly mislabeled as the cohort-sequential design) begins with a cross-section design and then follows all individuals for a number of measurement occasions. Here, measurement occasion is confounded with the cohort information, but age effects can be separated from the cohort effects once a sufficient amount of time has passed. The cohort-sequential design examines cohort differences for a specific period of the life course by repeatedly enrolling new individuals at a given age and following them only up to a particular age. In Fig. 3, I have depicted a cohort-sequential design that is optimized for studying the period of adolescence. Finally, the time-sequential design optimizes the ability to estimate effects related to the time of measurement.

Inspired by Bell (1953), modern approaches to the accelerated longitudinal design use the cross-sequential design to transform the collected data into a sparse dataset with many missing cells (see also Duncan and Duncan 2012). This accelerated longitudinal design uses the cohort and time of measurement information to create dummy codes and interaction terms to recover the information that is associated with cohort and time of measurement differences and, in the analysis model, use these dummy codes to estimate and thereby control for the cohort and time of measurement influences. When specified properly, the accelerated longitudinal design provides an unbiased estimate of age-related changes and differences across the total age span represented in the sample. Table 2 shows an example of an accelerated longitudinal model for the period of adolescence.

Another related transformation that life course researchers can utilize is to center the data on a particular event. With a design such as this, the emphasis is on understanding the change processes up to an event and the change processes after an event. Using puberty as an example, Table 3 shows how data can be transformed into a sparse arrangement but where the measurement occasions are either the measurement before the event or after the event. In this example, data from a single age cohort are grouped into the six different possible patterns in which evidence of puberty appears at a given wave of measurement. The letter P refers to puberty. Variables such as age within cohort and gender can be included as time-invariant contextual variables to examine

Cohort-Sequential

Time Sequential

Cross-Sequential

Cohort (Birth Year)	Time of Measurement 1996	1997	1998	1999	2000	2001	2002	2003	2004	2005	2006	2007	2008	2009	2010
1980	16	17	18	19	20	21	22	23	24	25	26	27	28	29	30
1981	15	16	17	18	19	20	21	22	23	24	25	26	27	28	29
1982	14	15	16	17	18	19	20	21	22	23	24	25	26	27	28
1983	13	14	15	16	17	18	19	20	21	22	23	24	25	26	27
1984	12	13	14	15	16	17	18	19	20	21	22	23	24	25	26
1985	11	12	13	14	15	16	17	18	19	20	21	22	23	24	25
1986	10	11	12	13	14	15	16	17	18	19	20	21	22	23	24
1987	9	10	[illegible]	12	13	14	15	16	17	18	19	20	21	22	23
1988	8	9	10	11	12	13	14	15	16	17	18	19	20	21	22
1989	7	8	[illegible]	[illegible]	11	12	13	14	15	16	17	18	19	20	21
1990	6	7	8	9	10	11	12	13	14	15	16	17	18	19	20
1991	5	6	7	8	9	10	11	[illegible]	[illegible]	[illegible]	[illegible]	[illegible]	[illegible]	18	19
1992	4	5	6	7	8	9	10	11	12	13	14	15	16	17	18
1993	3	4	5	6	7	8	9	10	11	12	13	14	15	16	17
1994	2	3	4	5	6	7	8	9	10	11	12	13	14	15	16
1995	1	2	3	4	5	6	7	8	9	10	11	12	13	14	15

Fig. 3 Traditional sequential designs (*Note*. Ages are entered in grey in the body of the table. Any given row would be an example of a longitudinal design and any given column would be an example of across-sectional study. A cohort-sequential design would be starting a new cohort at a certain age and then following longituidinally. A cross-sequential design starts with a traditional cross-sectional study and then follows all participants longitudinally. A time-squential design is a repeated cross-sectional design, with some participants followed longitudinally. From Little (2013) and copyright Todd D. Little. Reproduced with permission).

their influence on the change trends that would be modeled after the data transformation.

Life course health development researchers would do very well to incorporate the above design elements into the conduct of life course health development studies. Life course researchers are also keenly interested in the context effects and environmental influences in which the person is engaged. The person ←→ environment interactions across ages are central to life course theory. The various designs described above are also capable of including and modeling the dynamics of contextual interactions. Modeling contextual influences is primarily a measurement issue rather than a statistical or analytics issue.

Contextual influences can be represented analytically in various statistical forms, depending on how the contextual influence is expected to impact the person (Little et al. 2006c). These ways are as (a) direct effects, (b) indirect/mediating effects, (c) reciprocal/feedback effects, (d) moderating effects, and (e) hierarchically nested effects. In the parlance of multilevel modeling (Bickel 2007), the first four ways of including context variables would be as level 1 effects that are measured at the person level and are characterized as features of the person. For example, current health status is an environment of the person. The fifth way of including context variables would be as level 2 (or higher-level) influences if more than one person is measured within that context. For example, family health practices create a health environment that influences the members of the family. Context variables can be considered even higher levels of influence. For example, community health systems that support family health needs can vary across communities and influence family practices differentially, which in turn, influence individual health characteristics.

Hierarchically nested contextual influences can be modeled in an SEM framework using the power and the flexibility of multilevel SEM (Bovaird 2007; Bovaird and Shaw 2012). Multilevel SEM involves specifying any form of a SEM model and adding a multilevel component on top of it. New software such as xxM (Mehta 2013) allows any number of levels of nested data structures. With longitudinal studies of context, person-level contextual variables can also be included as either time-varying or time-invariant influences. The context of gender or race is an example of a time-invariant effect. The size of a

Table 2 Transforming a cross-sequential design into an accelerated longitudinal design

	Age in years; months for each cohort at each assessment					
Age/Cohort	0 Mos	4 Mos	8 Mos	12 Mos	16 Mos	20 Mos
Age 11 yrs	11;0	11;4	11;8	12;0	12;4	12;8
Age 12 yrs	12;0	12;4	12;8	13;0	13;4	13;8
Age 13 yrs	13;0	13;4	13;8	14;0	14;4	14;8
Age 14 yrs	14;0	14;4	14;8	15;0	15;4	15;8
Age 15 yrs	15;0	15;4	15:8	16;0	16;4	16;8
Age 16 yrs	16;0	16;4	16;8	17;0	17;4	17;8

	Full span of the ages covered																				
	11;0	11;4	11;8	12;0	12;4	12;8	13;0	13;4	13;8	14;0	14;4	14;8	15;0	15;4	15;8	16;0	16;4	16;8	17;0	17;4	17;8
Age 11 yrs	Wl	W2	W3	W4	W5	W6															
Age 12 yrs				Wl	W2	W3	W4	W5	W6												
Age 13 yrs							Wl	W2	W3	W4	W5	W6									
Age 14 yrs										Wl	W2	W3	W4	W5	W6						
Age 15 yrs													Wl	W2	W3	W4	W5	W6			
Age 16 yrs																Wl	W2	W3	W4	W5	W6

Note. Multiple cohorts could also be transformed in such a manner. A dummy code to represent age-cohort would be included within each pattern to account for potential cohort differences. The missing data are treated as missing at random and imputed. Mos refers to months, yrs. refers to years, and WB refers to wave of data collection (Copyright Todd D. Little)

Table 3 Transforming a longitudinal design into episodic time

Data Collection Wave Crossed with Episode Occurance											
Pattern	Wave 1	Wave 2		Wave 3	Wave 4		Wave 5	Wave 6			
Pattern 1	P	P + 1		P + 2	P + 3		P + 4	P + 5			
Pattern 2	P – 1	P		P + 1	P + 2		P + 3	P + 4			
Pattern 3	P – 2	P – 1		P	P + 1		P + 2	P + 3			
Pattern 4	P – 3	P – 2		P – 1	P		P + 1	P + 2			
Pattern 5	P – 4	P – 3		P – 2	P – 1		P	P + 1			
Patterns	P – 5	P – 4		P – 3	P – 2		P – 1	P			
	Episodic Occurence Crossed with Data Collection Wave										
	P – 5	P – 4	P – 3	P – 2	P – 1	P	P + 1	P + 2	P + 3	P + 4	P + 5
Pattern 1						Wl	W2	W3	W4	W5	W6
Pattern 2					Wl	W2	W3	W4	W5	W6	
Pattern 3				Wl	W2	W3	W4	Wf	W6		
Pattern 4			Wl	W2	W3	W4	W5	W6			
Pattern 5		Wl	W2	W3	W4	W5	W6				
Pattern 6	Wl	W2	W3	W4	W5	W6					

Note. Multiple cohorts could also be transformed in such a manner. A dummy code to represent age-cohort would be included within each pattern to account for potential cohort differences. The missing data are treated as missing at random and imputed (From Little (2013). Copyright Todd D. Little)

participant's social network is an example of a time-varying context effect. See Little et al. (2007c) for an edited volume dedicated to modeling contextual effects in longitudinal research.

Mediation and Moderation Mediation and moderation are critical statistical concepts for the field of life course health development research. These two concepts are consistently confused and often inappropriately tested. Mediation, for example, is a strict causal model of how one variable imparts its influence on another variable. It addresses the "how" of a causal chain. Like falling dominos, the linkage from one variable to the next as a causal impact must be established. In this regard, the only appropriate test for mediation must be longitudinal in nature (Cole and Maxwell 2003; Little et al. 2007; Maxwell and Cole 2007; Wu and Zumbo 2008).

At a minimum, two measurement occasions are needed to even implicate a mediation effect. Because mediation is a causal hypothesis about change, to implicate mediation involves demonstrating that a predictor, X, is able to predict *changes* in a mediator, M. To show that X is related to the change in M, prior levels of the mediator variable must be controlled. That is, the autoregressive influence of M on itself at a second time point must be estimated in order to show that X can predict changes in M. Similarly, a mediation analysis must be able to show that a mediator can predict changes in the outcome variable, Y. As with the mediator, the prior levels of the outcome variable, Y, must be entered into a model in order to demonstrate that M can predict changes in Y. Figure 3 shows an example of the simplest model for testing mediation. This figure depicts the half longitudinal design for testing mediation. In Fig. 3, the path labeled *a* is the first essential element of a mediation effect. It is the magnitude of the effect of X on the change in M. The second essential element of a mediation effect is labeled *b* in Fig. 3. It is the effect of M on the change in Y. Since mediation is a multiphase process, the joint effect must be calculated and tested for significance. Here, mediation is evident if the product of path *a* and path *b* is significant. To appropriately test with this product term is significant; either bootstrap estimation of the standard error of *ab* or a Monte Carlo simulation approach is used (McKinnnon 2008; Preacher and Hayes 2008a, b; Preacher and Selig 2012) Fig. 4.

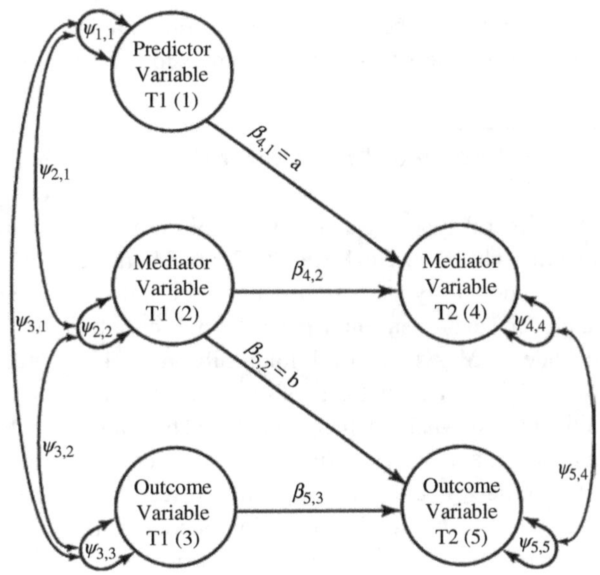

Fig. 4 *The half longitudinal design for testing mediation.* (*Note.* The representation of the measurement model is removed from the diagram. This design is the minimum required in order to empirically demonstrate mediation as a causal hypothesis. From Little (2013) and copyright Todd D. Little. Reproduced with permission)

Moderation is a quintessential context hypothesis. It addresses the conditions in which an effect between two variables is stronger or weaker. Tap water flows from the pipes to the glass at a flow rate determined by the context of the faucet valve. A moderator is like a valve, wide open and water flows freely and partly closed and the flow of water is restricted. Moderation is often confused with multivariate questions, for example, does one glass become fuller than another glass when the same amount of time has passed? The degree to which the water valve is open causes these differences. A question like how did my glass get half full is not a question of moderation. Here, many different liquids can combine or work in isolation to make the glass half full. Mostly juice and some water lead to a half-full glass. Mostly water and some milk also lead to a half-full glass. The type of liquid is not a moderator of the amount of water in the glass. Each liquid is an additive unique contribution to the height of the water in the glass.

Tests of mediation, moderation, and the unique and additive effects of a set of variables are each undermined when measurement error is involved. As I have been emphasizing, a latent variable SEM approach to conducting these tests provides the maximum accuracy and generalizability of inference. Moderation in particular is a notoriously underpowered procedure when tested as a manifest variable interaction term. Testing moderation in the latent space is a bit more complex. Three general approaches exist for testing moderation. A model-based approach is available in the Mplus software (using the LMS approach; Klein and Moosbrugger 2000; Muthén and Asparouhov 2003). Two indicator-based approaches can also be used: the double mean-centering approach forwarded by Marsh and colleagues (see Lin et al. 2010) and the orthogonalizing approach (Little et al. 2006). For more details on testing moderation in general, see Marsh et al.(2012), and for more details on testing both mediation and moderation in longitudinal models, see Little (in press; particularly Chap. 9).

Tests of moderation are also muddied by the fact that a significant interaction term cannot speak to which variable is moderating the other. A significant interaction term only indicates that the regression effect of the outcome on one of the two predictors varies as a function of the other. Although the example of a valve as the moderator of the water flow to a glass seems clear as to its role as a moderating influence, a third variable could potentially confound this conclusion. The amount of water pressure, for example, could cause the value to be open more when pressure is high and open less when the pressure is low.

4 Choice of Analysis Model

Two general types of analysis model dominate longitudinal research (Little 2013). For both of these model types, a mixture distribution approach and/or a multilevel kernel can be included (Masyn and Nylund-Gibson 2012; Mehta 2013). The first analysis model is the traditional cross-lagged panel model. The panel model remains an essential analysis model for life course health development researchers because it addresses key questions about what predicts change controlling for prior levels. Mediation and moderation hypotheses are readily addressed in the basic panel model. The panel model is fundamentally a question about individual differences standings at specific points in time. These models can be made more refined by incorporating lag at each wave as a moderator or using the recent models of continuous time modeling.

The second popular model for the analysis of longitudinal data is the growth curve model. The growth curve model is a model for the mean-level changes. It decomposes the mean and covariance information into a set of constructs to represent the change over time for each of the individuals in the sample. The set of constructs is usually an intercept construct, which usually represents the initial levels of the participants at the first measurement occasion, and a slope construct, which represents the shape of the growth/change over time for the sample. These two constructs have variances that reflect the individual differences in the intraindividual change trajectories. These models and their variants address the change trajectories and what predicts standing in the modeled trajectories.

As should be clear, each of these analysis models addresses distinctly different questions. Life course health development researchers need to be clear to match the correct model with the particular research question at hand. Too often, researchers are tempted to fit the more popular model (i.e., the growth curve model) when the question is fundamentally about the individual differences relationships and changes in those patterns. In the field of life course methodology and analytics, both techniques are undergoing developments and refinements (e.g., Grimm and Ram 2012; Little et al. 2007a; Selig and Little 2012; Wu et al. 2012), and as such, researchers need to stay on top of recent developments in their application to data.

Because life course health development is complex, nonlinear, multidimensional, multidirectional, and multilevel by its nature, the choice of analysis model must accurately correspond to the life course change process under scrutiny. That is, not only are hierarchical nested models (i.e., multilevel models) often needed, but also mixture distribution models bring the ability to discover and model the unobserved heterogeneity inherent in life course health development.

As mentioned the popularity of adding a mixture distribution component to a given model is very attractive to many life course researchers. Such models appeal to the person-centered views of many life course researchers. These techniques, however, are not always appropriate for the data or the research question and should be avoided unless the study and the data were designed to examine archetypes and latent subgroups. Some statisticians would have these techniques buried and a tombstone with R.I.P. placed upon it. Others would have the techniques resurrected and use R.I.P. as the mantra for how the techniques should be used. Namely, replicability, interpretability, and predictability are the three core validity criteria to pass when using these techniques (see Little 2013). For recent discussions of the issues, see Ram et al. (2012), Nagin and Odgers (2012), and Masyn and Nylund-Gibson (2012).

5 Conclusions

The craft of life course health development methodology and analytics requires dedication, sophistication, and a knack for molding the analysis tool to the research question at hand. For life course health development research to be at its most effective, utilizing the expertise of collaborative teams is essential. The days of one person being both expert theoretician and methodologist are waning. Partnering with dedicated experts on the various issues that I have outlined here will bring the needed sophistication and knack to execute research at its finest and most impactful levels.

References

Bandalos, D. L., & Finney, S. J. (2001). Item parceling issues in structural equation modeling. In G. A. Marcoulides & R. E. Schumacker (Eds.), *New developments and techniques in structural equation modeling (chap. 10)* (pp. 269–296). Hillsdale: Lawrence Erlbaum Associates.

Bell, R. Q. (1953). Convergence: An accelerated longitudinal approach. *Child Development, 24*, 145–152.

Bickel, R. (2007). *Multilevel analysis for applied research: It's just regression!* New York: The Guilford Press.

Bovaird, J. A. (2007). Multilevel structural equation models for contextual factors. In T. D. Little, J. A. Bovaird, & N. A. Card (Eds.), *Modeling contextual effects in longitudinal studies* (pp. 149–182). LEA: Mahwah.

Bovaird, J. A., & Shaw, L. H. (2012). Multilevel structural equation modeling. In B. Laursen, T. D. Little, & N. A. Card (Eds.), *Handbook of developmental research methods* (pp. 501–518). New York: Guilford Press.

Brown, T. A. (2014). *Confirmatory factor analysis for applied research* (2nd ed.). New York: Guilford.

Cole, D. A., & Maxwell, S. E. (2003). Testing mediational models with longitudinal data: Questions and tips in the use of structural equation modeling. *Journal of Abnormal Psychology, 112*, 558–577.

de Ayala, R. J. (2007). *The theory and practice of item response theory*. New York: Guilford Press.

Duncan, S. C., & Duncan, T. E. (2012). Accelerated longitudinal designs. In B. Laursen, T. D. Little, & N. A. Card (Eds.), *Handbook of developmental research methods* (pp. 31–45). New York: Guilford Press.

Enders, C. (2010). *Applied missing data analysis*. New York, NY: Guildford Press.

Funke, F., & Reips, U.-D. (2012). Why semantic differentials in Web-based research should be made from visual analogue scales and not from 5-point scales. *Field Methods, 24*, 310–327.

Graham, J. W., Taylor, B. J., & Cumsille, P. E. (2001). Planned missing data designs in the analysis of change. In L. M. Collins & A. G. Sayer (Eds.), *New methods for the analysis of change* (pp. 335–353). Washington, DC: American Psychological Association.

Graham, J. W., Taylor, B. J., Olchowski, A. E., & Cumsille, P. E. (2006). Planned missing data designs in psychological research. *Psychological Methods, 11*, 323–343.

Grimm, K. J., & Ram, N. (2012). Growth curve modeling from a structural equation modeling perspective. In B. Laursen, T. D. Little, & N. A. Card (Eds.), *Handbook of developmental research methods* (pp. 411–431). New York: Guilford Press.

Harel, O., Stratton, J., & Aseltine, R. (2011). Designed missingness to better estimate efficacy of behavioral studies. *Tenth conference on health survey research methods,* pp. 153–158.

Jia, F., Moore, E. W. G., Kinai, R., Crowe, K. S., Schoemann, A. M., & Little, T. D. (2014). Planned missing data design on small sample size: How small is too small? *International Journal of Behavioral Development, 38*, 1–18.

Jorgensen, T. D., Rhemtulla, M., Schoemann, A., McPherson, B., Wu, W., & Little, T. D. (2014). Optimal assignment methods in three-form planned missing data designs for longitudinal panel studies. *International Journal of Behavioral Development, 38*, 397–410.

Klein, A., & Moosbrugger, H. (2000). Maximum likelihood estimation of latent interaction effects with the LMS method. *Psychometrika, 65*, 457–474.

Likert, R. (1932). A technique for the measurement of attitudes. *Archives of Psychology, 22*, 1–55.

Lin, G.-C., Wen, Z., Marsh, H. W., & Lin, H.-S. (2010). Structural equation models of latent interactions: Clarification of orthogonalizing and double-mean-centering strategies. *Structural Equation Modeling, 17*, 374–391.

Little, T. D. (1997). Mean and covariance structures (MACS) analyses of cross-cultural data: Practical and theoretical issues. *Multivariate Behavioral Research, 32*, 53–76.

Little, T. D. (2013). *Longitudinal structural equation modeling*. New York: Guilford Press.

Little, T. D., & Rhemtulla, M. (2013). Planned missing data designs for developmental researchers. *Child Development Perspectives, 7*, 199–204.

Little, R. J., & Rubin, D. (2002). *Statistical analysis with missing data* (2nd ed.). New York: Wiley.

Little, T. D., Cunningham, W. A., Shahar, G., & Widaman, K. F. (2002). To parcel or not to parcel: Exploring the question, weighing the merits. *Structural Equation Modeling, 9*, 151–173.

Little, T. D., Bovaird, J. A., & Slegers, D. W. (2006a). Methods for the analysis of change. In D. K. Mroczek & T. D. Little (Eds.), *Handbook of personality development* (pp. 181–211). Mahwah: LEA.

Little, T. D., Bovaird, J. A., & Widaman, K. F. (2006b). On the merits of orthogonalizing powered and product terms: Implications for modeling interactions among latent variables. *Structural Equation Modeling, 13*, 497–519.

Little, T. D., Bovaird, J. A., & Card, N. A. (Eds.). (2006c). *Modeling contextual effects in longitudinal studies*. Mahwah: LEA.

Little, T. D., Card, N. A., Bovaird, J. A., Preacher, K., & Crandall, C. S. (2007a). Structural equation modeling of mediation and moderation with contextual factors. In T. D. Little, J. A. Bovaird, & N. A. Card (Eds.), *Modeling contextual effects in longitudinal studies* (pp. 207–230). Mahwah, LEA.

Little, T. D., Preacher, K. J., Selig, J. P., & Card, N. A. (2007c). New developments in SEM panel analyses of longitudinal data. *International Journal of Behavioral Development, 31*, 357–365.

Little, T. D., Rhemtulla, M., Gibson, K., & Schoemann, A. M. (2013a). Why the items versus parcels controversy needn't be one. *Psychological Methods, 18*, 285–300.

Little, T. D., Jorgensen, T. D., Lang, K. M., & Moore, E. W. G. (2013b). On the joys of missing data. *Journal of Pediatric Psychology, 39*(2), 151–162. doi:10.1093/jpepsy/jst048.

Little, T. D., Jorgensen, T. D., Lang, K. M., & Moore, E. W. G. (2014). On the joys of missing data. *Journal of Pediatric Psychology, 39*, 151–162.

MacKinnon, D. P. (2008). *Introduction to statistical mediation analysis*. Mahwah: Erlbaum.

Marsh, H. W., Hau, K.-T., Wen, Z., & Nagengast, B. (2012). Moderation. In T. D. Little (Ed.), *The Oxford handbook of quantitative methods* (Vol. 2, pp. 361–386). New York: Oxford University Press.

Masyn, K. E., & Nylund-Gibson, K. (2012). Mixture modeling. In T. D. Little (Ed.), *The Oxford handbook of quantitative methods* (Vol. 2, pp. 551–611). New York: Oxford University Press.

Maxwell, S. E., & Cole, D. A. (2007). Bias in cross sectional analysis of longitudinal mediation. *Psychological Methods, 12*, 23–44.

McDonald, R. (1999). *Test theory: A unified treatment*. Mahwah: Erlbaum.

Mehta, P. (2013). *xxM user's guide, version 1.0*. University of Houston: Author.

Meredith, W. (1993). Measurement invariance, factor analysis and factorial invariance. *Psychometrika, 58*, 525–543.

Milsap, R. E., & Cham, H. (2012). Investigating factorial invariance in longitudinal data. In B. Laursen, T. D. Little, & N. A. Card (Eds.), *Handbook of developmental research methods* (pp. 109–126). New York: Guilford Press.

Mistler, S. A., & Enders, C. K. (2012). Planned missing data designs for developmental research. In B. Laursen, T. D. Little, & N. A. Card (Eds.), *Handbook of developmental research methods* (pp. 742–775). New York: Guilford Press.

Muthén, B., & Asparouhov, T. (2003). *Modeling interactions between latent and observed continuous variables using maximum-likelihood estimation in Mplus*. Mplus Web Notes: No. 6.

Nagin, D. S., & Odgers, C. L. (2012). Group-based trajectory modeling in developmental science. In B. Laursen, T. D. Little, & N. A. Card (Eds.), *Handbook of developmental research methods* (pp. 464–480). New York: Guilford Press.

Preacher, K. J., & Hayes, A. F. (2008a). Asymptotic and resampling strategies for assessing and comparing indirect effects in multiple mediator models. *Behavior Research Methods, 40*, 879–891.

Preacher, K. J., & Hayes, A. F. (2008b). Contemporary approaches to assessing mediation in communication research. In A. F. Hayes, M. D. Slater, & L. B. Snyder (Eds.), *The Sage sourcebook of advanced data analysis methods for communication research* (pp. 13–54). Thousand Oaks: Sage.

Preacher, K. J., & Selig, J. P. (2012). Advantages of Monte Carlo confidence intervals for indirect effects. *Communication Methods and Measures, 6*, 77–98.

Ram, N., Grimm, K. J., Gatzke-Koop, L. M., & Molenaar, P. C. M. (2012). Longitudinal mixture models and the identification of archetypes. In B. Laursen, T. D. Little, & N. A. Card (Eds.), *Handbook of developmental research methods* (pp. 481–500). New York: Guilford Press.

Reips, U.-D. (2006). Web-based methods. In M. Eid & E. Diener (Eds.), *Handbook of multimethod measurement in psychology* (pp. 73–85). Washington, DC: American Psychological Association.

Reips, U.-D., & Funke, F. (2008). Interval level measurement with visual analogue scales in Internet-based research: VAS generator. *Behavior Research Methods, 40*, 699–704.

Rhemtulla, M., & Little, T. D. (2012). Planned missing data designs for research in cognitive development. *Journal of Cognition and Development, 13*, 425–438.

Rhemtulla, M., Brosseau-Liard, P., & Savalei, V. (2012). How many categories is enough to treat data as continuous? A comparison of robust continuous and categorical SEM estimation methods under a range of non-ideal situations. *Psychological Methods, 17*, 354–373.

Selig, J. P., & Little, T. D. (2012). Autoregressive and cross-lagged panel analysis for longitudinal data. In B. Laursen, T. D. Little, & N. A. Card (Eds.), *Handbook of developmental research methods* (pp. 265–278). New York, NY: Guilford Press.

Selig, J. P., Preacher, K. J., & Little, T. D. (2012). Modeling time-dependent association in longitudinal data: A lag as moderator approach. *Multivariate Behavioral Research, 47*, 697–716.

van Buuren, S. (2012). *Flexile imputation of missing data*. Boca Raton: CRC Press.

Widaman, K. F., & Reise, S. P. (1997). Exploring the measurement invariance of psychological instruments: Applications in the substance use domain. In K. J. Bryant, M. Windle, & S. G. West (Eds.), *The science of prevention: Methodological advances from alcohol and substance abuse research* (pp. 281–324). Washington, DC: APA.

Wu, A. D., & Zumbo, B. D. (2008). Understanding and using mediators and moderators. *Social Indicators Research, 87*, 367–392.

Wu, W., Selig, J. P., & Little, T. D. (2012). Longitudinal data analysis. In T. D. Little (Ed.), *The Oxford handbook of quantitative methods* (Vol. 2, pp. 387–410). New York: Oxford University Press.

4

Pregnancy Characteristics and Women's Cardiovascular Health

Abigail Fraser, Janet M. Catov, Deborah A. Lawlor, and Janet W. Rich-Edwards

1 Introduction

Growing evidence suggests that pregnancy is a "critical period" in a woman's life when her health development is especially sensitive to certain internal and external stimuli. As a normal response to pregnancy and in order to support the developing fetus, women become more insulin resistant and hyperlipidemic and experience an increase in blood pressure (BP; after an initial drop) and upregulation of coagulation factors and the inflammatory cascade (Sattar 2004). This is perhaps the prime example of health as an emergent property as it is one that enables the bearing of offspring and thus the perpetuation of humanity. While for a majority of women, this adaptation to pregnancy remains "healthy," in some women it develops into a complication of pregnancy such as gestational diabetes mellitus (GDM), preeclampsia, fetal growth restriction (FGR), and preterm delivery.

It has long been understood that pregnancy complications are important for the life course health development of offspring, but much less appreciated that these complications also have key implications for the long-term health development of the mother. An accumulating body of research has shown that these common pregnancy

This chapter contains a modified version of a previously published review and analysis of existing research that appeared in *Epidemiologic Reviews*. Reprinted with permission from:
Janet W. Rich-Edwards, Abigail Fraser, Deborah A. Lawlor, Janet M. Catov; Pregnancy Characteristics and Women's Future Cardiovascular Health: An Underused Opportunity to Improve Women's Health?. Epidemiol Rev 2014;36(1):57–70. doi: 10.1093/epirev/mxt006
AF and DAL work in a unit that receives infrastructure funding from the United Kingdom Medical Research Council (MC_UU_12013), and AF is funded by a United Kingdom Medical Research Council fellowship (MR/M009351/1). A grant to DAL from the Wellcome Trust also supports this collaborative work (WT094529MA). JMC is funded by RO1HL103825 and K12HD43441. JRE is supported by an American Heart Association Founder's Grant (13GRNT17070022). The authors have no relevant disclosures, financial or otherwise.

A. Fraser (✉) • D.A. Lawlor
Medical Research Council Integrative Epidemiology Unit at the University of Bristol, University of Bristol, Bristol, UK BS8 2BN
e-mail: abigail.fraser@bristol.ac.uk

J.M. Catov
Department of Obestetrics and Gynecology, University of Pittsburgh, Pittsburgh, PA 15213, USA

University of Pittsburgh, Department of Epidemiology, Pittsburgh, PA 15261, USA

Magee-Womens Research Institute, Pittsburgh, PA 15213, USA

J.W. Rich-Edwards
Connors Center for Women's Health and Gender Biology, Brigham and Women's Hospital, Boston, MA 02120, USA

Harvard Medical School, Boston, MA 02115, USA

Harvard School of Public Health, Boston, MA 02120, USA

complications predict the future risk of chronic diseases in women, including cardiovascular disease, diabetes, and breast cancer (Rich-Edwards 2009). In this chapter we use life course health development theoretical principles as a lens for an examination of the implications of pregnancy history for cardiovascular disease (CVD), a leading cause of female mortality (Oblast 1999; Yusuf et al. 2001).

Globally, one out of three women dies from CVD (Shah et al. 2009; Mathers et al. 2008). We do a worse job of recognizing and predicting CVD in women than in men, in part because CVD presents itself differently between the sexes (Mosca et al. 2011; Shaw et al. 2006). This has important implications for the prevention of CVD. Primary prevention, if applied to high risk populations early enough to avert the cumulative damage of chronic disease, can reduce CVD incidence (Scarborough and Weissberg 2011; Shay et al. 2012; MMWR 1989). In response to the growing appreciation that many preventive efforts start too late to be effective, there has been a call for "primordial prevention"—the prevention of the major CVD risk factors themselves (Labarthe 1999; Weintraub et al. 2011). In this context, pregnancy complications have the potential to be effective CVD risk "stress tests" to identify women who would most benefit from primordial or primary prevention efforts to reduce CVD risk (Sattar and Greer 2002). The concept of primordial prevention is consistent with the life course health development principle that health development is an emergent phenomenon and the best way to prevent future disease is to build health assets that have long-term salutary benefits.

On average, more than 80% of women in high-income countries bear at least one child (Martinez et al. 2012; OECD Family D 2014), as do upward of 90% of women in most lower- and middle-income nations (United Nations DoEaSA, Population Division 2009). A high proportion of women will, in the course of their reproductive career, have a pregnancy complicated by GDM, a hypertensive disorder of pregnancy, FGR macrosomia, or preterm delivery. The prevalence of any one of these conditions in any given pregnancy ranges from 2% to greater than 12%. In one UK study, 36% of singleton pregnancies were complicated by at least one of these factors (Fraser et al. 2012). In the U.S. national Nurses' Health Study 2, we estimated that 29% of parous study participants have had one of these pregnancy complications. As reviewed below, each of these complications has been associated with roughly a twofold increase in the risk of CVD events. If 80% of women are parous and 30% of them have had a pregnancy complication predictive of CVD, then about 25% of women are at heightened risk for future CVD risk.

We begin with a review of the evidence for associations of parity and common pregnancy complications (low birth weight, fetal growth restriction, preterm delivery, hypertensive disorders of pregnancy, and GDM) with future CVD risk. We conducted MEDLINE searches for English-language cohort and case-control studies published in the peer-reviewed literature through December 2012, as described in detail elsewhere (Rich-Edwards et al. 2014). Whether pregnancy is a sensitive period in terms of cardiovascular health development across the life course and complications per se contribute to long term CVD risk, whether they simply unmask women with an underlying propensity for CVD, or whether both pathways are in play remains unclear. As suggested by life course health development, longitudinal studies are needed to untangle these temporal effects. In the second part of the chapter, we further explore the physiologic mechanisms that might explain the associations between pregnancy complications and CVD. Finally, we discuss the implications of these findings for future research as well as for health care design and policy.

2 Associations of Parity and Pregnancy Complications with CVD Risk in Mothers

2.1 Parity and CVD

Most (Green and Moser 1988; Ness et al. 1993) but not all studies (Steenland et al. 1996) have found a positive association between parity (number of children) and later CVD. In the largest study to date, the association was examined in

1.3 million with a median follow-up time of 9.5 years (range 0–24) women using Swedish registry data (Parikh et al. 2010). Parity was associated with CVD in a J-shaped fashion, with two births representing the nadir of risk. Compared with women with two births, the multivariable-adjusted hazard ratios (95% confidence interval (CI)) for women with 0 and ≥5 births were 1.11 (1.09–1.14) and 1.57 (1.52–1.64), respectively.

Desired family size may affect the shape of the parity-CVD risk distribution in different societies and is an example of how societal norms and social structures may affect health development and its determinants. In Sweden, the modal family size (two children) coincides with the nadir of maternal cardiovascular risk (Parikh et al. 2010). This suggests that many women who bore only one child suffered from secondary infertility, first pregnancy complications that precluded further pregnancies, or severe neonatal outcomes that discouraged further childbearing. To the extent that subfertility and severe pregnancy complications predict future CVD risk, they may explain the low-parity "hook" of the J-shaped association of parity and maternal CVD. The increase in CVD risk with increasing parity after two children may be the result of different phenomena. These include rival, but not mutually exclusive, theories that (1) adverse physiologic change accumulates over pregnancies; (2) adverse lifestyle habits accrue with more children; and/or (3) selection bias in which women at higher CVD risk opt for larger families. Thus, it is unclear whether the association of higher parity with CVD risk is causal or correlational.

Some insight into the association of parity with maternal CVD risk may be gleaned by examining the association of number of children with paternal CVD risk. Similar associations for mothers and fathers would suggest that the association between parity and maternal CVD is not causal, but is more likely a result of confounding by socioeconomic position and/or behaviors related to child-rearing. Three reports examined associations of number of children with CVD in fathers. In general, men who have fathered the most children appear to have small increased CVD risk, though this association is not always statistically significant and is weaker than the associations observed among mothers (Dekker and Schouten 1993; Lawlor et al. 2003; Ness et al. 1995). Adjustment for lifestyle factors tends to reduce the associations in both mothers and fathers (Lawlor et al. 2003; Catov et al. 2007a). These results suggest that the association between high parity and CVD in later life may be largely the result of socioeconomic position and/or behavioral risk factors associated with child-rearing that are shared by both parents.

2.2 Common Pregnancy Complications and CVD in Mothers

Offspring birth weight predicts maternal lifespan (Catov et al. 2007a; Davey Smith et al. 1997, 2000a, b, 2007). Figure 1 presents the findings from studies that have examined associations of offspring birth weight or fetal growth—a function of birth weight and gestation length—with maternal CVD risk (Davey Smith et al. 1997, 2007, 2000a, b, 2005; Bellamy et al. 2007, 2011; Friedlander et al. 2007; Lykke et al. 2010a; Mongraw-Chaffin et al. 2010; Smith et al. 2001; Wikström et al. 2005; Fraser et al. 2012; Ness et al. 1993). One meta-analysis has calculated that, for every standard deviation (roughly 500 g) higher birth weight of the firstborn child, maternal CVD mortality is decreased by 25% (Davey Smith et al. 2007). It is unclear whether the inverse association of offspring birth weight with mortality is constant across the entire range of birth weight, as the association of high birth weight with maternal CVD risk varies by study. In some populations, the mothers of the largest infants (>4000 g or >4500 g) have the lowest risks of CVD (Davey Smith et al. 1997, 2000b), while in other populations there is an uptick in CVD risk for the mothers of macrosomic newborns (Davey Smith et al. 2007; Bonamy et al. 2011; Friedlander et al. 2007; Lykke et al. 2012). Given the strong associations of macrosomia with GDM and later type 2 diabetes (Metzger et al. 1993), the presence and magnitude of the association of large birth weight with future CVD risk may depend on the population prevalence of GDM and chronic diabetes during pregnancy (in other words,

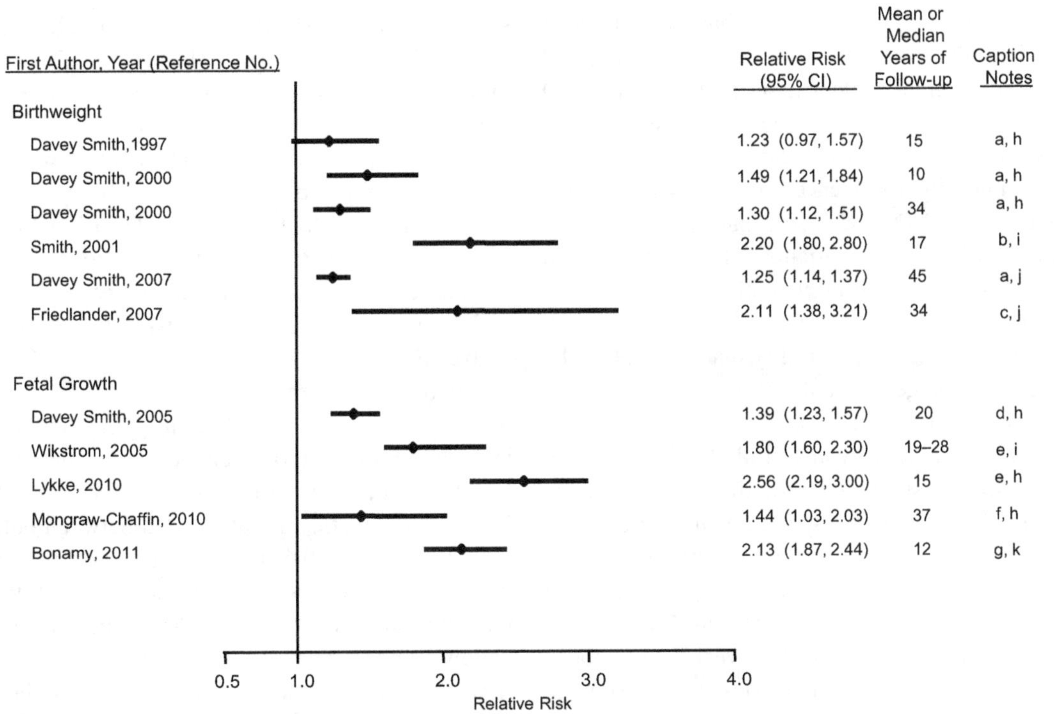

Fig. 1 Results from studies of offspring birth weight or fetal growth and relative risk of maternal cardiovascular disease (CVD). *a* Per 1 standard deviation (SD) lower birth weight; *b* lowest birth weight quintile compared to all others; *c* <2500 g compared to 1500–3999 g birth weight; *d* per 1 SD lower birth weight, adjusted for gestational age; *e* small for gestational age; *f* intrauterine growth retardation; *g* ~2 SD below mean birth weight adjusted for gestational age; *h* CVD mortality; *i* coronary heart disease (CHD) events ; *j* CHD mortality; *k* CVD events (*CI* confidence interval)

the extent to which large infant size is pathological). Indeed, the association of macrosomia with CVD risk is attenuated by adjustment for GDM(36) (Bonamy et al. 2011), indicating that a substantial portion of the association of macrosomia and CVD is explained by metabolic risk.

It is abundantly clear, however, that the 8% of deliveries that are low birth weight (<2500 g) are associated with twice the maternal CVD incidence and mortality of other deliveries (Davey Smith et al. 1997, 2000a, b, 2007). Associations of offspring birth weight with maternal CVD are only modestly diminished by adjustment for cigarette smoking and not affected by control for prepregnancy body mass index (Bonamy et al. 2011; Davey Smith et al. 2005).

Birth weight is the product of fetal growth rate and gestation length. Fetal growth, represented as birth weight corrected for gestation length, predicts maternal CVD risk (Bonamy et al. 2011; Lykke et al. 2012), as does gestation length (discussed below). In fact, the coincidence of restricted fetal growth and prematurity yields a more than threefold increased CVD risk (Bonamy et al. 2011). The curvilinear association of offspring birth weight with maternal CVD risk observed in many populations may be the product of competing pathological phenomena. At one end of the birth weight spectrum, the association of macrosomia with maternal CVD risk may be explained by underlying metabolic risk; at the other end of the spectrum, the association of low birth weight with maternal CVD risk may be driven by endothelial dysfunction and other pathologies associated with restricted fetal growth and preterm birth.

First offspring birth weight also predicts paternal CVD, although the magnitude of the positive association of offspring birth weight with paternal

CVD risk is less than a third of that for the infant's mother (Davey Smith et al. 2007). The fact that the birth weight of their first child predicts CVD events in both parents suggests that shared lifestyle or environmental factors, such as cigarette smoking, might influence both the growth of the fetus and CVD risk in the parents and/or that pleiotropic genetic variants affect both growth and CVD risk. Birth weight is passed down through maternal and paternal lines (Lie et al. 2006), opening the possibility that paternal CVD/fetal growth genes could affect both the pregnancy outcome and long-term chronic disease risk in the father (Freathy et al. 2007). However, the stronger association in mothers than in fathers suggests either parent-specific genomic imprinting or—as seems more parsimonious—that maternal health during pregnancy affects fetal growth and is a marker of her future CVD risk.

Preterm delivery (<37 weeks' gestation) accounts for 6–12% of deliveries in the developed world (Beck et al. 2010). The hazard ratios for CVD associated with total preterm delivery are depicted in Fig. 2 and are on the order of 1.3–2.6 for births <37 completed weeks compared with term births (Davey Smith et al. 2000b, 2005; Bonamy et al. 2011; Lykke et al. 2010a, b; Smith et al. 2001; Wikström et al. 2005; Catov et al. 2010a; Irgens et al. 2001; Nardi et al. 2006; Pell et al. 2004; Rich-Edwards et al. 2012). There is a greater range of relative risk when distinct preterm phenotypes are examined separately. While most preterm deliveries follow spontaneous labor or preterm premature rupture of membranes, a significant and growing fraction results from medically induced labor or Caesarean section without labor. The chief reasons for these medically indicated deliveries include preeclampsia and FGR, both of which have been associated with increased maternal CVD risk. In studies that have distinguished them, hypertensive preterm deliveries consistently have a stronger association with maternal CVD outcomes than do normotensive preterm deliveries, though the latter are still associated with a 1.2- to threefold increased risk compared with term deliveries (Catov et al. 2010a; Irgens et al. 2001). In the two studies that have contrasted CVD risk among mothers with spontaneous versus indicated preterm deliveries (Rich-Edwards et al. 2012; Hastie et al. 2011a), indicated delivery was associated with higher risks of CVD mortality than spontaneous preterm delivery. Nevertheless, spontaneous preterm delivery—compared with term delivery—was associated with doubling of CVD risk (Rich-Edwards et al. 2012; Hastie et al. 2011a).

Unlike the associations of parity or birth weight with paternal CVD risk, two studies (Davey Smith et al. 2005; Irgens et al. 2001) have reported that preterm delivery is not associated with paternal risk of CVD, implying that the association of preterm delivery with maternal CVD risk is not the product of a high-CVD risk lifestyle or genetic variants shared between both parents and their offspring. Of relevance, preterm birth risk appears to be passed only through the maternal line (Wilcox et al. 2008). These observations suggest that maternal intrauterine environment and health determine the risk of preterm delivery and explain its association with maternal CVD risk, rather than shared lifestyle or environment of the mother and father.

Gestational diabetes mellitus is a common and growing pregnancy complication that affects as many as 5% of pregnancies. It is well established that women with GDM are at increased risk of developing diabetes later in life (Bellamy et al. 2009); between 3% and 70% of women with a history of GDM will develop type 2 diabetes within three decades of the pregnancy (Kim et al. 2002), with a meta-analysis of 675,455 women finding a sevenfold increase in risk of later type 2 diabetes (Bellamy et al. 2009). Type 2 diabetes is an important CVD risk factor, having a markedly higher relative and absolute association with CVD in women than it does in men (Sarwar et al. 2010). Given these associations, it seems self-evident that a history of GDM would be associated with increased CVD risk. However, due largely to the fact that GDM screening during pregnancy was neither routine nor standardized until recent decades, there are few cohorts with long enough follow-up of screened populations to detect CVD incidence or mortality among women with a history of GDM (Shah et al. 2008; Carr et al. 2006). These are displayed in Fig. 3. The only large population-based study of this topic is a

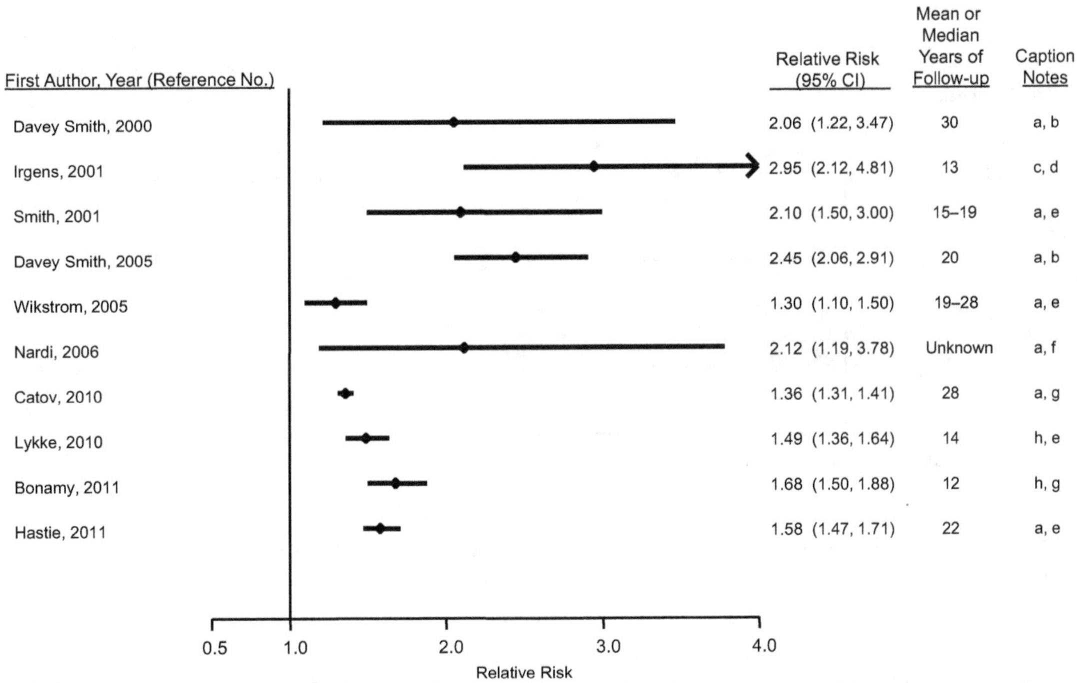

Fig. 2 Results from studies of preterm delivery and relative risk of maternal cardiovascular disease (CVD). *a* <37 weeks' gestation weeks compared with term; *b* CVD mortality; *c* <37 weeks' gestation length compared with term normotensive pregnancies; *d* CVD mortality, excluding stroke mortality; *e* coronary heart disease (CHD) events; *f* myocardial infarction; *g* CVD events; *h* 32–36 weeks' gestation length compared with term (*CI* confidence interval)

record linkage study conducted in Ontario, Canada, with a median follow-up of 11.5 years (Shah et al. 2008). In that study, a history of GDM was associated with a greater risk of hospital admission for acute myocardial infarction, coronary bypass, coronary angioplasty, stroke, or carotid endarterectomy (hazard ratio (HR) = 1.71; 95% CI, 1.08–2.69). Upon adjustment for diabetes after pregnancy, the association was attenuated toward the null (adjusted HR, 1.13; 0.67–1.89). A smaller, cross-sectional study found that women with a history of GDM had a higher CVD risk than women without a history of GDM (adjusted OR = 1.85, 1.21–2.82) and experienced CVD events 7 years earlier, on average (Carr et al. 2006).

Lesser degrees of antepartum hyperglycemia have also been associated with an elevated risk of subsequent diabetes and CVD. In the Ontario study, women with evidence of elevated glycemia short of GDM criteria were at an increased risk of diabetes (HR = 2.56, 2.28–2.87) (Retnakaran and Shah 2009a) and CVD (HR = 1.19, 1.02–1.39) (Retnakaran and Shah 2009b) compared to normoglycemic women.

Hypertensive disorders of pregnancy (HDPs) are common pregnancy complications that presage CVD. *Preeclampsia*, the combination of hypertension and proteinuria, affects approximately 2–5% of pregnancies, with a predominance among first pregnancies (Fraser et al. 2012; Wallis et al. 2008; North et al. 2011). Estimates of the prevalence of *gestational hypertension*, new-onset hypertension without proteinuria, vary from 3% to 14% (Fraser et al. 2012; Wallis et al. 2008; Roberts et al. 2005). Women with a history of preeclampsia have roughly fourfold higher incidence of hypertension and twofold elevated risks of heart disease, stroke, and venous thromboembolism (Bellamy et al. 2007; McDonald et al. 2008). Two systematic reviews, one of cohort studies (n = 25) and the other of both cohort (n = 10) and case-control (n = 5) studies,

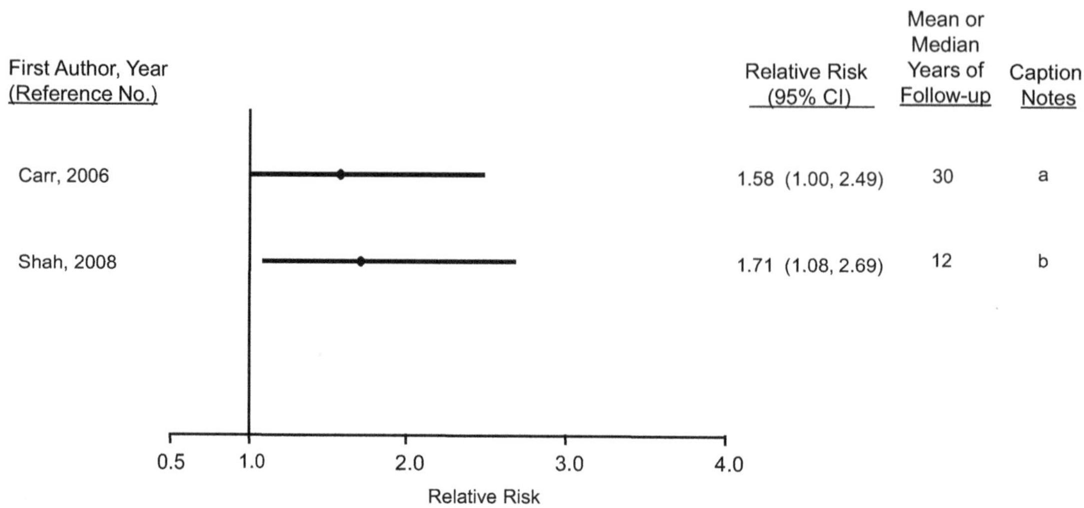

Fig. 3 Results from studies of gestational diabetes mellitus and relative risk of maternal cardiovascular disease (CVD). *a* Self-reported coronary artery disease, *b* CVD events (*CI* confidence interval)

have both reported a doubling of risk for different measures of CVD comparing women with preeclampsia to normotensive women over a median of 10–12-year follow-up (Bellamy et al. 2007; McDonald et al. 2008). Figure 4 depicts the relative risk of coronary heart disease (CHD) and CVD outcomes among mothers with a history of preeclampsia (Mongraw-Chaffin et al. 2010; Smith et al. 2001; Wikström et al. 2005; Irgens et al. 2001; Funai et al. 2005; Hannaford et al. 1997; Jónsdóttir et al. 1995; Kestenbaum et al. 2003; Lin et al. 2011; Lykke et al. 2009; Wilson et al. 2003).

Publications from three cohort studies published since those reviews give some insight into the onset and duration of CVD risk following HDP (Mongraw-Chaffin et al. 2010; Smith et al. 2001; Lin et al. 2011; Lykke et al. 2009). In a short-term follow-up of over 1,000,000 pregnancies in Taiwan, women with preeclampsia/eclampsia were at double the risk of major CVD from the third trimester of pregnancy up to three years postpartum, with particularly high relative risks for stroke (HR = 14.5, 1.3–165.1) and myocardial infarction (HR = 13.0, 4.6–6.3) (Lin et al. 2011). While these results suggest a high relative risk immediately following HDP, the confidence intervals are wide, and the absolute risk of CVD events is very small at this age, so that this immediate risk is unlikely to account for a large number of CVD events. The Child Health and Development Study in California has provided some of the longer follow-up; over 37 years after pregnancy, women with a history of preeclampsia in any pregnancy had double the risk of CVD death (HR = 2.14; 1.29–3.57) (Mongraw-Chaffin et al. 2010). This doubling of risk is consistent with studies with shorter duration of follow-up. Considering the exponential increase in the absolute numbers of CVD events with increasing age, this suggests that the elevated risk of CVD among women with a history of HDP is not limited to the early years postpartum.

Thus, studies repeatedly report a doubling of CVD risk among women with a history of preeclampsia and suggest lesser degrees of excess risk among women with a history of gestational hypertension, despite the strong association of gestational hypertension with development of chronic hypertension (Lykke et al. 2009). The combination of preterm delivery and preeclampsia—a likely marker of the severity of preeclampsia—is a particularly potent predictor of CVD risk. Compared to normotensive term pregnancies, women delivering preterm preeclamptic pregnancies have very high relative risks of future

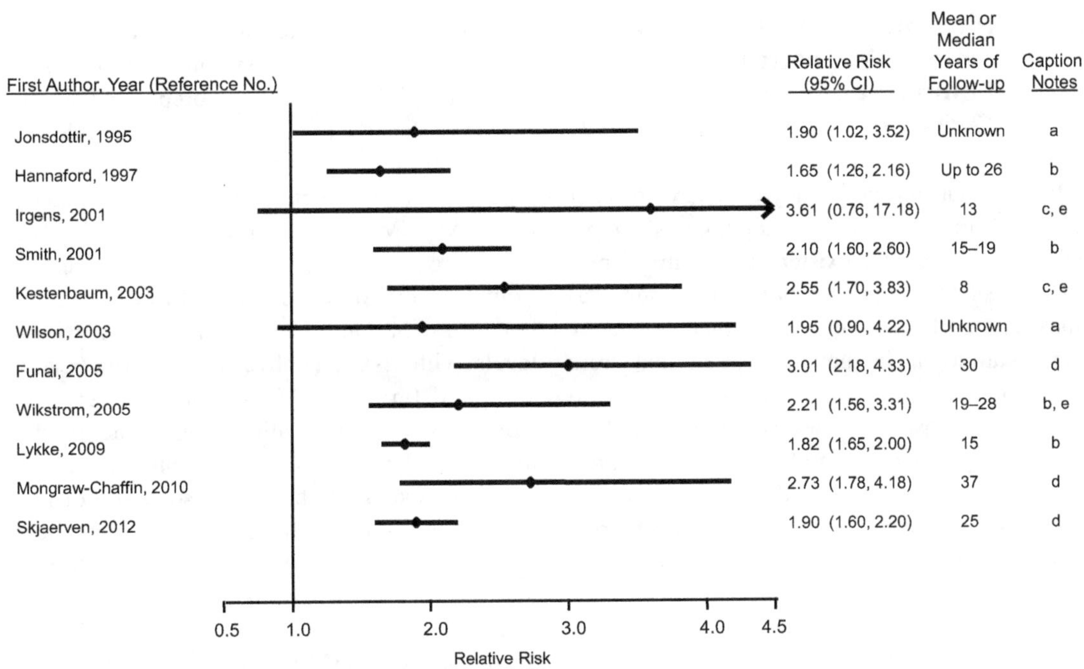

Fig. 4 Results from studies of hypertensive disorders of pregnancy and relative risk of maternal cardiovascular disease (CVD). *a* Coronary heart disease (CHD) mortality, *b* CHD events, *c* CVD events, *d* CVD mortality, *e* composite estimate provided by Bellamy review (18). A 2011 study by Lin (62) reported a relative risk of 23.0 (95% confidence interval (CI), 5.1–103.7) for CVD events (except stroke) during pregnancy and up to three years after delivery. We omitted that study from the figure so that we could keep the relative risk scale consistent across figures

CVD ranging from 2.5 to 9.5. (Mongraw-Chaffin et al. 2010; Smith et al. 2001; Lin et al. 2011; Skjaerven et al. 2012)

2.3 Recurrent Pregnancy Complications, Last Pregnancy Complications, and Maternal CVD Risk

Much of the literature is based on first pregnancies, precluding examination of the association of recurring pregnancy complications with CVD risk. There is evidence that recurrent preeclampsia (Lykke et al. 2009) and preterm delivery(Catov et al. 2010a; Lykke et al. 2010b) are associated with a greater risk of CVD than a single complicated pregnancy in multiparous women. Although the association of recurrent GDM with CVD risk has not been studied, after a first GDM pregnancy, each subsequent GDM pregnancy has been associated with a modestly increased risk of type 2 diabetes (adjusted HR = 1.16, 1.01–1.34) and each non-GDM pregnancy with a reduced risk of diabetes (HR = 0.34, 0.27–0.41) (Retnakaran et al. 2011). In fact, this highlights an intriguing pattern that is emerging with respect to last births: having preeclampsia (Skjaerven et al. 2012), preterm delivery (Rich-Edwards et al. 2012), or GDM (Retnakaran et al. 2011) in the last pregnancy appears to be associated with especially high risk of future CVD in mothers. Perhaps reflecting the same phenomenon, women who have one preterm delivery and one term delivery in their first two births appear to be at higher risk of CHD if the preterm delivery was the second birth (Catov et al. 2010a; Lykke et al. 2010b). This suggests that pregnancy complications severe enough to contraindicate or discourage a subsequent pregnancy may be particularly potent predictors of future CVD risk.

3 Physiological Mechanisms Linking Pregnancy Complications to Maternal CVD Risk

Pathways that link pregnancy exposures to later life CVD are not well understood. Considerable evidence supports the existence of common predisposing factors for both pregnancy complications and CVD risk suggesting that pregnancy complications can be thought of as a failed stress test, with pregnancy being the stressor. There have been almost no studies examining the alternative that pregnancy complications might *cause* increased CVD risk. To address this issue, we summarize evidence that compares CVD risk before, during, and after pregnancies with and without complications.

3.1 Cardiovascular Risk Factors Preceding Pregnancy Complications

Higher *prepregnancy blood pressure* is a risk factor for preeclampsia (Magnussen et al. 2007) and preterm delivery (Catov et al. 2013). Chronic hypertension has a well-established relation to increased risk of preeclampsia—known as "superimposed" preeclampsia. Even within the normotensive range, there is a positive dose-response association of prepregnancy systolic and/or diastolic blood pressure with preeclampsia, (Magnussen et al. 2007) and women who develop hypertensive disorders of pregnancy have higher blood pressure at 8 weeks' gestation than normotensive (Macdonald-Wallis et al. 2012). Preexisting hypertension has also been associated with FGR, especially in cases that were also preterm (Catov et al. 2008a). Risks for these complications also rise with increasing maternal age, suggesting that the aging endothelium may less successfully adapt to the profound vascular demands of pregnancy.

Prepregnancy lipid concentrations are also associated with pregnancy complications and offspring birth weight; the nature of the association varies with the pregnancy outcome in question. Lipid profiles consistent with elevated CVD risk, including higher prepregnancy triglyceride levels, total cholesterol, and lower HDL cholesterol, have been associated with preeclampsia and preterm delivery in the study in Norway (Magnussen et al. 2007, 2011). The US Coronary Artery Risk Development in Young Adults Study (CARDIA) found a curvilinear association of prepregnancy cholesterol levels with risk of delivering preterm (Catov et al. 2010b). With respect to fetal growth, women with a more atherogenic lipid profile may bear larger infants (Romundstad et al. 2007); this suggests that the association of low birth weight—at least the fetal growth component of low birth weight—with maternal CVD risk may not operate via dyslipidemia.

Prepregnancy adiposity and glucose/insulin dysregulation is strongly implicated in the etiology of GDM, based on the observation that women with GDM tend to have a family history of type 2 diabetes and higher body mass index (BMI) before pregnancy (Solomon et al. 1997), as well as higher levels of glucose and insulin and lower levels of adiponectin before the onset of the midpregnancy hyperglycemia that defines GDM (Nanda et al. 2011; Riskin-Mashiah et al. 2010; Sacks et al. 2003; Williams et al. 2004). Higher BMI and family history of diabetes are also associated with increased risk of preeclampsia (Qiu et al. 2003; O'Brien et al. 2003). The risk of preeclampsia doubles with every 5–7 kg/m^2 increase in body mass index before pregnancy (O'Brien et al. 2003).

Thus, subclinical elevations in the classic CVD risk factors of blood pressure, lipid levels, elevated BMI, and glucose/insulin dysregulation appear to predate both preeclampsia and GDM. Less clear is the extent to which CVD risk factors precede spontaneous preterm deliveries or FGR in normotensive pregnancies. Furthermore, the roles of prepregnancy inflammatory and coagulation factors with respect to pregnancy complications remain to be elucidated, despite the importance of these systems for both reproduction and CVD risk (Romero et al. 2007).

3.2 Cardiovascular Risk Factors During Pregnancy

3.2.1 Cardiovascular Adaptation in Normal Pregnancy

In normal gestation, maternal blood volume increases progressively from 6 to 8 weeks' gestation, peaking at an increase of 45% by 32 weeks (Monga and Creasy 1994). Cardiac output increases by 30–50%, with half of this increase occurring very early in gestation. Pulse rate increases 17%, and there are striking alterations in renal physiology. Although the insulin response to glucose is augmented in early pregnancy, insulin resistance emerges in the second half of pregnancy (Butte 2000). In addition, cholesterol and triglyceride profiles change after gestation week 9 to support steroid synthesis and fetal growth (Butte 2000). In uncomplicated pregnancy, there is a tendency for low-density lipoprotein (LDL) to shift across gestation from large, buoyant particles to smaller, denser, and more atherogenic particles (Hubel et al. 1998a). Fat is accumulated during the second trimester and then mobilized to support the dramatic fetal growth of the third trimester (Herrera 2000).

3.2.2 Cardiovascular Risk Factors During Pregnancy Complications

Vascular and endothelial dysfunction is characteristic of pregnancies complicated by preeclampsia or growth restriction. Placental underperfusion is common, and there are elevated markers of endothelial dysfunction in the maternal circulation. Women with hypertensive disorders of pregnancy demonstrate increased resistance in the uterine arteries (Ducey et al. 1987; Campbell and Griffin 1983), vascular stiffness, and impaired endothelial response (Savvidou et al. 2003, 2011). In addition, placental vascular lesions indicative of failed spiral artery remodeling, ischemia, or hemorrhage have also been reported in cases of both medically indicated and spontaneous preterm birth (Kelly et al. 2009).

During pregnancy, *lipid aberrations* accompany several pregnancy complications. Again, the direction of the associations appears to depend on the nature of the pregnancy complication. The dyslipidemias associated with atherosclerosis (hypertriglyceridemia, hypercholesterolemia, elevated free fatty acids, and excess oxidized LDL) are frequently seen during preeclampsia … (Clausen et al. 2001; Hubel et al. 1996, 1998b; Sattar et al. 1997). There is also emerging evidence to suggest that this atherogenic lipid profile is associated with both spontaneous and indicated preterm births (Edison et al. 2007; Catov et al. 2007b). Similarly, women with GDM exhibit elevations in triglycerides and, less consistently, total cholesterol and LDL during pregnancy (Enquobahrie et al. 2005). On the other hand, low maternal total and LDL-cholesterol concentrations appear in the third trimester in pregnancies complicated by FGR (Sattar et al. 1999). Placental studies are conflicting, with some suggesting reduced expression of lipoprotein receptors in placentas from FGR vs. appropriate weight for gestational age births (Wadsack et al. 2007) and others suggesting overexpression of these receptors (Stepan et al. 1999). FGR studies are hampered by nonstandard phenotyping, and thus findings may represent differing levels of severity. Despite these limitations, these data suggest that extremes of lipid concentrations are associated with adverse pregnancy outcomes. Longitudinal studies are needed to better understand how the relative contributions of low or high cholesterol are related to failed or compensatory lipid adaptation required to optimize fetal growth.

Metabolic dysregulation in pregnancy defines GDM and is a strong risk factor for preeclampsia; there is considerable overlap of the two conditions, with twice the rate of preeclampsia in diabetic versus nondiabetic pregnancies (Ostlund et al. 2004). However, GDM has only a modest association with spontaneous preterm birth (Hedderson et al. 2003). Higher early-pregnancy BMI is associated with increased risk of HDP and GDM (Solomon et al. 1997; O'Brien et al. 2003; Lawlor et al. 2012), but with reduced risk of SGA and spontaneous preterm birth in most studies (Smith et al. 2007).

Systemic inflammation during pregnancy may be important in the pathogenesis of several pregnancy complications. Elevated serum levels of C-reactive protein and/or leukocytes have been detected in women who experience GDM, FGR, and both spontaneous and indicated preterm deliveries (Catov et al. 2007c; Ernst et al. 2011; Freeman et al. 2004; Pitiphat et al. 2005; Wolf et al. 2001). However, neither mid-gestation circulating levels of C-reactive protein nor pro-inflammatory cytokines have proven to have prognostic value for specific pregnancy outcomes (Curry et al. 2007; Gammill et al. 2010).

Normal pregnancy is a state of *hypercoagulability*, and complications such as preeclampsia and preterm birth are characterized by particularly high biomarkers of an activated fibrinolytic cascade, as well as perhaps an impaired ability to mount this response appropriately (Catov et al. 2008b; Hackney et al. 2010; Heilmann et al. 2007). It has been hypothesized that aberrations in the cross talk between inflammation and the coagulation cascades could contribute to the pathophysiology of these pregnancy complications (Girardi 2011).

3.3 Cardiovascular Risk Factors After Pregnancy

3.3.1 Enduring Cardiovascular Impact of Normal Pregnancy

Most of the cardiovascular adaptations to normal pregnancy resolve in the postpartum period, although there are some detectable and lasting pregnancy effects. Blood pressure is modestly decreased in the postpartum period after a first uncomplicated pregnancy (Hackney et al. 2010). However, other lingering effects are not as salutary. Importantly, women retain, on average, 0.5–5.0 kg of weight following each pregnancy (Heilmann et al. 2007; Girardi 2011). Lactation may help resolve the cardiometabolic adaptations and fat accumulation associated with pregnancy (Agatisa et al. 2004; Berends et al. 2008; Catov et al. 2011).

The first birth may be a sentinel marker for complications in later pregnancies and future CVD risk (Lauenborg et al. 2005; Meyers-Seifer and Vohr 1996; Verma et al. 2002). Several factors distinguish first births. First, longitudinal studies suggest that the lasting blood pressure and lipid changes associated with pregnancy occur after first but not subsequent births (Hackney et al. 2010). In addition, first births are at higher risk for the major obstetric complications of preterm delivery, HDP, FGR, and stillbirth. Women with any of these complications are at higher risk in subsequent pregnancies for recurrence of the same complication as well as the onset of other complications. Importantly, complications during a first pregnancy impact the likelihood of having a subsequent pregnancy. As noted above, complications in a last pregnancy appear to be associated with especially high relative risks of CVD events. Thus, health status of the first and last pregnancies may be particularly telling of future maternal health.

The cumulative effect of these adaptations and resolutions and risks may contribute to the above-noted J-shaped association between parity and maternal CVD risk, with lowest risk for women who have delivered two infants. It is not clear whether pregnancies exert a cumulative cardiovascular burden with increasing parity, whether higher-order pregnancies at more advanced maternal age exert more cardiovascular risk, or whether women at high cardiovascular risk bear more children.

3.3.2 Cardiovascular Risk After Pregnancy Complications

The association of *vascular and endothelial dysfunction* with pregnancy complications continues after delivery. Women with preeclampsia have impaired endothelial function after pregnancy (Agatisa et al. 2004). This may also be true, although to a lesser extent, of women who deliver small babies due to FGR or preterm delivery. For example, lower offspring birth weight is associated with higher maternal blood pressure in the years after pregnancy (Davey Smith et al. 2005). Some (Catov et al. 2013; Berends et al. 2008) but not all (Catov et al. 2011) studies report higher blood pressure and atherosclerotic carotid vessel remodeling among women who have delivered an FGR neonate. Although studies are not unanimous (Macdonald-

Wallis et al. 2012; Lauenborg et al. 2005), women with a history of GDM are more likely to have hypertension (Meyers-Seifer and Vohr 1996; Verma et al. 2002), vascular dysfunction (Heitritter et al. 2005), impaired endothelium-dependent vasodilatation (Anastasiou et al. 1998), and higher carotid artery intima-media thickness (Tarim et al. 2006). These differences are not fully explained by the higher BMI typical of women with a history of GDM.

Studies of *lipid profiles after pregnancies* complicated by preeclampsia are consistent with increased atherogenesis risk, including consistently reported higher total cholesterol, LDL cholesterol, and triglycerides, although these differences are not always statistically significant (Fraser et al. 2012; Manten et al. 2007; Hubel et al. 2008; Laivuori et al. 1996; Magnussen et al. 2009; Romundstad et al. 2010; Sattar et al. 2003; Smith et al. 2009). Associations of reduced HDL cholesterol after preeclampsia have been reported by some (Fraser et al. 2012; Magnussen et al. 2009; Romundstad et al. 2010; Smith et al. 2009) but not all (Manten et al. 2007; Laivuori et al. 1996; Sattar et al. 2003) studies. One study has reported dyslipidemia among women with a history of spontaneous and indicated preterm births (Catov et al. 2011). Some (Lauenborg et al. 2005; Meyers-Seifer and Vohr 1996; Verma et al. 2002; Di Cianni et al. 2007) but not all (Schwarz et al. 2009) have reported elevated total cholesterol, LDL cholesterol, and/or triglycerides in women with a history of GDM. As with the studies of lipid concentrations before and during pregnancy, studies of lipid concentrations in women in the years after FGR are conflicting, with some reporting hyperlipidemia (Kanagalingam et al. 2009) and others reporting no differences compared to women with uncomplicated births (Catov et al. 2011).

It is now firmly established that women with a history of GDM have a manifold higher risk of developing *type 2 diabetes* than women with normoglycemic pregnancies (Bellamy et al. 2009). It is less widely appreciated that women with a history of preeclampsia are also at high risk of type 2 diabetes. After preeclampsia, mothers are three times more likely to develop diabetes within 16 years (Lykke et al. 2009), an observation bolstered by evidence of dysregulated glucose and insulin, as well as insulin resistance as early as 2 years after preeclamptic pregnancy (Fraser et al. 2012; Manten et al. 2007; Laivuori et al. 1996; Magnussen et al. 2009; Smith et al. 2009; Wolf et al. 2004). However, not all pregnancy complications are associated with risk of future metabolic disorder: in the Nurses' Health Study 2, although 2% of women who delivered a very preterm infant (<32 weeks' gestation) had a 35% higher risk of developing type 2 diabetes, moderate preterm delivery was not associated with increased diabetes risk (James-Todd et al. 2010).

After pregnancy, plasma C-reactive protein is elevated among women with prior eclampsia and indicated preterm births suggesting that systemic low-grade *inflammation* may link some adverse pregnancy outcomes and later CVD (Hastie et al. 2011b; Hubel et al. 2006). Several studies have documented higher C-reactive protein levels among women with a history of GDM (Heitritter et al. 2005; Di Cianni et al. 2007; Winzer et al. 2004). Although inflammation seems a likely culprit to explain the association of spontaneous preterm delivery with CVD risk, the only study to date that has examined this question has reported no differences in plasma C-reactive protein levels of women with a history of spontaneous preterm delivery compared to term delivery (Hastie et al. 2011b).

Women with a history of pregnancies complicated by preeclampsia may maintain a *procoagulation state* in the years after pregnancy, predisposing them to vascular and thrombotic events (Portelinha et al. 2009), although this pathway is less studied than others linking pregnancy complications to maternal CVD risk.

Thus, the associations of pregnancy complications with future CVD events in women are likely explained, at least in part, by their associations with classic CVD risk factors of hypertension, dyslipidemia, type 2 diabetes, and perhaps inflammation and thrombosis, which are evident before, during, and after such complicated pregnancies. Pregnancy provides a challenge to women's cardiovascular system, and pregnancy complications may serve as precursors, i.e., early indications that a woman is on a high-CVD risk trajectory, before these classic CVD risk factors are clinically detected. That said, this trajectory is complex and likely to be nonlinear. Given that most pregnancies occur in early adulthood, long before most CVD events occur, there is ample opportunity to influence that trajectory by recognizing that health develops continuously over the lifespan and that health development is a process resulting from the ongoing interactions between person and environment.

4 Recommendations for Future Research

4.1 Major Themes and Findings

The associations of pregnancy complications with CVD events are remarkably consistent.

Several pregnancy complications are more common among racial minority groups, who are also at higher risk of metabolic and cardiovascular disease. Although untested, the use of pregnancy complication history to screen women for targeted CVD prevention has potential to improve public health, given the magnitude of the associations, the prevalence of the pregnancy complications, and the importance of CVD in women. Pregnancy complications occur early enough in a woman's life course to offer a significant meaningful "runway" for primordial CVD prevention by lifestyle intervention and primary prevention by statins and antihypertensive drugs. In 2011, both the American Heart Association and the European Society of Cardiology included histories of preeclampsia and (in the case of the American Heart Association) GDM as part of CVD risk assessment that would trigger closer monitoring and control of CVD risk factors (Mosca et al. 2011; Regitz-Zagrosek et al. 2011). Pregnancy appears to be a critical transition period for a woman that stresses her cardiovascular system in ways that may shed light on future disease risk.

4.2 Research Priorities

(a) Epidemiologic research
- Establishing whether pregnancy complications per se contribute to CVD risk

We need to establish whether pregnancy complications act as stress tests to unmask women who are already at increased risk of CVD in later life and/or whether (and which) pregnancy complications have a causal, direct contribution to a woman's CVD risk. If pregnancy complications per se contribute to CVD risk independently of prepregnancy cardiovascular health, prevention strategies and treatment of pregnancy complications could be important not only for women and their offspring during the pregnancy but also later in life.

(b) Mechanism research
- Identifying mechanistic pathways to pregnancy complications and CVD

Should epidemiologic evidence suggest that pregnancy complications are causally associated with greater future CVD risk, it will be important to ascertain the underlying pathways responsible for these effects in order to identify potential treatment pathways. Gaining better understanding of the mechanisms underlying pregnancy complications themselves will also be important in informing prevention strategies.

(c) Translational research
- Improving risk stratification

Irrespective of whether pregnancy complications causally contribute to future CVD risk, a key question is the extent to which pregnancy history can be used to improve CVD risk scoring systems for women, such as the Framingham Risk Score. At present, these scoring systems are of debatable utility for women under age 70 (Greenland et al. 2010), and addition of pregnancy complications to prediction at these relatively younger ages may be particularly important. Several pregnancy complications are more common among racial minority groups, who are also at higher risk of metabolic and cardiovascular disease. Pregnancy history may be of particular importance in identifying risk in these groups.

- Establishing strategies to mitigate future CVD risk in women with pregnancy complications

If pregnancy complications are useful for early CVD risk prediction, the next question is whether earlier risk identification—as early as at the time of pregnancy—is a cost-effective way of reducing future risk. To do so it is important to examine whether women who experienced pregnancy complications should undergo more intense or earlier screening and monitoring in the postpartum years in order to determine whether they cross thresholds for treatment (e.g., with statins) earlier than women without pregnancy complications. We would also need to test the extent to which different lifestyle or pharmacologic preventions are effective at preventing future CVD in young or middle-aged women with a history of pregnancy complications. Key to this is identifying stages in the lifespan when women are (or are not) receptive to CVD prevention, including the postpartum year.

4.3 Data and Methods Development Priorities

(a) Importance of linking research across life stages: need for extended follow-up of women with known reproductive histories

The bulk of the research associating pregnancy history to CVD risk is derived from the linkage of large, often national, vital statistics registries for birth, hospitalization, and mortality statistics. These exercises have yielded consistent associations of pregnancy complications with CVD risk. However, as most registries were founded in the 1950s or 1960s, the longest-running has been able to follow women only into the early postmenopausal years. The data on GDM are further limited by the lack of consistent methods for screening and diagnosing GDM. Further follow-up will determine the extent to which the associations of pregnancy complications are maintained into the age range at which CVD events are most common in women. In the meantime, the stratification of risk by time since pregnancy is a helpful way to examine the extent to which risk associated with pregnancy complications changes over time (Hastie et al. 2011a). Although relative risk of CVD events may weaken with time, the absolute risks associated with a history of pregnancy complications is likely to grow with time since pregnancy, as women age. In addition, we should incorporate pregnancy history data into existing CVD cohorts with decades of follow-up. By illuminating the *timing* with which *particular CVD risk factors* emerge in the wake of specific pregnancy complications, we may be able to leverage the information contained by pregnancy history to predict CVD risk *earlier* than conventional risk screening protocols.

(b) Importance of linking research across life stages: need for studies with established CVD risk factors measured before, during, and after pregnancy

To understand the trajectory of CVD risk and the role of pregnancy complications in that trajectory, we need more studies to measure CVD risk factors prior to conception, particularly as evidence suggests that changes in blood pressure, augmentation index, and pulse wave velocity occur as early as 6 weeks' gestation, indicating that maternal adaptations occur very early in gestation (Mahendru et al. 2014). This raises the question of whether "booking" first trimester measures that are available in several birth cohorts is representative of prepregnancy values and emphasizes the importance of ascertaining cardiovascular health trajectories from pre- to postpartum.

(c) Need for innovative analytical approaches to improve causal inference

Methods for improving our understanding of whether pregnancy complications are causally related to later maternal health need to go beyond conventional multivariable approaches in prospective cohorts. For example, if it is found that genetic variants associated with high blood pressure and glucose intolerance/type 2 diabetes in general populations of men and nonpregnant women are also associated with HDP and GDM, this would lend some support to the hypothesis of a common etiology and pregnancy unmasking a preexisting (genetic) risk. There is some evidence that several type 2 diabetes mellitus variants from genome-wide association studies show robust associations with GDM (Karlsson et al. 2007; Lauenborg et al. 2009; Cho et al. 2009; Kwak et al. 2012).

Although it is not feasible to randomize women to pregnancy complications, long-term follow-up of women who have been in randomized controlled trials that have effectively prevented or treated the pregnancy complication will also address some of the research questions above. Lastly, experimental induction of pregnancy complications in animal models and following the mothers after delivery to examine whether vascular damage was sustained or metabolic risk increased are important for examining the question of a pregnancy causal effect (Bytautiene et al. 2010). However, the generalizability of the animal models depends on the fidelity with which the human pregnancy complications, such as preeclampsia, can be mimicked in other species, where they may not occur naturally.

4.4 Translational Priorities

We are just beginning to investigate the clinical implications of this growing body of research. First, we need to establish the role of pregnancy complications in determining maternal chronic disease risk. Independently of that, we also need to determine our ability to change the health trajectories of women with histories of complicated pregnancy. We will then have to consider the many issues of integrating the findings into clinical and public health systems. Some potential clinical implications include the need to link prenatal with primary care medical records, development of clinical screening strategies, prevention and treatment protocols after pregnancy complications, and increasing awareness among clinicians of these associations that span typical clinical silos between obstetrics and medicine (Rich-Edwards et al. 2010).

5 Conclusions

The stress test of pregnancy provides glimpses into the otherwise silent early adult years in which health development and chronic disease trajectories are set. Research to characterize the ways in which pregnancy complications inform us about subclinical and clinical vascular and metabolic risk in the mother is in its infancy. Future research will require large datasets that have prospectively collected accurate data on cardiovascular risk factors before, during, and after pregnancy, into middle age and beyond, when disease begins to emerge; data on pregnancy complications is also required. Only with such detailed information can we determine the extent to which specific pregnancy complications are related to future CVD, over and above prepregnancy risk factors, and whether they add to established risk factor scores calculated in middle age. With large birth cohorts increasingly recognizing the importance of long-term follow-up of the mother as well as their infant, the potential for this research is increasing. Ultimately, randomized controlled trials will be necessary to establish whether pregnancy advice and/or continued monitoring and early treatment of women identified as at risk during pregnancy is a cost-effective way of reducing CVD risk in women. Research in this area will require integration across such diverse specialties including obstetrics, primary care, pediatrics, endocrinology, and cardiology. This broader perspective may yield novel insights into the determinants of pregnancy outcomes and health development across the lifespan, perhaps creating a large shift in the ways in which we promote the health of women and children.

References

Agatisa, P. K., Ness, R. B., Roberts, J. M., Costantino, J. P., Kuller, L. H., & McLaughlin, M. K. (2004). Impairment of endothelial function in women with a history of preeclampsia: An indicator of cardiovascular risk. *American Journal of Physiology – Heart and Circulatory Physiology, 286*, H1389–H1393.

Anastasiou, E., Lekakis, J. P., Alevizaki, M., et al. (1998). Impaired endothelium-dependent vasodilatation in women with previous gestational diabetes. *Diabetes Care, 21*, 2111–2115.

Beck, S., Wojdyla, D., Say, L., et al. (2010). The worldwide incidence of preterm birth: A systematic review of maternal mortality and morbidity. *Bulletin of the World Health Organization, 88*, 31–38.

Bellamy, L., Casas, J. P., Hingorani, A. D., & Williams, D. J. (2007). Pre-eclampsia and risk of cardiovascular disease and cancer in later life: Systematic review and meta-analysis. *British Medical Journal, 335*, 974.

Bellamy, L., Casas, J. P., Hingorani, A. D., & Williams, D. (2009). Type 2 diabetes mellitus after gestational diabetes: A systematic review and meta-analysis. *Lancet, 373*, 1773–1779.

Berends, A. L., de Groot, C. J., Sijbrands, E. J., et al. (2008). Shared constitutional risks for maternal vascular-related pregnancy complications and future cardiovascular disease. *Hypertension, 51*, 1034–1041.

Bonamy, A. K., Parikh, N. I., Cnattingius, S., Ludvigsson, J. F., & Ingelsson, E. (2011). Birth characteristics and subsequent risks of maternal cardiovascular disease: Effects of gestational age and fetal growth. *Circulation, 124*, 2839–2846.

Butte, N. F. (2000). Carbohydrate and lipid metabolism in pregnancy: Normal compared with gestational diabetes mellitus. *The American Journal of Clinical Nutrition, 71*, 1256S–1261S.

Bytautiene, E., Lu, F., Tamayo, E. H., et al. (2010). Long-term maternal cardiovascular function in a mouse model of sFlt-1-induced preeclampsia. *American Journal of Physiology. Heart and Circulatory Physiology, 298*, H189–H193.

Campbell, S., Griffin, D. R., Pearce, J. M., et al. (1983). New doppler technique for assessing uteroplacental blood flow. *Lancet, 321*, 675–677.

Carr, D. B., Utzschneider, K. M., Hull, R. L., et al. (2006). Gestational diabetes mellitus increases the risk of cardiovascular disease in women with a family history of type 2 diabetes. *Diabetes Care, 29*, 2078–2083.

Catov, J., Newman, A., Roberts, J., et al. (2007a). Association between infant birth weight and maternal cardiovascular risk factors in the health, aging, and body composition study. *Annals of Epidemiology, 17*, 36–43.

Catov, J. M., Bodnar, L. M., Kip, K. E., et al. (2007b). Early pregnancy lipid concentrations and spontaneous preterm birth. *American Journal of Obstetrics and Gynecology, 197*, 610. e611–610. e617.

Catov, J. M., Bodnar, L. M., Ness, R. B., Barron, S. J., & Roberts, J. M. (2007c). Inflammation and dyslipidemia related to risk of spontaneous preterm birth. *American Journal of Epidemiology, 166*, 1312–1319.

Catov, J. M., Nohr, E. A., Olsen, J., & Ness, R. B. (2008a). Chronic hypertension related to risk for preterm and term small-for-gestational-age births. *Obstetrics and Gynecology, 112*, 290.

Catov, J., Bodnar, L., Hackney, D., Roberts, J., & Simhan, S. (2008b). Activation of the fibrinolytic cascade early in pregnancy among women with spontaneous preterm birth. *Obstetrics and Gynecology, 112*, 1116–1122.

Catov, J. M., Wu, C. S., Olsen, J., Sutton-Tyrrell, K., Li, J., & Nohr, E. A. (2010a). Early or recurrent preterm birth and maternal cardiovascular disease risk. *Annals of Epidemiology, 20*, 604–609.

Catov, J. M., Ness, R. B., Wellons, M. F., Jacobs, D. R., Roberts, J. M., & Gunderson, E. P. (2010b). Prepregnancy lipids related to preterm birth risk: The coronary artery risk development in young adults study. *Journal of Clinical Endocrinology and Metabolism, 95*, 2009–2028.

Catov, J. M., Dodge, R., Yamal, J. M., Roberts, J. M., Piller, L. B., & Ness, R. B. (2011). Prior preterm or small-for-gestational-age birth related to maternal metabolic syndrome. *Obstetrics and Gynecology, 117*, 225–232.

Catov, J. M., Dodge, R., Barinas-Mitchell, E., et al. (2013). Prior preterm birth and maternal subclinical cardiovascular disease 4 to 12 years after pregnancy. *Journal of Women's Health, 22*(2002), 835–843.

Cho, Y. M., Kim, T. H., Lim, S., et al. (2009). Type 2 diabetes-associated genetic variants discovered in the recent genome-wide association studies are related to gestational diabetes mellitus in the Korean population. *Diabetologia, 52*, 253–261.

Clausen, T., Djurovic, S., & Henriksen, T. (2001). Dyslipidemia in early second trimester is mainly a feature of women with early onset pre-eclampsia. *BJOG, 108*, 1081–1087.

Curry, A., Vogel, I., Drews, C., et al. (2007). Mid-pregnancy maternal plasma levels of interleukin 2, 6, and 12, tumor necrosis factor-alpha, interferon-gamma, and granulocyte-macrophage colony-stimulating factor and spontaneous preterm delivery. *Acta Obstetricia et Gynecologica Scandinavica, 86*, 1103–1110.

Davey Smith, G., Hart, C., Ferrell, C., et al. (1997). Birth weight of offspring and mortality in the Renfrew and Paisley study: Prospective observational study. *British Medical Journal, 315*, 1189–1193.

Davey Smith, G., Harding, S., & Rosato, M. (2000a). Relation between infants' birth weight and mothers' mortality: Prospective observational study. *British Medical Journal, 320*, 839–840.

Davey Smith, G., Whitley, E., Gissler, M., & Hemminki, E. (2000b). Birth dimensions of offspring, premature birth, and the mortality of mothers. *Lancet, 356*, 2066–2067.

Davey Smith, G., Sterne, J., Tynelius, P., Lawlor, D. A., & Rasmussen, F. (2005). Birth weight of offspring and subsequent cardiovascular mortality of the parents. *Epidemiology, 16*, 563–569.

Davey Smith, G., Hypponen, E., Power, C., & Lawlor, D. A. (2007). Offspring birth weight and parental mortality: Prospective observational study and meta-analysis. *American Journal of Epidemiology, 166*, 160–169.

Dekker, J. M., & Schouten, E. G. (1993). Number of pregnancies and risk of cardiovascular disease. *The New England Journal of Medicine, 329*, 1893–1894. author reply 1894–1895.

Di Cianni, G., Lencioni, C., Volpe, L., et al. (2007). C-reactive protein and metabolic syndrome in women with previous gestational diabetes. *Diabetes/ Metabolism Research and Reviews, 23*, 135–140.

Ducey, J., Schulman, H., Farmakides, G., et al. (1987). A classification of hypertension in pregnancy based on Doppler velocimetry. *American Journal of Obstetrics and Gynecology, 157*, 680–685.

Edison, R. J., Berg, K., Remaley, A., et al. (2007). Adverse birth outcome among mothers with low serum cholesterol. *Pediatrics, 120*, 723–733.

Enquobahrie, D. A., Williams, M. A., Qiu, C., & Luthy, D. A. (2005). Early pregnancy lipid concentrations and the risk of gestational diabetes mellitus. *Diabetes Research and Clinical Practice, 70*, 134–142.

Ernst, G. D. S., de Jonge, L. L., Hofman, A., et al. (2011). C-reactive protein levels in early pregnancy, fetal growth patterns, and the risk for neonatal complications: The Generation R Study. *American Journal of Obstetrics and Gynecology, 205*, 132.e131–132.e112.

Fraser, A., Nelson, S. M., Macdonald-Wallis, C., et al. (2012). Associations of pregnancy complications with calculated cardiovascular disease risk and cardiovascular risk factors in middle age/clinical perspective. *Circulation, 125*, 1367–1380.

Freathy, R. M., Weedon, M. N., Bennett, A., et al. (2007). Type 2 diabetes TCF7L2 risk genotypes alter birth weight: A study of 24,053 individuals. *American Journal of Human Genetics, 80*, 1150–1161.

Freeman, D. J., McManus, F., Brown, E. A., et al. (2004). Short-and long-term changes in plasma inflammatory markers associated with preeclampsia. *Hypertension, 44*, 708–714.

Friedlander, Y., Paltiel, O., Manor, O., et al. (2007). Birthweight of offspring and mortality of parents: The Jerusalem perinatal study cohort. *Annals of Epidemiology, 17*, 914–922.

Funai, E. F., Friedlander, Y., Paltiel, O., et al. (2005). Long-term mortality after preeclampsia. *Epidemiology, 16*, 206–215.

Gammill, H. S., Powers, R. W., Clifton, R. G., et al. (2010). Does C-reactive protein predict recurrent preeclampsia? *Hypertension in Pregnancy, 29*, 399–409.

Girardi, G. (2011). Role of tissue factor in pregnancy complications: Crosstalk between coagulation and inflammation. *Thrombosis Research, 127*(Suppl 3), S43–S46.

Green, A. B. V., & Moser, K. (1988). Mortality in women in relation to their childbearing history. *BMJ (Clinical research ed), 297*, 391–395.

Greenland, P., Alpert, J. S., Beller, G. A., et al. (2010). 2010 ACCF/AHA guideline for assessment of cardiovascular risk in asymptomatic adults: A report of the American College of Cardiology Foundation/ American Heart Association Task Force on Practice Guidelines. *Circulation, 122*, e584–e636.

Hackney, D. N., Catov, J. M., & Simhan, H. N. (2010). Low concentrations of thrombin-inhibitor complexes and the risk of preterm delivery. *American Journal of Obstetrics and Gynecology, 203*, 184.e181–184.e186.

Hannaford, P., Ferry, S., & Hirsch, S. (1997). Cardiovascular sequelae of toxaemia of pregnancy. *Heart, 77*, 154–158.

Hastie, C. E., Smith, G. C., MacKay, D. F., & Pell, J. P. (2011a). Maternal risk of ischaemic heart disease following elective and spontaneous pre-term delivery: Retrospective cohort study of 750 350 singleton pregnancies. *International Journal of Epidemiology, 40*, 914–919.

Hastie, C. E., Smith, G. C. S., Mackay, D. F., & Pell, J. P. (2011b). Association between preterm delivery and subsequent C-reactive protein: A retrospective cohort study. *American Journal of Obstetrics and Gynecology, 205*, 556.e551–556.e554.

Hedderson, M. M., Ferrara, A., & Sacks, D. A. (2003). Gestational diabetes mellitus and lesser degrees of pregnancy hyperglycemia: Association with increased risk of spontaneous preterm birth. *Obstetrics and Gynecology, 102*, 850–856.

Heilmann, L., Rath, W., & Pollow, K. (2007). Hemostatic abnormalities in patients with severe preeclampsia. *Clinical and Applied Thrombosis/Hemostasis, 13*, 285–291.

Heitritter, S. M., Solomon, C. G., Mitchell, G. F., Skali-Ounis, N., & Seely, E. W. (2005). Subclinical inflammation and vascular dysfunction in women with previous gestational diabetes mellitus. *Journal of Clinical Endocrinology and Metabolism, 90*, 3983–3988.

Herrera, E. (2000). Metabolic adaptations in pregnancy and their implications for the availability of substrates to the fetus. *European Journal of Clinical Nutrition, 54*, S47.

Hubel, C. A., McLaughlin, M. K., Evans, R. W., Hauth, B. A., Sims, C. J., & Roberts, J. M. (1996). Fasting serum triglycerides, free fatty acids, and malondialdehyde are increased in preeclampsia, are positively correlated, and decrease within 48 hours post partum. *American Journal of Obstetrics and Gynecology, 174*, 975–982.

Hubel, C., Shakir, Y., Gallaher, M., McLaughlin, M., & Roberts, J. (1998a). Low-density lipoprotein particle size decreases during normal pregnancy in association with triglyceride increases. *Journal of the Society for Gynecologic Investigation, 5*, 244–250.

Hubel, C. A., Lyall, F., Weissfeld, L., Gandley, R. E., & Roberts, J. M. (1998b). Small low-density lipoproteins and vascular cell adhesion molecule-1 are increased in association with hyperlipidemia in preeclampsia. *Metabolism, 47*, 1281–1288.

Hubel, C. A., Powers, R., Snaedal, S., et al. (2006). C-reactive protein is increased 30 years after eclamptic pregnancy. *J Soc Gynecol Invest, 13*(2 Suppl), 292A.

Hubel, C. A., Powers, R. W., Snaedal, S., et al. (2008). C-reactive protein is elevated 30 years after eclamptic pregnancy. *Hypertension, 51*, 1499–1505.

Irgens, H. U., Reisaeter, L., Irgens, L. M., & Lie, R. T. (2001). Long term mortality of mothers and fathers after pre-eclampsia: Population based cohort study. *BMJ (Clinical research ed), 323*, 1213–1217.

James-Todd, T. K. A., Hibert, E., Mason, S., Vadnais, M., Hu, F., & Rich-Edwards. J. (2010). Gestation length, birth weight and subsequent risk of type 2 diabetes in mothers. Oral presentation. *Presented at American Diabetes Association's 70th Scientific Sessions*, June 2010, Orlando, FL.

Jónsdóttir, L., Arngrimsson, R., Geirsson, R. T., Slgvaldason, H., & Slgfússon, N. (1995). Death rates from ischemic heart disease in women with a history of hypertension in pregnancy. *Acta Obstetricia et Gynecologica Scandinavica, 74*, 772–776.

Kanagalingam, M. G., Nelson, S. M., Freeman, D. J., et al. (2009). Vascular dysfunction and alteration of novel and classic cardiovascular risk factors in mothers of growth restricted offspring. *Atherosclerosis, 205*, 244–250.

Kelly, R., Holzman, C., Senagore, P., et al. (2009). Placental vascular pathology findings and pathways to preterm delivery. *American Journal of Epidemiology, 170*, 148–158.

Kestenbaum, B., Seliger, S. L., Easterling, T. R., et al. (2003). Cardiovascular and thromboembolic events following hypertensive pregnancy. *American Journal of Kidney Diseases, 42*, 982–989.

Kim, C., Newton, K. M., & Knopp, R. H. (2002). Gestational diabetes and the incidence of type 2 diabetes a systematic review. *Diabetes Care, 25*, 1862–1868.

Kwak, S. H., Kim, S. H., Cho, Y. M., et al. (2012). A genome-wide association study of gestational diabetes mellitus in Korean women. *Diabetes, 61*, 531–541.

Labarthe, D. R. (1999). Prevention of cardiovascular risk factors in the first place. *Preventive Medicine, 29*, S72–S78.

Laivuori, H., Tikkanen, M. J., & Ylikorkala, O. (1996). Hyperinsulinemia 17 years after preeclamptic first pregnancy. *The Journal of Clinical Endocrinology and Metabolism, 81*, 2908–2911.

Lauenborg, J., Mathiesen, E., Hansen, T., et al. (2005). The prevalence of the metabolic syndrome in a danish population of women with previous gestational diabetes mellitus is three-fold higher than in the general population. *The Journal of Clinical Endocrinology and Metabolism, 90*, 4004–4010.

Lauenborg, J., Grarup, N., Damm, P., et al. (2009). Common type 2 diabetes risk gene variants associate with gestational diabetes. *The Journal of Clinical Endocrinology and Metabolism, 94*, 145–150.

Lawlor, D. A., Emberson, J. R., Ebrahim, S., et al. (2003). Is the association between parity and coronary heart disease due to biological effects of pregnancy or adverse lifestyle risk factors associated with child-rearing? *Circulation, 107*, 1260–1264.

Lawlor, D. A., Relton, C., Sattar, N., & Nelson, S. M. (2012). Maternal adiposity—a determinant of perinatal and offspring outcomes? *Nature Reviews Endocrinology, 8*, 679–688.

Lie, R. T., Wilcox, A. J., & Skjaerven, R. (2006). Maternal and paternal influences on length of pregnancy. *Obstetrics and Gynecology, 107*, 880–885.

Lin, Y.-S., Tang, C.-H., Yang, C.-Y. C., et al. (2011). Effect of pre-eclampsia–eclampsia on major cardiovascular events among peripartum women in Taiwan. *The American Journal of Cardiology, 107*, 325–330.

Lykke, J. A., Langhoff-Roos, J., Sibai, B. M., Funai, E. F., Triche, E. W., & Paidas, M. J. (2009). Hypertensive pregnancy disorders and subsequent cardiovascular morbidity and type 2 diabetes mellitus in the mother. *Hypertension, 53*, 944–951.

Lykke, J. A., Langhoff-Roos, J., Lockwood, C. J., Triche, E. W., & Paidas, M. J. (2010a). Mortality of mothers from cardiovascular and non-cardiovascular causes following pregnancy complications in first delivery. *Paediatric and Perinatal Epidemiology, 24*, 323–330.

Lykke, J., Paidas, M., Damm, P., Triche, E., Kuczynski, E., & Langhoff-Roos, J. (2010b). Preterm delivery and risk of subsequent cardiovascular morbidity and type-II diabetes in the mother. *BJOG: An International Journal of Obstetrics & Gynaecology, 117*, 274–281.

Lykke, J. A., Paidas, M. J., Triche, E. W., & LANGHOFF-ROOS, J. (2012). Fetal growth and later maternal death, cardiovascular disease and diabetes. *Acta Obstetricia et Gynecologica Scandinavica, 91*, 503–510.

Macdonald-Wallis, C., Lawlor, D. A., Fraser, A., May, M., Nelson, S. M., & Tilling, K. (2012). Blood pressure change in normotensive, gestational hypertensive, preeclamptic, and essential hypertensive pregnancies. *Hypertension, 59*, 1241–1248.

Magnussen, E. B., Vatten, L. J., Lund-Nilsen, T. I., Salvesen, K. A., Smith, G. D., & Romundstad, P. R. (2007). Prepregnancy cardiovascular risk factors as predictors of pre-eclampsia: Population based cohort study. *BMJ (Clinical research ed), 335*, 978.

Magnussen, E. B., Vatten, L. J., Smith, G. D., & Romundstad, P. R. (2009). Hypertensive disorders in pregnancy and subsequently measured cardiovascular risk factors. *Obstetrics and Gynecology, 114*, 961–970.

Magnussen, E. B., Vatten, L. J., Myklestad, K., Salvesen, K. Å., & Romundstad, P. R. (2011). Cardiovascular risk factors prior to conception and the length of pregnancy: Population-based cohort study. *American Journal of Obstetrics and Gynecology, 204*, 526. e521–526.e528.

Mahendru, A. A., Everett, T. R., Wilkinson, I. B., Lees, C. C., & McEniery, C. M. (2014). A longitudinal study of maternal cardiovascular function from preconception to the postpartum period. *Journal of Hypertension, 32*, 849–856.

Manten, G. T., Sikkema, M. J., Voorbij, H. A., Visser, G. H., Bruinse, H. W., & Franx, A. (2007). Risk factors for cardiovascular disease in women with a history of pregnancy complicated by preeclampsia or intrauterine growth restriction. *Hypertension in Pregnancy, 26*, 39–50.

Martinez, G., Daniels, K., & Chandra, A. (2012). Fertility of men and women aged 15–44 years in the United States: National survey of family growth, 2006–2010. *Natl Health Stat Report, 12*, 1–28.

Mathers, C., Boerma, J. T., Fat, D. M., & World Health Organization. (2008). *The global burden of disease : 2004 update*. Geneva: World Health Organization.

McDonald, S. D., Malinowski, A., Zhou, Q., Yusuf, S., & Devereaux, P. J. (2008). Cardiovascular sequelae of preeclampsia/eclampsia: A systematic review and meta-analyses. *American Heart Journal, 156*, 918–930.

Metzger, B. E., Cho, N. H., Roston, S. M., & Radvany, R. (1993). Prepregnancy weight and antepartum insulin secretion predict glucose tolerance five years after gestational diabetes mellitus. *Diabetes Care, 16*(1wik), 42–1605.

Meyers-Seifer, C. H., & Vohr, B. R. (1996). Lipid levels in former gestational diabetic mothers. *Diabetes Care, 19*, 1351–1356.

MMWR. (1989). Chronic disease reports in the Morbidity and Mortality Weekly Report (MMWR). *MMWR Morb Mortal Wkly Rep, 38*, 1–8.

Monga, M., & Creasy, R. (1994). Cardiovascular and renal adaptation to pregnancy. In R. Creasy, R. Resnik, J. D. Iams, et al. (Eds.), *Maternal-fetal medicine: Principles and practice* (pp. 758–767). Philadelphia: WB Saunders.

Mongraw-Chaffin, M. L., Cirillo, P. M., & Cohn, B. A. (2010). Preeclampsia and cardiovascular disease death. *Hypertension, 56*, 166–171.

Mosca, L., Benjamin, E. J., Berra, K., et al. (2011). Effectiveness-based guidelines for the prevention of cardiovascular disease in women – 2011 update: A guideline from the american heart association. *Circulation, 123*, 1243–1262.

Nanda, S. S. M., Syngelaki, A., Akolekar, R., & Nicolaides, K. H. (2011). Prediction of gestational diabetes mellitus by maternal factors and biomarkers at 11 to 13 weeks. *Prenatal Diagnosis, 31*, 135–141.

Nardi, O., Zureik, M., Courbon, D., Ducimetière, P., & Clavel-Chapelon, F. (2006). Preterm delivery of a first child and subsequent mothers' risk of ischaemic heart disease: A nested case–control study. *European Journal of Cardiovascular Prevention & Rehabilitation, 13*, 281–283.

Ness, R. B., Harris, T., Cobb, J., et al. (1993). Number of pregnancies and the subsequent risk of cardiovascular disease. *The New England Journal of Medicine, 328*, 1528–1533.

Ness, R. B., Cobb, J., Harm, T., & D'Agostino, R. B. (1995). Does number of children increase the rate of coronary heart disease in men? *Epidemiology, 6*, 442–445.

North, R. A., McCowan, L. M., Dekker, G. A., et al. (2011). Clinical risk prediction for pre-eclampsia in nulliparous women: Development of model in international prospective cohort. *BMJ (Clinical research ed), 342*, d1875.

O'Brien, T. E., Ray, J. G., & Chan, W. S. (2003). Maternal body mass index and the risk of preeclampsia: A systematic overview. *Epidemiology, 14*, 368–374.

Oblast, T. I. (1999). Decline in deaths from heart disease and stroke—United States, 1900–1999. *Heart Disease and Stroke, 63*(1900), 593–597.

OECD Family D. (2014). Childlessness (SF 2.5) In: *Social Policy Division, Organisation for Economic Co-operation and Development*. Paris, France: 2010. SF2.5 report on childlessness. www.oecd.org/social/family/database. Accessed 24 June, 2013.

Ostlund, I., Haglund, B., & Hanson, U. (2004). Gestational diabetes and preeclampsia. *European Journal of Obstetrics, Gynecology, and Reproductive Biology, 113*, 12–16.

Parikh, N. I., Cnattingius, S., Dickman, P. W., Mittleman, M. A., Ludvigsson, J. F., & Ingelsson, E. (2010). Parity and risk of later-life maternal cardiovascular disease. *American Heart Journal, 159*, 215–221. e216.

Pell, J. P., Smith, G. C., & Walsh, D. (2004). Pregnancy complications and subsequent maternal cerebrovascular events: A retrospective cohort study of 119,668 births. *American Journal of Epidemiology, 159*, 336–342.

Pitiphat, W., Gillman, M. W., Joshipura, K. J., Williams, P. L., Douglass, C. W., & Rich-Edwards, J. W. (2005). Plasma C-reactive protein in early pregnancy and preterm delivery. *American Journal of Epidemiology, 162*, 1108–1113.

Portelinha, A., Cerdeira, A. S., Belo, L., et al. (2009). Haemostatic factors in women with history of Preeclampsia. *Thrombosis Research, 124*, 52–56.

Qiu, C., Williams, M. A., Leisenring, W. M., et al. (2003). Family history of hypertension and type 2 diabetes in relation to preeclampsia risk. *Hypertension, 41*, 408–413.

Regitz-Zagrosek, V., Lundqvist, C. B., Borghi, C., et al. (2011). ESC Guidelines on the management of cardiovascular diseases during pregnancy. The Task Force on the Management of Cardiovascular Diseases during Pregnancy of the European Society of Cardiology (ESC). *European Heart Journal, 32*, 3147–3197.

Retnakaran, R., & Shah, B. R. (2009a). Abnormal screening glucose challenge test in pregnancy and future risk of diabetes in young women. *Diabetic Medicine, 26*, 474–477.

Retnakaran, R., & Shah, B. R. (2009b). Mild glucose intolerance in pregnancy and risk of cardiovascular disease: A population-based cohort study. *Canadian Medical Association Journal, 181*, 371–376.

Retnakaran, R., Austin, P. C., & Shah, B. R. (2011). Effect of subsequent pregnancies on the risk of developing diabetes following a first pregnancy complicated by gestational diabetes: A population-based study. *Diabetic Medicine, 28*, 287–292.

Rich-Edwards, J. W. (2009). Reproductive health as a sentinel of chronic disease in women. *Women's Health (London, England), 5*, 101–105.

Rich-Edwards, J. W., McElrath, T. F., Karumanchi, S. A., & Seely, E. W. (2010). Breathing life into the lifecourse approach: Pregnancy history and cardiovascular disease in women. *Hypertension, 56*, 331–334.

Rich-Edwards, J. W. K. K., Wilcox, A., & Skjaerven, R. (2012). Duration of first pregnancy predicts maternal cardiovascular death, whether delivery was medically indicated or spontaneous. *American Journal of Epidemiology, 175*(Suppl 11), S64.

Rich-Edwards, J. W., Fraser, A., Lawlor, D. A., & Catov, J. M. (2014). Pregnancy characteristics and women's future cardiovascular health: An underused opportunity to improve women's health? *Epidemiologic Reviews, 36*, 57–70.

Riskin-Mashiah, S., Damti, A., Younes, G., & Auslender, R. (2010). First trimester fasting hyperglycemia as a predictor for the development of gestational diabetes mellitus. *European Journal of Obstetrics, Gynecology, and Reproductive Biology, 152*, 163–167.

Roberts, C. L., Algert, C. S., Morris, J. M., Ford, J. B., & Henderson-Smart, D. J. (2005). Hypertensive disorders in pregnancy: A population-based study. *The Medical Journal of Australia, 182*, 332–335.

Romero, R., Espinoza, J., Gonçalves, L. F., Kusanovic, J. P., Friel, L., & Hassan, S. (2007). The role of inflammation and infection in preterm birth. *Seminars in Reproductive Medicine, 25*, 021–039.

Romundstad, P. R., Davey Smith, G., Nilsen, T. I., & Vatten, L. J. (2007). Associations of prepregnancy cardiovascular risk factors with the offspring's birth weight. *American Journal of Epidemiology, 166*, 1359–1364.

Romundstad, P. R., Magnussen, E. B., Smith, G. D., & Vatten, L. J. (2010). Hypertension in pregnancy and later cardiovascular risk: Common antecedents? *Circulation, 122*, 579–584.

Sacks DA, C. W., Wolde-Tsadik, G., & Buchanan, T. A. (2003). Fasting plasma glucose test at the first prenatal visit as a screen for gestational diabetes. *Obstetrics and Gynecology, 101*, 1197–1203.

Sarwar, N., Gao, P., Seshasai, S. R., et al. (2010). Diabetes mellitus, fasting blood glucose concentration, and risk of vascular disease: A collaborative meta-analysis of 102 prospective studies. *Lancet, 375*, 2215–2222.

Sattar, N. (2004). Do pregnancy complications and CVD share common antecedents? *Atherosclerosis Supplements, 5*, 3–7.

Sattar, N., & Greer, I. A. (2002). Pregnancy complications and maternal cardiovascular risk: Opportunities for intervention and screening? *British Medical Journal, 325*, 157–160.

Sattar, N., Bendomir, A., Berry, C., Shepherd, J., Greer, I. A., & Packard, C. J. (1997). Lipoprotein subfraction concentrations in preeclampsia: Pathogenic parallels to atherosclerosis. *Obstetrics and Gynecology, 89*, 403–408.

Sattar, N., Greer, I., Galloway, P., et al. (1999). Lipid and lipoprotein concentrations in pregnancies complicated by intrauterine growth restriction. *Journal of Clinical Endocrinology and Metabolism, 84*, 128–130.

Sattar, N., Ramsay, J., Crawford, L., Cheyne, H., & Greer, I. A. (2003). Classic and novel risk factor parameters in women with a history of preeclampsia. *Hypertension, 42*, 39–42.

Savvidou, M. D., Hingorani, A. D., Tsikas, D., Frölich, J. C., Vallance, P., & Nicolaides, K. H. (2003). Endothelial dysfunction and raised plasma concentrations of asymmetric dimethylarginine in pregnant women who subsequently develop pre-eclampsia. *The Lancet, 361*, 1511–1517.

Savvidou, M. D., Kaihura, C., Anderson, J. M., & Nicolaides, K. H. (2011). Maternal arterial stiffness in women who subsequently develop pre-eclampsia. *PLoS ONE, 6*, e18703.

Scarborough, P., & Weissberg, P. (2011). *Trends in coronary heart disease, 1961–2011*. London: British Heart Foundation.

Schwarz, E. B., Ray, R. M., Stuebe, A. M., et al. (2009). Duration of lactation and risk factors for maternal cardiovascular disease. *Obstetrics and Gynecology, 113*, 974–982.

Shaat, N. L. A., Karlsson, E., Ivarsson, S., Parikh, H., Berntorp, K., & Groop, L. (2007). A variant in the transcription factor 7-like 2 (TCF7L2) gene is associated with an increased risk of gestational diabetes mellitus. *Diabetologia, 50*, 972–979.

Shah, B. R., Retnakaran, R., & Booth, G. L. (2008). Increased risk of cardiovascular disease in young women following gestational diabetes mellitus. *Diabetes Care, 31*, 1668–1669.

Shah, R. U., Klein, L., & Lloyd-Jones, D. M. (2009). Heart failure in women: Epidemiology, biology and treatment. *Women's Health (London, England), 5*, 517–527.

Shaw, L. J., Bairey Merz, C. N., Pepine, C. J., et al. (2006). Insights from the NHLBI-Sponsored Women's Ischemia Syndrome Evaluation (WISE) Study: Part I: Gender differences in traditional and novel risk factors, symptom evaluation, and gender-optimized diagnostic strategies. *Journal of the American College of Cardiology, 47*, S4–S20.

Shay, C. M., Ning, H., Allen, N. B., et al. (2012). Status of cardiovascular health in US adults clinical perspective prevalence estimates from the National Health and Nutrition Examination Surveys (NHANES) 2003–2008. *Circulation, 125*, 45–56.

Skjaerven, R., Wilcox, A. J., Klungsoyr, K., et al. (2012). Cardiovascular mortality after pre-eclampsia in one child mothers: Prospective, population based cohort study. *BMJ (Clinical research ed), 345*, e7677.

Smith, G. C., Pell, J. P., & Walsh, D. (2001). Pregnancy complications and maternal risk of ischaemic heart disease: A retrospective cohort study of 129,290 births. *Lancet, 357*, 2002–2006.

Smith, G. C. S., Shah, I., Pell, J. P., Crossley, J. A., & Dobbie, R. (2007). Maternal obesity in early pregnancy and risk of spontaneous and elective preterm deliveries: A retrospective cohort study. *American Journal of Public Health, 97*, 157–162.

Smith, G. N., Walker, M. C., Liu, A., et al. (2009). A history of preeclampsia identifies women who have underlying cardiovascular risk factors. *American Journal of Obstetrics and Gynecology, 200*(58), e51–e58.

Solomon, C. G., Willett, W. C., Carey, V. J., et al. (1997). A prospective study of pregravid determinants of gestational diabetes mellitus. *JAMA, 278*, 1078–1083.

Steenland, K., Lally, C., & Thun, M. (1996). Parity and coronary heart disease among women in the American Cancer Society CPS II population. *Epidemiology, 7*, 641–643.

Stepan, H., Faber, R., & Walther, T. (1999). Expression of low density lipoprotein receptor messenger ribonucleic acid in placentas from pregnancies with intrauterine growth retardation. *British Journal of Obstetrics and Gynaecology, 106*, 1221–1222.

Tarim, E., Yigit, F., Kilicdag, E., et al. (2006). Early onset of subclinical atherosclerosis in women with gestational diabetes mellitus. *Ultrasound in Obstetrics & Gynecology, 27*, 177–182.

United Nations DoEaSA, Population Division. (2009). *World fertility report*. New York: United Nations Publications.

Verma, A., Boney, C. M., Tucker, R., & Vohr, B. R. (2002). Insulin resistance syndrome in women with prior history of gestational diabetes mellitus. *The Journal of Clinical Endocrinology and Metabolism, 87*, 3227–3235.

Wadsack, C., Tabano, S., Maier, A., et al. (2007). Intrauterine growth restriction is associated with alterations in placental lipoprotein receptors and maternal lipoprotein composition. *American Journal of Physiology - Endocrinology and Metabolism, 292*, E476–E484.

Wallis, A. B., Saftlas, A. F., Hsia, J., & Atrash, H. K. (2008). Secular trends in the rates of preeclampsia, eclampsia, and gestational hypertension, United States, 1987–2004. *American Journal of Hypertension, 21*, 521–526.

Weintraub, W. S., Daniels, S. R., Burke, L. E., et al. (2011). Value of primordial and primary prevention for cardiovascular disease: A policy statement from the American Heart Association. *Circulation, 124*, 967–990.

Wikström, A. K., Haglund, B., Olovsson, M., & Lindeberg, S. N. (2005). The risk of maternal ischaemic heart disease after gestational hypertensive disease. *BJOG: An International Journal of Obstetrics & Gynaecology, 112*, 1486–1491.

Wilcox, A. J., Skjaerven, R., & Lie, R. T. (2008). Familial patterns of preterm delivery: Maternal and fetal contributions. *American Journal of Epidemiology, 167*, 474–479.

Williams, M. A., Qiu, C., Muy-Rivera, M., Vadachkoria, S., Song, T., & Luthy, D. A. (2004). Plasma adiponectin concentrations in early pregnancy and subsequent risk of gestational diabetes mellitus. *The Journal of Clinical Endocrinology and Metabolism, 89*, 2306–2311.

Wilson, B. J., Watson, M. S., Prescott, G. J., et al. (2003). Hypertensive diseases of pregnancy and risk of hypertension and stroke in later life: Results from cohort study. *British Medical Journal, 326*, 845.

Winzer, C., Wagner, O., Festa, A., et al. (2004). Plasma adiponectin, insulin sensitivity, and subclinical inflammation in women with prior gestational diabetes mellitus. *Diabetes Care, 27*, 1721–1727.

Wolf, M., Kettyle, E., Sandler, L., Ecker, J. L., Roberts, J., & Thadhani, R. (2001). Obesity and preeclampsia: The potential role of inflammation. *Obstetrics and Gynecology, 98*, 757–762.

Wolf, M., Hubel, C. A., Lam, C., et al. (2004). Preeclampsia and future cardiovascular disease: Potential role of altered angiogenesis and insulin resistance. *The Journal of Clinical Endocrinology and Metabolism, 89*, 6239–6243.

Yusuf, S., Reddy, S., Ôunpuu, S., & Anand, S. (2001). Global burden of cardiovascular diseases. *Circulation, 104*, 2746–2753.

5

Epidemiological Study Designs: Traditional and Novel Approaches to Advance Life Course Health Development Research

Stephen L. Buka, Samantha R. Rosenthal, and Mary E. Lacy

1 Introduction

1.1 Goals in Life Course Research

A life course approach to health and human development provides a conceptual and methodological framework to understand the multiple, multilevel, and synchronized (i.e. temporally integrated) determinants of health and disease across the lifespan. Theories underlying life course approaches are varied, but each emphasizes the importance of the occurrence and accrual of life events, plasticity, thriving, or risk over time and how these contribute to the development of particular outcomes of interest, including pathways associated with optimal health (George 1999; Kuh et al. 2003; Ben-Shlomo and Kuh 2002; Halfon et al. 2014). A number of key questions pertinent to the emergence of health development across the lifespan can be addressed using life course frameworks that would otherwise be difficult to ascertain. From furthering our understanding of familial and genetic contributions to the aetiology of health conditions to exploring the natural course of disorders in different populations and to examining the time-specific and cumulative impacts of social and environmental factors, the use of a life course framework has advanced our understanding of the systemic causes and course of multiple health conditions and positive health development.

The goal of the field of epidemiology is to advance the understanding of the determinants of health and disease among human populations. Consistent with the seven principles of LCHD (see Halfon and Forrest, Chap. 2), over the past few decades, there has been a growing recognition of the multiple determinants of most disorders and the need for a life course approach (Kuh et al. 2003; Ben-Shlomo and Kuh 2002; Halfon et al. 2014; Buka 2003; Buka and Lipsitt 1994; Angold and Costello 1995; Susser and Susser 1996). These developments in epidemiology were influenced by earlier and parallel advances in the field of human development (c.f., Baltes, Elder, Magnusson) (Baltes et al. 1998; Giele and Elder 1998; Magnusson 1996; Elder and Rockwell 1979). In epidemiology, as in other disciplines, we have come to understand that few, if any, events occur in isolation (Barker 2004; Elder and Shanahan 2007). Hence, the central focus in life course approaches to health development and life course epidemiology is on the complex process of occurrence and accrual of risks at multiple levels. For example, the probability that two identical twin infants will develop a substance use disorder may differ due to a number of subtle environmental differences

S.L. Buka (✉) • S.R. Rosenthal • M.E. Lacy
Department of Epidemiology, Brown University, Providence, RI, USA
e-mail: stephen_buka@brown.edu

that each encounters over the course of their life. In a recent editorial, Stephen Gilman described life course and developmental epidemiology as 'sharing the fundamental principles that health at any given point in time is substantially influenced by prior circumstances, and that disease processes unfold through a combination of risks operating at multiple levels—ranging from genetic inheritance and psychological vulnerability to social conditions' (Gilman 2002).

Epidemiological research shares basic goals with life course development concerning the origins, course, and prevention of health, disease, and disorder and, in turn, through the integration of the perspectives, the promotion of health development. Both advance through a variety of traditional and more recently developed study designs (Aschengrau and Seage 2008; Rothman et al. 2008). Each study design represents a different approach to common research questions and has implications for the ways in which study participants are selected and information is collected and analysed. The design chosen by an investigator is driven by the research question being posed along with considerations of cost, efficiency, and ethical and practical considerations (Aschengrau and Seage 2008; Woodward 2005). While many traditional epidemiological questions can be addressed through a number of alternative designs, some are of limited utility for issues at the core of a life course health development approach.

1.2 Framework for This Chapter

This chapter reviews the major design options for studying health and disease across the life course. The organization is by study design and describes major features of each design approach, key instances of each design, and potential challenges and limitations associated with each design. To limit the scope of this chapter, we take as an example the study of substance use and substance use disorder diagnosis as an instance of a complex health condition warranting investigation from a life course perspective. Study designs included are (i) cohort studies (general prospective cohort studies, perinatal/birth cohorts, twin studies, and high-risk cohort studies); (ii) case–control studies, including nested case–control studies within larger cohorts; (iii) cross-sectional studies; (iv) quasi-experimental designs; and (v) randomized controlled trials (RCTs). Although certain design strategies, namely, cohort studies, lend themselves more readily to the life course approach, we have chosen to describe other study designs that can also be used to further our understanding of health, disorder, and disease from the life course perspective. The chapter concludes with general considerations for designing life course studies, as well as recommendations for future directions of the field.

One frequent topic in life course epidemiology is the initiation, progression, and trajectories following substance use. Given the emphasis in the LCHD principles of the role of synchrony in the timing of developmental processes at multiple levels, ranging from the molecular through the historical (evolutionary), a life course approach has been useful in assessing the timing of substance use onset, the broader contexts that contribute to early use patterns, the progression from use to abuse or dependence, and the identification of intergenerational and early life experiences on substance use patterns (Magnusson 1996; Jablonka and Lamb 2005). One particular research question that has been examined extensively is the relationship between traumatic experience and the development of a substance use disorder. Over the past century, this question has been examined using a variety of different study designs in an effort to more thoroughly probe the potential causal link between trauma and the aetiology of substance use disorder. As the chapter progresses, we use this topic to illustrate the ways in which various threats to the validity of a claim for causality manifest under different study designs. For the purposes of a clear illustration, we focus on diagnosed substance use disorder as our outcome.

2 Major Design Options

In the epidemiological literature, studies are typically grouped into observational and experimental studies (Ahern and Leslie 2014; Pickles et al. 2007).

2.1 Observational

The majority of life course studies are observational studies (Pickles et al. 2007). As compared with experimental studies, in which exposures are randomly assigned to study participants, in observational designs, the investigator observes and records data on a group of people, with no active manipulation of exposure conditions, generating information on the relationships between exposure and disease as they naturally unfold. Whereas the causal inferences that can be derived from observational studies are typically not as strong as those in experimental studies, observational studies are free from the ethical dilemmas associated with allocating exposure in experimental designs. Observational studies typically take two forms, cohort studies or case–control studies; each form has a number of variations.

2.1.1 Cohort Studies

In epidemiology, a prospective cohort study[1] is one in which participants are enrolled before the outcome of interest has occurred and are then followed for a period of time. This is one of the preferred design options for studying substance use disorders across the life course because it allows for direct measurement of both exposures and outcomes as they occur, providing strong evidence for temporality of exposure–outcome relationships. These designs are also useful for illustrating the importance of the LCHD principle regarding the importance of the timing and social structure of exposure to environmental events, both normative and non-normative (Baltes et al. 2006). There remain, however, many important design considerations, challenges, and limitations in the design and conduct of such studies.

In a cohort study, participants are often selected to be representative of a larger population of interest—defining the relevant population of interest is central to designing a maximally informative cohort study. In some instances, the population may be defined by the set of key exposures of interest—e.g. a pregnancy, school-age, or midlife cohort. In others, the most informative population may be those at elevated risk of developing disease, e.g. family history of disorder and certain environmental exposures. If an investigator has multiple outcomes of interest, it can be difficult to identify specific subpopulations at risk of disease, in which case a more general population may be most appropriate.

Data are collected to provide information on the outcomes that are the focus for the study; the implications for this are particularly important in a prospective study because, as the cohort ages, an investigator may wish that additional data had been collected on another exposure or disease (Susser et al. 2000). Additionally, decisions related to study design and data collection are made relative to the science of the field when the study is initiated. This phenomenon is referred to as the scientific period effect (Susser et al. 2000; Wadsworth et al. 2003). Illustrating and reflecting how health development research is embedded in historically defined scientific periods, it has become a truism that many of the greatest discoveries of long-term prospective cohort studies were not anticipated at the time of initiation and that certain data (such as genetic material) that become relevant at a later scientific time may have been overlooked at the onset of earlier projects.

Another key consideration in designing a prospective cohort study is minimizing study dropout and loss to follow-up. Given the long periods of follow-up often involved in prospective cohort studies, it is especially important to consider procedures to minimize study dropout during the

[1]Epidemiology has traditionally made a distinction between prospective cohort studies and retrospective cohort studies, also called historic *cohort* studies, in which the primary outcomes of interest have occurred prior to the initiation of the study, but longitudinal data on both exposures and outcomes exist. Distinctions between prospective, retrospective, and even 'ambispective' cohort studies have become less prominent in more recent epidemiology texts.

planning phase. A number of strategies have been used to minimize study attrition: collection of detailed contact information, sending reminders of follow-up interviews, building rapport, and sharing study findings with participants in the form of newsletters or bulletins (Wadsworth et al. 2003; Stratford et al. 1999).

Challenges and Limitations of Cohort Studies

Cohort studies have contributed greatly to our understanding of the prevalence and distribution of substance use disorders, the course of disorders across time, and information related to utilization of substance use treatment services. They have also been useful in illustrating a number of the challenges and limitations associated with carrying out a long-term prospective cohort study. Considerable human and fiscal resources are needed to enrol, track, and retain participants and to carry out meaningful follow-up for such a long span of time. These challenges are especially prominent in life course studies on substance abuse, due to the time and effort needed to accurately assess outcomes and the multiple potential contributing risk and protective factors that operate at varied levels of influence (from molecular to societal) on the initiation and progression of substance abuse. In addition, as in all observational studies, the designers of cohort studies must anticipate concerns about both imprecisely measured and unmeasured confounding which can undermine the utility of such efforts. Faced with limited resources, investigators must balance the breadth, depth, and size of such cohorts: breadth in terms of the range of contributing conditions and potential confounders assessed, depth regarding the length and intensity of assessment, and size in terms of the number of participants enrolled. Informative cohort studies have ranged from hundreds to hundreds of thousands of participants with commensurate trade-offs between statistical power, on the one hand, and richness of data regarding the multiple complex developmental trajectories that may eventually manifest as disorder, on the other.

Finite resources demand additional trade-offs between cohort enrolment and retention. Successful cohort studies not only need a rich array of data regarding potential risk factors and outcomes, but meaningful inference also requires a high level of retention and protection against threats to validity resulting from attrition and resulting selection bias. While some attrition is inevitable, considerable creative effort and investment in subject retention is necessary to ensure that costly cohort studies yield data of maximal scientific utility. While this applies for cohort studies in general, the close relationship between many disorders and social engagement (such as participation in a prospective cohort study) poses a particularly serious challenge for life course studies. The extent to which attrition is also associated with risk conditions of interest may irrevocably reduce the potential of cohort studies to generate unbiased estimates of interest.

Despite these challenges, however, cohort studies will remain at the forefront of design options to advance the understanding of health development. The strength of a cohort in the LCHD context is primarily the ability to investigate prospectively the synergistic influences of multiple conditions (e.g. genetic, biological, behavioural, social, environmental)—both risk and protective—over time, compare influences at different phases of development, identify potentially sensitive developmental periods, and characterize longitudinal health trajectories as they unfold. They are clearly the method of choice to examine the impact of potentially adverse or risk conditions, which could not be manipulated through a randomized design, due to ethical considerations.

Major Prospective Cohort Studies of Substance Use Disorder

There are several important and well-known general prospective cohort studies examining substance use disorders across the life course. Due to space limitations, we summarize the considerations and decisions made for two of these study designs: Woodlawn Study (2017) and Monitoring the Future Study (2016). These studies serve as excellent examples of the unique type of question that can be answered, as well as the challenges that arise in conducting a prospective cohort study for life course health development. Both studies employed a multi-wave prospective cohort design, and the Monitoring the Future study was designed to enroll a nationally representative sample of the American young adult population. The Woodlawn Study, funded by the National Institute on Drug Abuse (NIDA) and initiated in 1966, recruited a high-risk community of African-American first graders from the same disadvantaged inner city community in Chicago to examine risk factors for substance use disorder. These first graders were followed for a total of four waves: first grade, adolescence, young adulthood, and midlife. This study collected data over the life course—from childhood through adulthood—and initiated data collection prior to the onset of drug use. This design approach allows investigators to compare the onset of substance use disorder and substance use trajectories among children who had similar early roots but disparate pathways to adulthood in terms of family relationships, school, work, peer relationships, religion, and community involvement—a very useful design for a life course health development approach (The Woodlawn Project: A Life Course Study 2017).

Monitoring the Future (MTF) project, also funded by NIDA, began in 1975 using a multi-stage, stratified random sampling framework to enroll a cohort of participants that were representative of American high school students; each year about 16,000 students in approximately 133 public and private high schools nationwide participate. Though many use this dataset as panel data, or annual cohorts of nationally representative data, there is potential to use MTF as a prospective cohort study. Beginning with the class of 1976, a randomly selected sample from each senior class has been followed up biannually after high school on a continuing basis. Twelve years past high school, participants receive their last young adult questionnaire and then follow-up procedures change to 5-year intervals to cover middle adulthood. This study design allows for investigators to examine (1) changes in particular years such as secular trends or 'period effects', (2) developmental changes that show up consistently for all cohort groups or 'age effects', (3) consistent differences among class cohorts through the life cycle or 'cohort effects', and (4) changes linked to different types of environments or role transitions (Rothman et al. 2008). Both of these cohorts span multiple decades and multiple life stages, providing detailed information on trends in substance use disorder over the life course.

Cohort Example: Trauma and Substance Use Disorder Across the Life Course

Using data from 5 years of follow-up, Chilcoat and Breslau examined the relationship between experiencing a traumatic event and the risk for drug abuse or dependence (Chilcoat and Breslau 1998). They found that participants who had a traumatic event had more than a fourfold increase in risk of drug abuse or dependence compared with those with no history of a traumatic event, after controlling for a number of potential confounders. This study exemplifies the value of prospective cohort studies to advance causal inference in the absence of experimentation: it clearly establishes temporality of exposure (traumatic event) and outcome (drug abuse or dependence), it uses a valid measure to identify diagnoses of drug abuse or dependence (DSM-III-R diagnoses), and it takes into account a number of important factors that could potentially confound the true association between trauma and drug abuse or dependence. However, despite the study's many strengths, because it is an observational study, there remain a number of potential threats to validity. Typically, selection bias is one of the greatest threats to the validity of an observational study. In this case, however, study participants were randomly selected from the membership list of a 400,000 member health maintenance organization in Southeast Michigan. Given all participants were likely from the same region, conclusions may not be generalizable to those in different parts of the

(continued)

(continued)

country. Thus, conclusions should be replicated elsewhere. Information bias is reduced in this example, as diagnoses of drug abuse or dependence were generated independent of knowledge of experiencing trauma. Finally, there remains the potential that there is residual and unmeasured confounding. It would be impossible to measure every potential confounder that occurs over the 5 years that the study spans, and, further, the study was not designed solely to address this particular research question. In any study with such a wide scope and with multiple years of follow-up, there is always the possibility that an important potential confounder was overlooked or was not adequately measured. Prospective cohort studies can span decades, which is very useful for a life course approach, but this comes with additional challenge.

2.1.2 Perinatal and Birth Cohorts

In addition to the general design features of a prospective cohort study, in a birth or perinatal cohort, there are additional challenges involved with recruiting and enrolling participants at or before birth. Parents are the primary target for recruitment, and, depending on the length of follow-up, parents may serve as the primary respondent even though the cohort of interest comprises the offspring generation. In a perinatal cohort study, the emphasis is on factors that occur in the months immediately prior to and following birth. Therefore, studies of this design typically will recruit and enroll parents (usually mothers) who are pregnant or planning to become pregnant in the near future. Data are typically collected on the mother and child throughout the pregnancy, at birth, and for a defined length of time following birth. In a birth cohort, investigators typically design a sampling scheme to target births that occur in a specific geographic region within a specified period of time. For both perinatal and birth cohorts, the length of follow-up is determined by the research questions being posed and the resources available for the study.

Issues related to data collection are another unique concern for perinatal and birth cohorts. While parents may serve as the primary respondent during the child's infancy and toddler years, it is possible to collect data directly on very young children. Special consideration, however, must be given to the length and appropriateness of data collection procedures, training of interviewers, and study consent and assent procedures to ensure adequate protection of human subjects.

Over the years, birth and perinatal cohorts have proved an invaluable source of information in the study of life course health development. Benefiting from the general strengths of cohort studies (e.g. exposure data unbiased by later health status, ability to distinguish cause from effect and temporal sequences), cohorts started at or before birth have the added value of assessing risk, protective variables, and developmental course at the earliest stages of human development. This study design enables investigators to examine the impact of the foetal, infant, and early childhood experience on health development across the life course. We now describe two influential perinatal and birth cohorts, again limiting our scope to studies that have generated substance use disorder diagnoses.

Major Birth Cohort Studies of Substance Use Disorder

There are several important birth cohorts that allow for the study of life course health development and assess substance use disorders. Some of these we describe in detail: the Collaborative Perinatal Project (CPP), New England Family Study (NEFS), and Dunedin Multidisciplinary Health and Development Study (DMHDS).

The CPP was initiated more than 50 years ago to investigate prospectively the prenatal and familial antecedents of paediatric, neurological, and psychological disorders of childhood. The CPP is, in fact, not a birth cohort but rather a prenatal cohort. Across the United States, 12 university-affiliated medical centres participated, including two in New England (in Boston and Providence). More than 50,000 pregnancies were enrolled between 2 January 1959 and 31 December 1965 (16,557 in the NEFS sites) (Broman 1984; Broman et al. 1985). The study followed up 88% of survivors at 1 year, 75% at 4 years, and 79% at 7 years.

Data from examinations and interviews were recorded by trained staff at each site beginning at the time of registration for prenatal care, using standardized protocols, forms, manuals, and codes. At the first prenatal visit, a complete reproductive and gynaecological history, recent and past medical history, socio-economic interview, and family history were recorded. Prenatal clinic visits were scheduled monthly during the first 7 months of pregnancy, every 2 weeks during the 8th month, and every week thereafter. Blood samples were collected for serology and for storage of frozen sera. After admission for delivery, trained observers recorded the events of labour and delivery, and the obstetrician completed labour and delivery protocols. Approximately 75% of subjects had cord blood samples drawn and stored. The neonate was observed in the delivery room, examined by a paediatrician at 24 h intervals in the newborn nursery, and received a neurological examination at 2 days. Study offspring received five subsequent assessments: at ages 4, 8, and 12 months and 4 and 7 years. At each follow-up examination, the mother was interviewed about the child's history, records of medical treatment were obtained if applicable, and physical measurements were taken. Paediatric–neurological examinations occurred at 4 and 12 months and at 7 years and psychological examinations at 8 months and at 4 and 7 years. Family and social history information was obtained from the mother at intake and at 7 years. Diagnostic summaries were prepared by study physicians following the 12-month and 7-year assessments.

Between 2001 and 2004, the New England Family Study was established to locate and interview a sample of the adult CPP offspring in Providence and Boston who lived beyond 7 years of age (15,721)—resulting in a multitude of birth cohort studies spanning more than 40 years. In recent years, this team has extended the follow-up and assessment of three-generation pedigrees in the NEFS, which is still ongoing (i.e. CPP mothers, their offspring who comprise the CPP cohort members, and the offspring of the CPP cohort members). These projects all seek to integrate family designs with early life risk conditions, capitalizing upon the large number of cohort members with multiple offspring. With the increased emphasis on family designs, the overall effort was renamed 'The New England Family Study' (NEFS) (Gilman et al. 2008).

A prominent birth cohort that measures substance use disorder and has taken a life course health development approach is the Dunedin Multidisciplinary Health and Development Study (DMHDS). Investigators enrolled children from 91% of consecutive births from 1 April 1972 through 13 March 1973 in Dunedin, New Zealand. Perinatal data were obtained at delivery, and follow-ups occurred at 3, 5, 7, 9, 11, 13, 15, 18, and 21 years of age. Future assessments are planned for ages 44 and 50 years. At each assessment, study members participated in physical tests, dental examinations, blood tests, and completed computer questionnaires and surveys. At the age 21 year assessment, 94% of cohort members remained in the study, showing no significant attrition effect—a remarkable feat in a longitudinal birth cohort of this nature. Investigators attribute this low attrition rate to aggressive retention measures such as flying participants who had moved away back to New Zealand and using interviewers in other locations such as Australia (Silva and Stanton 1997). Birth cohorts such as the CPP and the DMHDS are incredibly useful for life course health development research because they allow investigators to gain knowledge of developmental processes, as well as multilevel genetic and environmental risk factors.

Birth Cohort Example: Maternal Smoking and Alcohol Use Disorder Across the Life Course

Using the New England Family Study described above, second-generation individuals were followed from birth for more

(continued)

(continued)

than 40 years. Investigators examined the relationship between maternal smoking during pregnancy and lifetime risk for alcohol use disorder (DSM-IV) among 1625 offspring (aged 34–44 years) of 1254 mothers (Nomura et al. 2011). Exposure information was collected from pregnant women at their first prenatal visit, and these questions were repeated at each subsequent prenatal visit up until the time of delivery. Given the robust birth cohort design and long follow-up period, analyses were able to account for maternal mental health during pregnancy, birth weight, neurological abnormality at age 1, childhood behavioural regulation at age 7 years, and academic functioning at age 7 years. Adjusting for these developmental factors and additional demographic variables, results indicated that those with mothers who smoked at least 20 cigarettes per day during pregnancy had a 30% increased risk of lifetime alcohol use disorder. Despite the study's many strengths, there are also limitations inherent to birth cohorts of this type. First, the sample of this particular birth cohort is not representative of a broader population, and therefore external validity is potentially limited. Also, given the long period of follow-up, obstetric care at birth was very different than the modern level of care. Specifically, the mortality rate for those born prematurely was much higher in the late 1960s—thus many children suffering from behavioural regulation problems and poor academic functioning may be offered more effective assistance had they been born today. Finally, as with all observational study designs and those with long follow-up periods, there remains the potential that there is residual and unmeasured confounding. It would be impossible to measure every potential confounder that occurs over the 40 years of that the study.

2.1.3 Twin Studies

Due to their unique genetic status, twins play a valuable role in life course health development research. Using twins as study participants helps investigators advance understanding of genetic and environmental risks, differentiate between genetic influences in different subgroups of people (e.g. males versus females, different age groups, people of different race/ethnicities), and better understand gene–environment interactions. Ultimately, twin studies allow researchers to estimate the proportion of variance in a trait attributable to genetic variation versus the proportion that is due to shared environment or unshared environment (Bundey 1991). Twins are usually recruited from registries, which now exist across the globe. Twin studies can be conducted across study design types, thought the most robust would be longitudinal—similar to a prospective cohort design (Boomsma et al. 2002).

There are several important considerations in twin studies. First, studying twins who grow up in a shared environment does not allow the researcher to consider the effects of both shared environment and gene–environment interaction simultaneously. Rather, this can be addressed by including additional non-twin siblings in the design. Second, results from twin studies cannot be directly generalized to a broader population as there may be genetic factors that lead specifically to a higher incidence of twinning. This raises potential threats to external validity (Bundey 1991). Traditionally, the general consensus was that twin studies represented an optimal study design to examine gene–environment interactions across the life course. Recent criticisms of twin studies and, more generally, 'variation-partitioning' methods employed by behavioural geneticists have emerged, calling into question the extent to which such studies can shed light onto nuanced developmental processes involved in life course development (Tabery 2014; Moore 2015). Tabery (2014) posits that the traditional twin methods offer an overly 'black-box' view of development and are better for general predictions regarding future health outcomes than for nuanced 'mechanism elucidation' of the means by which such developmental processes unfold. This criticism may be unduly harsh as (1) with human populations, observation (rather than experimental manipulation) of gene–environment interactions is the only ethical option and (2) contemporary behavioural geneticists typically avoid simplistic black-box approaches, with hypotheses and analyses informed by other biological and developmental sciences. Recent developments in high-dimensional analysis of both genetic (e.g. GWAS) and environmental (EWAS) factors may help advance traditional approaches to understand the interactive influences of genetic and environmental influences on life course health development (Patel et al. 2010).

Major Twin Studies of Substance Use Disorder

There are many twin registries and twin studies around the world, most of which are in Europe. A few of these have been used to examine substance abuse, two of which we will highlight: the Danish Twin Registry and the Swedish Twin Registry. The Danish Twin Registry was established in the 1950s and is one of the oldest twin registries in the world. The registry now comprises information on almost all twins born in Denmark since 1870. It contains data from church books, the Central Office of Civil Registration, health behaviour and lifestyle variables, and clinical examinations for more than 88,000 twin pairs (Skytthe et al. 2011). Though substance use disorder is one of many outcomes assessed in the registry data, hundreds of other studies using this registry have examined ageing, age-related health, cardiovascular disease, and other rare diseases (Boomsma et al. 2002).

The Swedish Twin Registry contains three cohorts, each differing by ascertainment and extent of data collection. The first cohort was born between 1886 and 1925. Data for the first cohort was ascertained from all parishes across Sweden and contains information on demographics, risk behaviours, cardiovascular health, respiratory health, and environmental exposures. Information on the second cohort, born between 1926 and 1958, was ascertained using nationalized birth registrations and mailed questionnaires. Information covered similar domains as the first cohort and also collected an additional personality inventory. The third cohort, born between 1959 and 1990, was identified by birth registry and has been linked to the Medical Birth Registry. Researchers working with the Swedish Twin Registry have now begun an effort called Screening Across the Lifespan Twin (SALT) study in which investigators have identified subsamples of twins in the registry for more in-depth studies in which blood samples will be obtained; phenotyping and genotyping will be performed; detailed information on health behaviours, clinical diagnoses, and medications will be collected; and linkages will be made to medical records (Lichtenstein et al. 2002). Both of these registries, as well as twin cohorts generally, pose a unique opportunity to examine the multilevel and multidimensional genetic and environmental risks for health development across the life course.

Twin Cohort Example: Childhood Sexual Abuse and Substance Use Disorder

The research literature has consistently suggested a link between childhood sexual abuse and negative health outcomes, but there remain concerns for selection bias and confounding by family environment. To address this question while minimizing confounding by family environment, investigators derived a sample of 1159 female–female twin pairs and 832 male–male twin pairs from a young adult Australian volunteer twin panel. Structured psychiatric telephone interviews were conducted to assess childhood sexual abuse and adverse psychosocial outcomes including alcohol dependence (DSM-IV) and nicotine dependence (DSM-IV). Family background information was elicited including parental fighting, parental conflict, stepparent presence, neglect, and physical abuse. Results suggested that individuals with a history of childhood sexual abuse have increased risk

(continued)

(continued)

of developing alcohol and nicotine dependence. Results also showed that childhood sexual abuse is associated with substantial risk that is not explained by other family background factors. There is, however, a potential for bias. Selection bias may have arisen due to the fact that parents aware of abuse may have been less likely to volunteer their twins for research. Regardless, using a twin study approach allowed researchers to dissect the direct and correlated family background effects of childhood sexual abuse (Nelson et al. 2002).

2.1.4 High-Risk Cohort

The high-risk cohort study is a variation on the general cohort study described above, with the key distinction being that subjects are recruited because they have been selected on the basis of their exposure history. Often, subjects are identified as being at high risk for developing the outcome of interest based on particular behaviours and characteristics or manifestations of previous pathology in their parents.

Studies such as these allow researchers to better examine the natural history of disorders in relation to a particular high-risk population. One potential limitation of high-risk studies, however, is that their results, and, ultimately, the conclusions they draw, may only be applicable for high-risk populations. By contrast, high-risk studies do provide an efficient means of examining relatively rare disorders.

Major High-Risk Cohort of Substance Use Disorder

Though high-risk cohorts of substance use disorder tend to be smaller studies of very specific high-risk populations (e.g. injection-drug users, HIV-infected individuals, or the homeless), veterans have been identified as a high-risk group more likely than others to fall victim to substance abuse as a means of coping. Following the 1991 Gulf War, the US Congress and the Institute of Medicine recommended the US Department of Defense to conduct a high-risk cohort study of military personnel. This initiative was entitled the Millennium Cohort Study and is the largest prospective health study of military personnel including more than 200,000 participants. Data collection for the study began in 2001 with the 77,047 participants enrolled. Every 3 years additional participants are enrolled and an additional wave of data collection is conducted. The very first group recruited has completed five waves of data collection to date. Questionnaires at each wave assess general health, health behaviours, clinical diagnoses, physical symptoms, mental illness, health care utilization, and military life and experience. Many studies have already been conducted using this cohort and many focus on substance disorder and mental health (The Millenium Cohort Study 2010). This high-risk cohort allows researchers to better understand the risk associated with military service and seeing combat, but may not represent health development in the general population.

High-Risk Cohort Example: Posttraumatic Stress Disorder and Substance Abuse

An investigation into the relationship between posttraumatic stress disorder (PTSD) symptoms and substance abuse utilizing a high-risk cohort was conducted by Bremner et al. (1996). These investigators recruited Vietnam combat veterans with PTSD to study the effect of specific PTSD symptoms on substance abuse. Analyses examined the occurrence of substance abuse among veterans with respect to PTSD symptomology. The high-risk design ensured a large number of veterans with and without PTSD symptoms resulting in a powerful method to examine the influence of these symptoms on substance abuse. Analyses revealed a strong and consistent association between onset of PTSD symptoms and onset of substance abuse. Similarly, an increase of PTSD symptoms

(continued)

(continued)

predicted onset of substance abuse. This study allowed researchers to better examine the natural history of substance abuse among Vietnam War veterans with PTSD. However, the conclusions they draw may only be applicable for this high-risk population.

2.1.5 Case–Control Studies

Unlike the study designs we have described up to this point in which participants are recruited into the study and followed over time to ascertain their outcome status, in a case–control study, participants are selected based on the presence or absence of a disorder, and exposure data are obtained after the outcome has been ascertained. Although case–control studies are not the strongest design option for conducting life course research, this particular study design has a number of benefits (Schlesselman and Schneiderman 1982). Because participants are selected after the outcome of interest has occurred, case–control studies are typically extremely cost-effective, especially in studying rare diseases. As compared with cohort studies, in which the investigator may need to follow a large number of participants for years to identify the outcome of interest, in a case–control study, the outcome has already occurred, and the investigator seeks to determine those exposures or conditions that may have contributed to this occurrence.

Challenges and Limitations of Case–Control Studies

In a case–control study, the primary threats to study validity lie in the selection of controls and in the ascertainment of exposure status. Because in a case–control study, the outcome has occurred prior to the investigator's assessment, there is a threat of recall bias (Schlesselman and Schneiderman 1982; Lee et al. 2007; Berney and Blane 1997). Exposures, by definition, occurred in the past, and those collected through participant self-report introduce the possibility of people inaccurately recalling their exposure history. Often, those who have developed the outcome of interest are more likely to examine their past exposures more carefully in an attempt to find an explanation for why they developed the disease. In a case such as this, where cases are systematically reporting exposure differently from controls, recall bias has been introduced into the study, and, because it systematically differs among exposed and unexposed, this bias may potentially skew study findings. The challenge lies in identifying a way to measure past exposures without introducing bias or inconsistencies in their assessment.

In the trauma and substance abuse literature, reports of childhood sexual abuse and physical punishment were shown to be unreliable. Specifically, unreliability arose because those who were subject to abuse often provided false-negative reports. This could cause estimates of abuse prevalence based on a single report to seriously underestimate the true prevalence; however, estimates of the relative risk of psychiatric problems conditional on abuse are robust to the effects of these reporting errors (Fergusson et al. 2000). It is very important when using a case–control design to optimize the reliability of exposure measurements to minimize or avoid the potential of recall bias being introduced into the study.

Another important limitation is the potential for selection bias. In a case–control study, identification of cases is fairly straightforward; it is the identification of controls, however, that presents a challenge (Schlesselman and Schneiderman 1982; Wacholder et al. 1992). Cases and controls must arise from the same study base; if controls were to have developed the outcome of interest, they must have been eligible to be identified as cases. Although this sounds relatively straightforward, in practice it can be quite difficult to ensure that the controls properly represent the study base from which cases have been drawn. This is an especially important point because, in order to estimate accurately the effect of exposure on the outcome, the controls are being used to estimate the exposure distribution in the study population; therefore, a misrepresentative selection of controls could bias study results significantly (Lee et al. 2007).

Given case–control studies are conducted, retrospectively, there are not commonly ongoing examples of case–control studies as there are with cohorts. Therefore, we present a specific example of a case–control study of substance use disorder, but will not highlight any major case–control studies as we did with cohorts.

Case–Control Example: Traumas and Alcohol Abuse and Dependence

Investigators selected cases from area intervention programmes, 132 adolescents with alcohol dependence (DSM-IV) and 51 with alcohol abuse (DSM-IV), and controls by random-digit dialling and advertisement in the broader community, 73 adolescents. Questions were asked concerning lifetime traumatic events such as physical abuse, sexual abuse, violent victimization, witnessing violence, and other miscellaneous traumas. Results found that traumatic events in every category had higher rates of occurrence in the alcohol dependence and abuse groups than in the control group. Some limitations remain in this study: we cannot assume causality, adolescents with disorder may not be representative of all adolescents with disorder, community controls may not be representative of adolescents in the general population, and there may be reporting error in trauma reports (Clark et al. 1997).

2.1.6 Nested Case–Control Designs

A nested case–control study is a variation of the traditional case–control study design. In this study design, cases of a disease that occur in a defined cohort are identified, and often, a specified number of matched controls are selected from among those in the cohort who have not developed the disease. This design is advantageous when the exposure of interest is difficult or expensive to obtain and when the outcome is rare. A nested case–control design is particularly efficient due to reductions in recruitment and data collection costs with relatively minor loss in statistical efficiency (Ernster 1994). Yet, challenges and limitations of this design remain and are similar to those of a traditional case–control design.

Nested Case–Control Example: Trauma and Substance Use Disorder

Cutajar et al. (2010) investigated the relationship between childhood sexual abuse and the occurrence of substance use disorder. In this study, researchers drew cases from a pre-existing cohort of child sexual abuse victims compiled by the Victorian Institute of Forensic Medicine in Australia. This approach is referred to as a nested case–control study design. Researchers identified 2759 sexually abused children from the cohort (verified via forensic medical records assessed between 1964 and 1995). The control group was drawn from a random sample of Victorian residents from the national electoral database. This yielded 2677 age- and gender-matched controls from the general population. Both case and control participants were linked with a public psychiatric database, the Victorian Psychiatric Case Register, between 12 and 43 years later. Control subjects were matched on gender and age groupings drawn from the general population through a random sample of the national electoral database. The use of archival data from childhood to identify victims of sexual abuse lends strength to this study as it minimizes the introduction of recall bias. Yet, there is the potential for selection bias insofar as the comparison group may not be representative of the population from which the cases arose; for instance, there may be something systematically different between those with a history of childhood

(continued)

(continued)

sexual abuse and those in the general population. In a study such as this, where cases are identified from forensic medical records, it can be difficult to define clearly what constitutes the study base, i.e. what group of patients would have eventually been identified by forensic medical records had they experienced childhood sexual abuse. Results from this study suggest those with a history of childhood sexual abuse have almost six times the odds of substance abuse disorder compared to those with no sexual abuse history.

2.1.7 Cross-Sectional Studies

In life course research, cross-sectional studies provide information on both the prevalence of disease and associations between risk factors and disease but typically provide little definitive information to further understanding of causal relationships. In a typical cross-sectional study, participants are sampled and interviewed at a single time point (Gilman 2002). As compared to case–control studies described above, cross-sectional studies typically place less emphasis on reconstructing past exposure; rather they provide a snapshot of prevalence of disease and associations between exposure and disease in a given sample at a given time often limiting the inference we can make regarding the temporal sequence between exposure and disease. Another difference from case–control studies is the sampling framework. In case–control studies, a great deal of effort is placed on sampling an informative set of controls that are representative of the population that gave rise to the case. In cross-sectional studies, participants may include either a sample of convenience (based on their availability and willingness to participate) or they are often based on a representative sample of the general population (which allows for high generalizability). Cross-sectional studies, while not typically considered a strong design option for life course research, provide important insight into the prevalence of disorders in a population and can provide initial evidence as to potential associations that can be investigated further using a more stringent study design (Kraemer et al. 2000). Additionally, retrospective data can be collected from participants either using archival data or during the interview process in an attempt to reconstruct past exposure history.

Challenges and Limitations of Cross-Sectional Studies

Cross-sectional studies have a host of limitations. First, if the sample is a convenience sample, rather than representative of the population, threats to external validity exist. Second, non-response can result in bias of study measures. For example, despite trying to sample for a representative population, many individuals may not respond due to having severe negative health outcomes or being part of a high-risk, transient population; both of these examples would result in a loss of critical study information. Also, due to the cross-sectional nature of data collection, temporality of the exposure and outcome cannot be confirmed. Finally, cross-sectional designs are not suitable for studying rare diseases or diseases with short duration.

Major Cross-Sectional Studies of Substance Use Disorder

There are many publicly available, nationally representative cross-sectional surveys conducted in the United States. Of these, several include measures of substance use disorder. We will describe one of these: the National Survey on Drug Use and Health (NSDUH). The NSDUH provides national- and state-level data on substance use, disorder, and mental health in the United States. It is sponsored by the Substance Abuse and Mental Health Services Administration. The NSDUH is administrated annually to approximately 70,000 randomly selected individuals aged 12 years and older. The goals of NSDUH are to provide accurate prevalence estimates on the level and patterns of substance use and abuse, track trends in substance use, assess the consequences of substance use, and identify groups at high risk for substance disorder. Though this cross-sectional survey assesses different individuals over time, it provides useful information on secular trends of and consistent risk factors for substance use disorder (National Survey on Drug Use and Health 2017).

Cross-Sectional Example: Trauma and Substance Use Disorder

Returning to our examination of the relationship between trauma and substance use disorder, Molnar, Buka, and Kessler conducted a cross-sectional study using a US national household probability sample of 8098 participants aged 15 to 54 years from the National Comorbidity Survey (Molnar et al. 2001). Given the size and relatively low cost of a single cross-sectional assessment, researchers were able to account for age, race, parental divorce, parental psychopathology, parental verbal and physical abuse, and parental substance use problems while examining the association between childhood sexual abuse and substance use disorder (DSM-III-R). Results found those with a history of childhood sexual assault had about a twofold odds of drug dependence and 1.7 times the odds of alcohol dependence compared to those with no history of childhood sexual assault. However, cross-sectional data do not allow for causal inferences to be made about the relationship between being assaulted and substance use disorder; given that all data are from one time point, there is no evidence as to the temporality of the exposure–outcome relationship. Further, information bias can arise depending on how data are collected. In the example above, timing and characteristics of childhood sexual assault and substance use disorder were self-reported, introducing the possibility of reporting bias and recall bias. Cross-sectional studies also have the potential for unmeasured confounding. Given that all data are collected from one time point, many other factors that could be influencing the association of interest are not captured by the one-time assessment.

2.2 Quasi-Experimental Designs

Unlike true experiments, where the investigator manipulates the exposures or conditions affecting research participants, quasi-experiments are characterized by investigator manipulation of observations (not treatments). Given the focus of this chapter, observations would typically be assessments of substance use disorder, implemented after the occurrence of major events of relevance to life course theory—such as natural disasters (e.g. Hurricane Katrina), acts of terrorism, and events resulting from policy changes and the like, such as marijuana legalization. Such quasi- or natural experiments largely differ from traditional observational studies in that participants are largely 'selected' into exposed or unexposed groups by an event that is substantially not within their own control.

2.2.1 Challenges and Limitations of Quasi-Experimental Studies

As natural experiments, these studies are often less subject to selection bias than typical observational studies. However, at the same time, attempts to study the consequences of such quasi-experiments may be hampered by the challenges of responding quickly to initiate an investigation soon after a natural occurrence of interest has taken place. Poorly implemented efforts may introduce problems related to both information bias (where respondents are typically not blind to the event of interest and may provide non-comparable information) and confounding, where the investigation may not be able to assess the full relevant set of potential confounding factors.

Quasi-Experimental Example: Trauma and Substance Use Disorder

Returning to our example on trauma and substance use disorder, Reijneveld et al. found themselves in a position to examine the impact of trauma in a natural experiment (Reijneveld et al. 2003). In 2001, a fire in a café in Volendam, Netherlands, wounded 250 adolescents and killed 14.

(continued)

(continued)

Surprisingly, 15 months prior to the disaster, all students aged 12–15 years from a school in Volendam (of whom 31 had been in the café during the fire), and from two other schools, had been selected as controls for a study. Five months after the disaster, researchers obtained follow-up data from Volendam adolescents and controls from the other two schools. Contrary to previous study designs, which examined the impact of trauma on substance use, Reijneveld et al. were able to examine this relationship in a setting in which trauma, a potentially strong explanatory variable for substance use, was directly manipulated by forces outside the control of the researchers. The exposure (the disaster) was a horrific accident; yet, only adolescents living in Volendam were 'exposed'. Compared with an observational design, in which there are very many interrelated factors impacting an adolescent's likelihood of exposure to trauma, in this study, trauma was controlled by a force outside of the researchers' and participants' control (an 'exogenous' factor). It was not, however, randomly assigned; the exposure to the disaster was correlated with going to school in Volendam, raising potential concerns of remaining confounding. Therefore, any factors related to neighbourhood or town that differ between those exposed to the fire and those not exposed were not addressed. The authors observed that Volendam adolescents who were exposed to the disaster had almost fivefold the odds of excessive alcohol use compared to other adolescents, providing important new evidence supporting the causal relationship between trauma and excessive alcohol use among adolescents.

2.3 Experimental Designs

In experimental studies, such as randomized control trials (RCTs), participants are randomly assigned to receive exposure or not with the exposure being manipulated by study investigators. Given a large enough sample, the implications of this randomization and manipulation of exposure are related to the inferences that may be made about causality. When exposure is truly assigned at random to study participants, it is assumed that, on average, all known and unknown confounders are evenly distributed across the study arms and, therefore, that the two arms of the study are exchangeable. When these and other conditions are fulfilled (adequately large sample, effective randomization, reasonably representative sample, meaningful external validity/ generalizability), RCTs provide a unique opportunity to generate evidence of the causal impact of exposures on subsequent health and development. As discussed below, conventionally the major limitations raised regarding experimental studies concerned feasibility and ethics. More recent contributions from the developmental and social sciences raise more fundamental questions regarding the utility of experimental approaches in the context of rich and multifactorial developmental processes such as those involved with life course health development (Lerner and Callina 2014; Sampson 2010).

2.3.1 Challenges and Limitations of Experimental Studies

In substance abuse epidemiology, investigators typically examine the impact of harmful exposures or 'risk factors' on substance use disorders; obviously, the random allocation of harmful exposures to study participants is not ethically permissible. To illustrate, researchers have long wanted to understand the impact of trauma on the development of substance use disorder; nevertheless it would be unethical to randomly assign participants to undergo a traumatic life event so that investigators could study their response. Further, logistic considerations and the high cost associated with the long-term follow-up of subjects further limit the use of RCTs in life course research. As a result, due to the ethical considerations combined with practical constraints, experimental studies (in particular of potentially harmful conditions) are not often used in psychiatric or substance use research. Randomized controlled trials pertaining to trauma and substance use disorders are limited to those that assess the effectiveness of treatments or interventions such as cognitive behavioural therapy or sertraline administration (Cohen et al. 2007; Van Dam et al. 2012).

Randomized Controlled Trial Experimental Example: PTSD and Substance Use Treatment

A recent RCT by Mills et al. aimed to determine whether an integrated treatment for PTSD and substance dependence can achieve greater reductions in PTSD and substance dependence symptom severity compared with usual treatment for substance dependence (Mills et al. 2012). In 2007–2009 in Sydney, Australia, 103 adults with diagnoses of PTSD and substance dependence were recruited from substance use treatment services, media advertisements, and practitioner referrals. Fifty-five participants were randomized to receive Concurrent Treatment of PTSD and Substance Use Disorders Using Prolonged Exposure (COPE) in addition to usual treatment for substance dependence, and 48 were randomized to receive the usual treatment only. Participants were reinterviewed at 6 weeks, 3 months, and 9 months. Results suggested the treatment group had significant reductions in PTSD symptom severity relative to the control group, yet there was no significant difference in prevalence or severity of substance dependence between treatment and control groups. Whereas this study does not perfectly map on to previous examples examining the relationship between trauma and substance use disorder, it does illustrate the strengths of the RCT for life course research. In this study, the randomization of adults diagnosed with PTSD and substance dependence created groups that appear to be exchangeable at baseline. Exchangeability of the groups allows us to make comparisons between the groups under the assumption that the groups are identical with the exception of the treatment. Further, we would expect that randomization would eliminate the potential for selection bias to occur in the allocation of treatment, thus preventing systematic differences between the two groups (i.e. all participants have equal probability of receiving treatment or control). RCTs can be incredibly informative for establishing causation between an exposure and an outcome, though many exposures would be unethical for an investigator to administer. However, in assessing the impact of treatments for disorders throughout the life course, RCTs would be the gold standard.

3 Discussion

We close by revisiting several of the central principles of the life course health development framework introduced at the beginning of this volume (see Halfon and Forrest 2017) and discussing opportunities to advance understanding of the causes and promotion of health development through the various research design alternatives covered in this chapter. The current chapter discusses traditional epidemiologic designs and offers examples of how these have been altered and extended to contribute to our nascent understanding of how health and disease develop across the life course. However, the concept of ‘health development’ goes beyond traditional and often static definitions of ‘health’, ‘disease’, and ‘disorder’. Fully integrating the life course health development framework into study design selection requires new thinking and innovation from the epidemiology community. As outlined in Principle 1, health development—the focus of scientific inquiry in this field—is conceptualized as a dynamic process that ‘combines both health and development…blends a temporal dimension into our conceptualization of human health…{with} time-dependent and transactional connotations’ (p. 15). Designs that are faithful to this view will require new perspectives, measures, and analytic methods. Developments in latent class trajectory modelling (Nagin 2016), behavioural trajectories, and their investigation in multilevel contexts (Cerda et al. 2008) are all contributing to this extension of traditional design approaches.

Principle 3 in the LCHD framework addresses the topic of complexity. Complexity refers to how health development is dependent upon complex reciprocal interactions between individuals and their physical, natural, and social environments. To appropriately study complexity, a broad array of individual and environmental factors must be measured. Epidemiologic methods allow for the assessment of interactions and multiple interactions in studies; however, the number of variables and variable interactions assessed is inversely related to the resulting level of statistical power and directly related to the number of type II or false-positive findings. Similarly, understanding that interactions play an important role in health development, researchers should examine bidirectional relationships between individual and environmental characteristics. Future studies examining interactions should be designed as longitudinal studies (to determine temporality/causality), and large sample sizes should be used to increase power to detect important interactions. New efforts to develop 'environment-wide association study' (EWAS) methods, to parallel genome-wide association studies (GWAS) and new developments in machine learning, may provide additional solutions to the problem of sample size and growing numbers of potential risk and protective factors (Patel et al. 2010). Also, given the complexity of the life course approach, it is unlikely that a single study will definitively advance LCHD theory. Rather, a compilation of studies from different populations (or the same population over time) at different stages in the life course and across different realms of development (e.g. physical, social, environmental, genetic, epigenetic, etc.) and contexts will be necessary for advances regarding health development throughout the life course.

Another fundamental element principle of the LCHD framework is timing. This principle refers to the concept that there are specific developmental stages throughout the life course (e.g. in utero, pubescence) in which the impact of certain exposures on an individual can be greater than during other periods, with the attendant implications of the importance of nurturing children when they are most sensitive to these influences. Reflecting the importance of the time dimension for health development, this principle further underscores the value of prospective cohort designs, not only as these involve the study of time, but also, in contrast to retrospective or cross-sectional designs, they permit more accurate prospective assessment of multiple risk and protective conditions as these occur. For example, the landmark Adverse Child Experiences Survey has documented the association between childhood adversity and a range of poor health outcomes, using adult retrospective reports of child experiences (Felitti et al. 1998). Refined understanding of the impact and timing of such early adverse experiences will, however, require prospective studies that are less subject to potential recall, detection, and selection biases (Widom et al. 2015). Interest in 'timing' does not necessarily always imply the need for longitudinal designs. Cross-sectional studies conducted during particularly sensitive stages of the life course could also be informative, and preferable to cross-sectional studies during other, less impactful periods. Also, in longitudinal cohorts, researchers may want to consider giving more weight to exposures during these sensitive periods. Collaboration across disciplines will help suggest certain stages in the life course that are likely to have particular relevance for long-term health development, for example, due to a propensity for epigenetic alterations or other forms of biologic sensitivity (Moffitt 2013).

In closing, life course approaches to advance understanding of the causes and prevention of disorders are rich in both potential and challenges. Relatively rare disorders and outcomes require large sample sizes; complex conditions require considerable effort and resources for accurate assessment and characterization; multiple contributing factors from the molecular to the societal level require rich exposure assessments; and the complexity of the human condition introduces a range of potential confounding factors. Each of the study designs presented in this chapter has advanced our knowledge of how disorders originate, progress, may be treated, and may diminish over the life course. Yet they have been traditionally used to investigate relative static conditions, disorders, and disease states. Further work applying the principles of life course health development to study design, measurement, and analytic approaches are essential to help realize the goals and aspirations of the life course framework (Buka and Lipsitt 1994; Buka 2003).

References

Ahern, J., & Leslie, H. H. (2014). Life course approach to substance use. In K. C. Koenen, S. Rudenstine, S. Galea, & E. Susser (Eds.), *A life course approach to mental disorders* (pp. 133–140). Oxford: Oxford University Press.

Angold, A., & Costello, E. J. (1995). Developmental epidemiology. *Epidemiologic Reviews, 17*(1), 74–82.

Aschengrau, A., & Seage, G. R. (2008). *Essentials of epidemiology in public health* (2nd ed.). Sudbury: Jones & Bartlett.

Baltes, P. B., Lindenberger, U., & Staudinger, U. M. (1998). Life-span theory n developmental psychology. In W. Damon & R. M. Lerner (Eds.), *Handbook of child psychology volume 1: Theoretical models of human development* (pp. 1029–1143). New York: Wiley.

Baltes, P. B., Lindenberger, U., & Staudinger, U. M. (2006). Life span theory in developmental psychology. In W. Damon & R. M. Lerner (Eds.), *Handbook of child psychology: Vol. 1. Theoretical models of development* (6th ed., pp. 569–664). Hoboken: Wiley.

Barker, D. J. P. (2004). The developmental origins of adult disease. *Journal of the American College of Nutrition, 23*(Suppl 6), 588S–595S.

Ben-Shlomo, Y., & Kuh, D. (2002). A life course approach to chronic disease epidemiology: Conceptual models, empirical challenges and interdisciplinary perspectives. *International Journal of Epidemiology, 31*(2), 285–293.

Berney, L. R., & Blane, D. B. (1997). Collecting retrospective data: Accuracy of recall after 50 years judged against historical records. *Social Science & Medicine, 45*(10), 1519–1525.

Boomsma, D., Busjahn, A., & Peltonen, L. (2002). Classical twin studies and beyond. *Nature Reviews Genetics, 3*, 872–882.

Bremner, J. D., Southwick, S. M., Darnell, A., & Charney, D. S. (1996). Chronic PTSD in Vietnam combat veterans: Course of illness and substance abuse. *The American Journal of Psychiatry, 153*(3), 369–375.

Broman, S. (1984). *The collaborative perinatal project: An overview*. New York: Praeger.

Broman, S., Bien, E., & Shaughnessy, P. (1985). *Low achieving children: The first seven years*. Hillsdale: Lawrence Erlbaum Associates.

Buka, S. L. (2003). Principles of developmental epidemiology. In S. H. White & D. B. Pillemer (Eds.), *Developmental psychology and the social changes of our time*. Cambridge, MA: Harvard University Press.

Buka, S. L., & Lipsitt, L. P. (1994). Toward a developmental epidemiology. In S. L. Friedman & H. C. Haywood (Eds.), *Developmental follow-up: Concepts, domains and methods* (pp. 331–350). San Diego: Academic Press.

Bundey, S. (1991). Uses and limitations of twin studies. *Journal of Neurology, 238*(7), 360–364.

Cerda, M., Sánchez, B. N., Sandro, G., Tracy, M., & Buka, S. L. (2008). Estimating co-occurring behavioral trajectories within a neighborhood context: A case study of multivariate transition models for clustered data. *American Journal of Epidemiology, 168*(10), 1190–1203.

Chilcoat, H. W., & Breslau, N. (1998). Investigations of causal pathways between PTSD and drug use disorders. *Addictive Behaviors, 23*(6), 827–840.

Clark, D. B., Lesnick, L., & Hegedus, A. M. (1997). Traumas and other adverse life events in adolescents with alcohol abuse and dependence. *Journal of the American Academy of Child and Adolescent Psychiatry, 36*(12), 1744–1751.

Cohen, J. A., Mannarino, A. P., Perel, J. M., & Staron, V. (2007). A pilot randomized controlled trial of combined trauma-focused CBT and sertraline for childhood PTSD symptoms. *Journal of the American Academy of Child and Adolescent Psychiatry, 46*(7), 811–819.

Cutajar, M. C., Mullen, P. E., Ogloff, J. R. P., Thomas, S. D., Wells, D. L., & Spataro, J. (2010). Psychopathology in a large cohort of sexually abused children followed up to 43 years. *Child Abuse & Neglect, 34*(11), 813–822.

Elder, G. H., Jr., & Rockwell, R. C. (1979). The life-course and human development: An ecological perspective. *International Journal of Behavioral Development, 2*(1), 1–21.

Elder, G. H., & Shanahan, M. J. (2007). The life course and human development. In *Handbook of child psychology* (6th ed., pp. 665–715). New York: Wiley.

Ernster, V. L. (1994). Nested case-control studies. *Preventive Medicine, 23*(5), 587–590.

Felitti, V. J., Anda, R. F., Nordenberg, D., Williamson, D. F., Spitz, A. M., Edwards, V., Koss, M. P., & Marks, J. S. (1998). Relationship of childhood abuse and household dysfunction to many of the leading causes of death in adults. The Adverse Childhood Experiences (ACE) study. *American Journal of Preventative Medicine, 14*(4), 245–258.

Fergusson, D. M., Horwood, L. J., & Woodward, L. J. (2000). The stability of child abuse reports: A longitudinal study of the reporting behaviour of young adults. *Psychological Medicine, 30*(3), 529–544.

George, L. K. (1999). *Life-course perspectives on mental health* (pp. 565–583). New York: Springer.

Giele, J. Z., & Elder, G. H., Jr. (1998). Life course research: Development of a field. In J. Z. Giele & G. H. Elder Jr. (Eds.), *Methods of life course research: Qualitative and quantitative approaches* (pp. 5–27). Thousand Oaks, CA: Sage.

Gilman, S. E. (2002). Commentary: Childhood socioeconomic status, life course pathways and adult mental health. *International Journal of Epidemiology, 31*(2), 403–404.

Gilman, S. E., Martin, L. T., Abrams, D. B., Kawachi, I., Kubzansky, L., et al. (2008). Educational attainment and cigarette smoking: A causal association? *International Journal of Epidemiology, 37*, 615–624.

Halfon, N., & Forrest, C. B. (2017). The emerging theoretical framework of life course health development. In N. Halfon, C. B. Forrest, R. M. Lerner, & E. Faustman (Eds.), *Handbook of life course health-development science*. Cham: Springer.

Halfon, N., Larson, K., Lu, M., Tullis, E., & Russ, S. (2014). Lifecourse health-development: Past, present and future. *Matern Child Health, 18*(2), 344–365.

Jablonka, E., & Lamb, M. J. (2005). *Evolution in four dimensions: Genetic, epigenetic, behavioral, and symbolic variation in the history of life*. Cambridge, CA: The MIT Press.

Kraemer, H. C., Yesavage, J. A., Taylor, J. L., & Kupfer, D. (2000). How can we learn about developmental processes from cross-sectional studies, or can we? *The American Journal of Psychiatry, 157*(2), 163–171.

Kuh, D., Ben-Shlomo, Y., Lynch, J., Hallqvist, J., & Power, C. (2003). Life course epidemiology. *Journal of Epidemiology and Community Health, 57*(10), 778–783.

Lee, W., Bindman, J., Ford, T., et al. (2007). Bias in psychiatric case—Control studies. *The British Journal of Psychiatry, 190*(3), 204–209.

Lerner, R. M., & Callina, K. S. (2014). Relational developmental systems theories and the ecological validity of experimental designs: Commentary on Freund and Isaacowitz. *Human Development, 56*, 372–380.

Lichtenstein, P., De Faire, U., Floderus, B., Svartengren, M., Svedberg, P., & Pedersen, N. L. (2002). The Swedish twin registry: A unique resource for clinical, epidemiological and genetic studies. *Journal of Internal Medicine, 252*(3), 184–205.

Magnusson, D. (Ed.). (1996). *The lifespan development of individuals: Behavioral, neurobiological and psychosocial perspectives*. Cambridge, CA: Cambridge University Press.

Mills, K. L., Teesson, M., Back, S. E., Brady, K. T., Baker, A. L., et al. (2012). Integrated exposure-based therapy for co-occurring posttraumatic stress disorder and substance dependence. *JAMA, 308*(7), 690–699.

Moffitt, T. E. (2013). Childhood exposure to violence and lifelong health: Clinical intervention science and stress-biology research join forces. *Development and Psychopathology (Cambridge University Press), 25*, 1619–1634.

Molnar, B. E., Buka, S. L., & Kessler, R. C. (2001). Child sexual abuse and subsequent psychopathology: Results from the National Comorbidity Survey. *American Journal of Public Health, 91*(5), 753–760.

Monitoring the Future: a continuing study of American youth (2016). University of Michigan. http://www.monitoringthefuture.org/

Moore, D. S. (2015).The asymmetrical bridge: A review of James Tabery's book "Beyond versus." *Acta Biotheoretica*. doi: 10.1007/s10441–015-9270-z.

Nagin, D. S. (2016). Group-based trajectory modeling and criminal career research. *Journal of Research in Crime and Delinquency, 53*(3), 356–371.

National Survey on Drug Use and Health (2017). Substance Abuse and Mental Health Services Administration. U.S. Department of Health and Human Services. https://nsduhweb.rti.org

Nelson, E. C., Heath, A. C., Madden, P. A., Cooper, M. L., Dinwiddie, S. H., Bucholz, K. K., Glowinski, A., McLaughlin, T., Dunne, M. P., Statham, D. J., & Martin, N. G. (2002). Association between self-reported childhood sexual abuse and adverse psychosocial outcomes: Results from a twin study. *JAMA Psychiatry, 59*(2), 139–145.

Nomura, Y., Gilman, S. E., & Buka, S. L. (2011). Maternal smoking during pregnancy and risk of alcohol use disorders among adult offspring. *Journal of Studies on Alcohol and Drugs, 72*, 199–209.

Patel, C. J., Bhattacharya, J., & Butte, A. J. (2010). An environment-wide association study (EWAS) on type 2 diabetes mellitus. *PloS One, 5*(5), e10746. doi:10.1371/journal.pone.0010746.

Pickles, A., Maughan, B., & Wadsworth, M. (2007). *Epidemiological methods in life course research*. New York: Oxford University Press.

Reijneveld, S. A., Crone, M. R., Verhulst, F. C., & Verloove-Vanhorick, S. P. (2003). The effect of a severe disaster on the mental health of adolescents: A controlled study. *Lancet, 362*(9385), 691–696.

Rothman, K. J., Greenland, S., & Lash, T. L. (2008). *Modern epidemiology* (3rd ed.). Philadelphia: Lippincott Willams & Wilkins.

Sampson, R. J. (2010). Gold standard myths: Observations on the experimental turn in quantitative criminology. *Journal of Quantitative Criminology, 26*(4), 489–500.

Schlesselman, J. J., & Schneiderman, M. A. (1982). Case control studies: Design, conduct, analysis. *Journal of Occupational and Environmental Medicine, 24*(11), 879.

Silva, P. A., & Stanton, W. R. (1997). *From child to adult: The Dunedin Multidisciplinary health and development study*. New York: Oxford University Press.

Skytthe, A., Kyvik, K. O., Holm, N. V., & Christensen, K. (2011). The Danish twin registry. *Scandinavian Journal of Public Health, 39*(7 Suppl), 75–78.

Stratford, R., Mulligan, J., Downie, B., & Voss, L. (1999). Threats to validity in the longitudinal study of psychological effects: The case of short stature. *Child: Care, Health and Development, 25*(6), 401–419.

Susser, M., & Susser, E. (1996). Choosing a future for epidemiology: II. From black box to Chinese boxes and eco-epidemiology. *American Journal of Public Health, 86*(5), 674–677.

Susser, E., Terry, M. B., & Matte, T. (2000). The birth cohorts grow up: New opportunities for epidemiology. *Paediatric and Perinatal Epidemiology, 14*(2), 98–100.

Tabery, J. (2014). *Beyond versus: The struggle to understand the interaction of nature and nurture*. Cambridge: MIT Press.

The Millenium Cohort Study (2010). Department of Defense. https://www.millenniumcohort.org/

The Woodlawn Project: A Life Course Study (2017). Johns Hopkins Bloomberg School of Public Health. http://www.jhsph.edu/research/affiliated-programs/woodlawn-study/

Van Dam, D., Vedel, E., Ehring, T., & Emmelkamp, P. M. G. (2012). Psychological treatments for concurrent posttraumatic stress disorder and substance use disorder: A systematic review. *Clinical Psychology Review, 32*(3), 202–214.

Wacholder, S., Silverman, D. T., McLaughlin, J. K., & Mandel, J. S. (1992). Selection of controls in case-control studies. II. Types of controls. *American Journal of Epidemiology, 135*(9), 1029–1041.

Wadsworth, M. E. J., Butterworth, S. L., Hardy, R. J., et al. (2003). The life course prospective design: An example of benefits and problems associated with study longevity. *Social Science & Medicine, 57*(11), 2193–2205.

Widom, C. S., Zaja, C., & Du Mont, K. A. (2015). Intergenerational transmission of child abuse and neglect: Real or detection bias? *Science, 347*(27), 1480–1485.

Woodward, M. (2005). *Epidemiology: Study design and data analysis* (2nd ed.). Boca Raton: Chapman & Hall/CRC Press.

6

Using the National Longitudinal Surveys of Youth (NLSY) to Conduct Life Course Analyses

Elizabeth C. Cooksey

1 Introduction

The National Longitudinal Surveys of Youth (NLSY) include two separate youth cohorts in the United States: the NLSY79 that started in 1979 and the NLSY97 that began in 1997. Each is a nationally representative, longitudinal study with high response rates and frequent follow-ups. Also under the NLSY family of studies are the NLSY79 Child and Young Adult surveys, which follow all children born to female NLSY79 respondents. Data from the NLSY are used by researchers from a wide variety of disciplines including sociology, economics, geography, public health, nursing, psychology, statistics, education, maternal and child health, public policy, and political science. Data are free and easy to access and have also been utilized in cross-national research and policy studies.

Another indicator of the importance of the NLSY is the number of publications written by researchers. As of August 2015, 2892 articles, 188 book chapters, and 131 monographs were listed in the NLS bibliography as using at least one of the three NLSY surveys, along with 862 PhD dissertations. In 2014 there were 2250 registered users who downloaded NLSY data, and many others did so as non-registered guests.

In this chapter I begin with a brief history of the National Longitudinal Surveys. I then provide more in-depth information on the three NLSY surveys: the NLSY79, the NLSY79 Child and Young Adult Surveys, and the NLSY97. Next I illustrate some of the ways in which the NLSY provides unique opportunities for researchers. I then present an overview of information pertaining to health that is available in each of the surveys and highlight some of the health-related life course research that has been undertaken using one or more of the NLSY datasets. I conclude with information on how NLSY data may be obtained.

2 A Brief History of the NLS: The Original Cohorts

2016 marked the 50th anniversary of the first National Longitudinal Survey (NLS) interview and 50 years of involvement in the NLS project by the Center for Human Resource Research (CHRR) at The Ohio State University. Sponsored by the US Department of Labor, the first cohort of *Older Men* consisted of 5020 males born

E.C. Cooksey (✉)
Center for Human Resource Research, The Ohio State University, Suite 200, 921 Chatham Lane, Columbus, OH 43221, USA
e-mail: Cooksey.1@osu.edu

between 1906 and 1921 who were ages 45–59 when first interviewed by the Census Bureau in 1966. This cohort was selected to enable research on the employment patterns of men as they neared the completion of their careers and answer questions regarding their plans for retirement. An oversample of black respondents was included, and 13 interviews were conducted over a span of 24 years. A total of 2092 Older Men were interviewed in 1990 when they were ages 71–83 years old, and interviews were also conducted with 2206 widows or other family members of deceased respondents. Although primarily focused on aspects of employment income and retirement, the survey also collected information on health and physical condition.

The NLS of *Young Men*, a sample of 5225 males born between 1941 and 1952, was also started in 1966 when they were 14–24 years old. The Young Men's cohort chronicled the employment patterns of men transitioning from school and into the work force or joining the military, i.e., making initial career and job decisions that would impact their employment in the decades to follow. Twelve interviews were conducted between 1966 and 1981 when the study ended. As with the Older Men, young black men were oversampled, and information was collected on health and physical condition.

The following year, 1967, a sample of 5083 *Mature Women* born between 1922 and 1937 was drawn to study the return of women to the labor force as their children grew up, and to investigate how women balanced the roles of homemaker, mother, and labor force participant. A total of 22 surveys were undertaken with these women, with their first interview at ages 30–44 and their last interview in 2003, at ages 63–77. Finally, in 1968, 5159 *Young Women* were interviewed at ages 14–24 as they were completing school, making career and job decisions, and starting families. Twenty-two interviews were undertaken with the Young Women's cohort, ending in 2003. As with both Original Cohorts of males, the two cohorts of female respondents again included oversamples of blacks and survey questions on health and physical condition.

3 The National Longitudinal Surveys of Youth

The *NLSY79* originally comprised a sample of 12,686 men and women born between 1957 and 1964 who were living in the United States when the survey began. When first interviewed in 1979, they were ages 14–22 years. This time CHRR partnered with the National Opinion Research Center (NORC) to undertake the fielding of the survey, which was conducted primarily with funds from the Bureau of Labor Statistics at the US Department of Labor, although other agencies provided funding for various purposes. For example, the National Institute of Child Health and Human Development (NICHD) has supported the collection of a wide range of data in the NLSY79, including marriage and fertility histories for all respondents as well as comprehensive pre- and postnatal data relating to each child born to female NLSY79 respondents and information pertaining to child health and childcare from the early survey years. The Armed Services Vocational Aptitude Battery (ASVAB) was administered to both the civilian and military youth samples interviewed in 1980 ($N = 11{,}914$) with sponsorship from the Department of Defense (DoD). These data include respondent raw scores, standard scores, scale scores, and standard errors for each of the ten test sections, including general science, arithmetic reasoning, work knowledge, mechanical comprehension, and two constructed Armed Forces Qualifications Test (AFQT) scores. The AFQT has been shown to be a significant predictor of later life course outcomes across a whole range of social, economic, educational, and health domains. Support from the DoD also made possible the 1979–1984 interviews of 1280 youth enlisted in the military.

Beginning in 1979, a 5-year collaborative effort between CHRR and the National Center for Research in Vocational Education resulted in a survey of the high schools civilian NLSY79 respondents attended, along with the collection of detailed transcript information, for 8778 NLSY79 respondents expected to complete high school during the 1980–1983 survey years.

Information on up to 64 high school courses, including course descriptions, final grades, and credit received, was collected. Moreover, data were gathered from the record of the last secondary school attended by the NLSY79 respondents. These variables include both respondent-specific and school-specific information on such factors as (a) the respondent's school enrollment status, highest grade attended, remedial classes taken, and scores/percentiles/grade levels for various intelligence and aptitude tests administered during the youth's schooling and (b) each school's total enrollment, grading system, types of curricula offered, dropout rate, student body composition, and staffing characteristics. In addition, the National Institute of Education sponsored a set of time-use questions in 1981, and a self-report supplement to the 1980 survey was funded by the US Department of Justice to collect data on respondents' participation in, and income from, various delinquent and criminal activities. Lastly, funding from the National Institute on Alcohol Abuse and Alcoholism and the National Institute on Drug Abuse has made possible expanded sets of alcohol and substance use questions.

The NLSY79 cohort was selected to replicate the NLS of Young Women and Young Men cohorts and was also designed to help researchers and policymakers evaluate the expanded employment and training programs for youths legislated by the 1977 amendments to the Comprehensive Employment and Training Act. Survey respondents have been interviewed every year through 1994 and every other year since then. The 2014/2015 survey marked the 26th round of data collection, with respondents ages 50–58 at the start of the round.

Interviews are conducted either face to face or by telephone, with telephone mode increasing with each subsequent round as respondents have become more geographically dispersed or expressed a preference for phone interviews. In recent rounds more than 90% have been conducted by telephone.

The initial sample of 12,686 youth interviewed in 1979 comprised a cross-sectional sample of 6111 respondents designed to represent the noninstitutionalized civilian segment of people living in the United States in 1979 and born between January 1, 1957, and December 31, 1964, along with a supplemental sample of 5295 civilian Hispanic or Latino/Latina, black, and economically disadvantaged nonblack/non-Hispanic respondents of the same ages. Also included was a sample of 1280 respondents designed to represent the population serving in one of the four branches of the US military as of September 30, 1978, who were born between January 1, 1957, and December 31, 1961, and who were therefore ages 17–21 as of December 31, 1978. The initial sample was evenly divided by gender and had 7510 nonblack/non-Hispanic respondents, 3174 black respondents, and 2002 Hispanic or Latino/Latina respondents. Due to budget constraints, 1079 members of the supplemental sample of armed forces youth were discontinued after the 1984 survey, and the economically disadvantaged nonblack/non-Hispanic supplemental sample of 1643 individuals was discontinued after 1990. In Round 25 (completed in 2013), over 80% of respondents in the remaining sample types were interviewed; of these respondents, 69% had answered every survey round since 1979 with a further 14% answering all but one.

The oversamples of black and Hispanic respondents and the fact that data have been collected either every year or every other year from the same set of people over such a long period of time, so many of them answering questions at 24 or more separate survey points, make the NLSY79 a remarkable panel study of individuals ideally suited for life course studies. Beginning in their teenage years, these individuals were followed as they left secondary school, entered college or training programs, moved into their first jobs, moved in with partners, got married, had children (although not necessarily in that order), lost jobs, changed jobs, had more children, bought and sold houses, progressed into middle age, began to think that they might like to retire one day, and paid into pension plans. And throughout these years, NLSY79 respondents answered not only questions about work, marriage, and family activities but also about beliefs, hopes, and expectations for the future, mental and physical health, alcohol and drug use, and sexual activity and contraceptive use. Although at its heart the NLSY79 remains a labor survey, its breadth of topics covered ensures that the nuances of people's work lives can be placed into the much larger context within which people actually live their lives. And as I describe later, the NLSY79 has also collected information on a host of healthy and unhealthy behaviors and a range of mental and physical health antecedents and outcomes that are not only important in terms of people's work lives but provide unique opportunities for health researchers who wish to study health over the life course.

Although the NLSY79 is a survey of individuals rather than a survey of households, respondents interviewed in 1979 originated from 8770 unique households out of which 2862 households included more than one NLSY79 respondent. The most common relationships between respondents living in multiple respondent households at this time were those of sibling or spouse: 5863 respondents were members of a household containing multiple interviewed siblings (biological, step, or adopted), and 334 respondents were members of a household in which their spouse was also interviewed (see Table 1).

The NLSY79 Child and Young Adult Surveys The NLSY79 Child study began in 1986 with funding from NICHD; at that time there were 5255 children reported by 2922 interviewed mothers. Designed to obtain comprehensive information on the experiences of children born to female NLSY79 respondents, a battery of cognitive, socioemotional, and physiological assessments has been administered biennially to all children of selected ages through 1992 and to children below the age of 15 since 1994. Some of these assessments directly assess each child's development using nationally normed tests such as the Peabody Picture Vocabulary Test-Revised (PPVT-R) which measures a child's hearing vocabulary; the Digit Span subscale of the Wechsler Intelligence Scale for Children-Revised (WISC-R) which measures short-term memory (Wechsler 1974); the Peabody Individual Achievement Test (PIAT): math, reading recognition, and reading comprehension assessments which measure ability in mathematics, oral reading, and the ability to derive meaning from printed words (Dunn and Dunn 1981); and Harter's Self-Perception Profile for Children (SPPC) that measures a child's perceived competence in academics and sense of general self-worth (Harter 1985). Although all of these tests have been administered to children of the NLSY79 biennially, the ages at which they were given have sometimes changed, and users of the data are advised to check the user's guide at https://www.nlsinfo.org. As shown in Table 2, other tests such as the McCarthy Scale of Children's Abilities: Verbal Memory subscale, Memory for Location Assessment, and Body Parts Assessment were only administered in early rounds of the survey.

The number of children assessed during a given child survey year is a function of the number of children born to interviewed NLSY79 mothers, the number of children living in the homes of those mothers, and, finally, the number of those children actually interviewed. Of the 5842 NLSY79 females eligible for the first child interview in 1986, 2922 mothers and 4971 children were interviewed. From this sample of eligible children, assessment data were collected for 4786 of them.

Each mother also provides reports on her children's temperament, motor and social development, behavior problems, and home environment. Three age-specific versions of the temperament scale assess such factors as activity, predictability, positive affect, fearfulness, compliance, and insecure attachment among young children; the motor and social development scale measures milestones in the areas of motor, cognitive, communication, and social development for children

Table 1 Number of NLSY79 civilian respondents by type of single/multiple sibling household, 1979

Type of household	Number of respondents	Number of households
Single respondent	5908	5908
Multiple siblings		
Two siblings	3386	1693
Three siblings	1725	575
Four siblings	604	151
Five siblings	130	26
Six siblings	18	3
Total multiple siblings	**5863**	**2448**

Table 2 Child assessments by year of survey

Child assessment	1986	1988	1990	1992	1994	1996-2014
Parts of the body: number of body parts child can identify by common names	*	*				
Memory for locations: how long child remembers the location of the doll	*	*				
Verbal memory test: ability to remember and repeat word sequences	*	*	*	*	*	
Peabody Picture Vocabulary Test (PPVT)	*	*	*	*	*	*
Memory for Digit Span test (WISC-R): memory for number order	*	*	*	*	*	*
PIAT math subtest	*	*	*	*	*	*
PIAT reading: recognition and comprehension subtests	*	*	*	*	*	*
SPPC: what child thinks he or she is like, how he or she thinks and feels	*	*	*	*	*	*
Temperament scales	*	*	*	*	*	*
Motor and social development scale (not administered in 2004)	*	*	*	*	*	*
Behavior problems index	*	*	*	*	*	*
Interviewer evaluation of testing conditions	*	*	*	*	*	*
HOME-SF inventory	*	*	*	*	*	*

*Signifies that those questions were asked in that particular survey round

under age four; and one of the most widely used scales in research on children using the NLSY79 is the Behavior Problems Index (BPI) which is completed for all children ages four and over. The BPI consists of an overall behavior problem score that is comprised of six subscales (antisocial, anxious or depressed, hyperactive, headstrong, dependent, and peer conflicts), and individual items may also be classified as internality and externality scales. Interviewer assessments of children's shyness, cooperation, interest, and persistence during the interview, as well as their attitude about and rapport with the interviewer, are also collected. The final measure in Table 2, the Home Observation Measurement of the Environment-Short Form (HOME-SF), is a modification of the HOME inventory (Caldwell and Bradley 1984) and is a unique measure of the quality of the cognitive stimulation and emotional support provided by a child's family. This measure has also been extensively used in research as both an input in helping to explain other child characteristics or behaviors and as an outcome to explain associations between the quality of a child's home environment and earlier familial and maternal traits and behaviors.

The NLSY79 Child surveys have also gathered substantial information about the educational experiences of each child. Mothers have provided information about preschool and regular school attendance, type of school attended, grades skipped or repeated, and how well the child performs in class. Since 1988, children ages 10 and over have supplied information on characteristics of their school, the involvement of their parents in their education, and their educational expectations. In 1995–1996 a one-time school survey—funded by a grant through the National Institute of Child Health and Human Development—was conducted to collect information from school officials at schools attended by NLSY79 child respondents in grades 1 through 12 during either the 1993–1994 or 1994–1995 school year. This effort gathered information about the characteristics of the school and standardized test scores recorded from student transcripts.

Each child survey from 1988 onward has also collected self-reported information from children age 10 and older about child-parent interactions, responsibilities at home, attitudes toward school, time use, employment, religious attendance, alcohol and drug use, sexual activity (at age 13 and older), dating and friendship patterns, and various other attitudes and behaviors.

In 1994, the NLSY79 data collection was again expanded to incorporate extensive interviews with NLSY79 *Young Adults*. This is not a new cohort but rather what NLSY79 Children are called when they turn age 15 (technically, the young adult sample is defined as children who have their 15th birthday in the year they are interviewed; thus, some of them are still age 14 when interviewed as young adults). In 1994, 6109 children under age 15 and 980 young adults reported by 3464 mothers were interviewed. In 1994 and 1996, the young adult data collection effort was part and parcel of the child data collection effort under a contract with the US Department of Labor with funds provided by NICHD. In 1998, because of funding constraints, interviews were limited to young adults under age 21. Since 2000, however, CHRR has obtained separate funds through the NICHD grant process to continue to interview young adults aged 21 and over and hence expand the analytical value of these data. All young adults ages 15–30 are interviewed biennially, and after age 30, they are interviewed every other survey round or roughly every 4 years.

In 1994, 1996, and 1998, the interviews were mainly conducted in person and included two parts. First was a computer-assisted personal interview that largely paralleled the main NLSY79 data collection but with a greater focus on youth issues. This included detailed employment, education, and family/relationship profiles, income, training, military service, and attitudinal measures and assessments such as the Rosenberg Self-Esteem Scale and the CESD depression scale. Second, young adults completed a confidential self-report questionnaire which focused on more sensitive issues including sexual activity, contraception, expectations for the future, dating and relationship experiences, political attitudes, pro-social behaviors, substance use, and risk-taking attitudes.

Other questions continued or were parallel to questions from the Child survey such as data on routine health checks, accidents and injuries, dating behaviors, the respondent's relationship with his or her parents, risk-taking behaviors, and school experiences and satisfaction.

The 2000 and later data collection efforts shifted to focus more heavily on recent mainstream employment and family experiences for the older grant-age young adults, many of whom had completed their schooling. Examples of more tailored questions for this older age group include the timing of and reasons for leaving home, the contact young adults had with their parents when they left home, their marriage and cohabitation histories, and (as they entered parenthood) the different kinds of childcare facilities they used and how much their childcare arrangements cost. In 2004 a series of questions on asthma was added, and the Ten-Item Personality Inventory (TIPI) was included in 2006. In 2008 the survey incorporated a six-item anger scale and questions on whether or not respondents had seen action in combat zones, with whom their biological children lived at the time of their birth, and more details about healthy activities. Also, building from qualitative research done by Wendy Manning and Pamela Smock (2005), new questions were designed to get a better handle on the types of relationships and dating activities that youth engaged in during their teens and twenties. Additional health-related questions were included between 2010 and 2014 and these are described in more detail in the health section.

At the start of the 2014 field period for round 26 of the NLSY79, female respondents were ages 50–57 and had essentially completed their fertility. At this time a total of 11,512 children were known to have been born to the original 6283 NLSY79 female respondents. Most of these births occurred during the years this cohort has been interviewed although a modest number of children were born prior to 1979. An unknown number of additional children will have been born to women who have left the survey (mostly as a result of being part of the economically disadvantaged oversample that was dropped after 1990) subsequent to their attrition. Fifty-one percent are sons and 49% are daughters, and based on the race/ethnicity of their mothers, 53% would be classified as nonblack/non-Hispanic, 28% as black, and 19% as Hispanic. The oldest child was born in 1970 to a teenage mother. The youngest child was born in 2011 to a mother in the older childbearing years. At the time of the first interview in 1986, child ages ranged from 0 to 15 years of age. In 2014/2015 NLSY79 Children were 0–14 years old and Young Adults were ages

14–44 years. Finally, retention rates have again been very high: at the end of fielding in 2013, 81% of young adults and 90% of children eligible to be fielded during this survey round had been interviewed. Of these respondents, close to 77% of young adults had been interviewed either every time or all but once which translates into 13 or 14 different data points over a 28-year period.

The *NLSY97* is the newest survey in the NLS program and comprises a sample of 8984 young men and women born between 1980 and 1984 who were ages 12–17 when first interviewed in 1997. As with the NLSY79, the NLSY97 also had a cross-sectional sample of respondents designed to be representative of people at those ages and living in the United States at the time (N = 6748) and a supplemental sample of 2236 black and Hispanic respondents, which resulted in a total sample that was 52% nonblack/non-Hispanic, 26% black, 21% Hispanic or Latino/Latina, and just under 1% mixed race. Because all household residents in the appropriate age range were selected, again some households included more than one NLSY97 respondent, the most common relationship being that of siblings. The original sample in 1997 was 51% male and 49% female.

CHRR and NORC again partnered to undertake the study which was also primarily funded by the BLS. Other agencies have contributed to the project over the years, however. For example, in Round 1, a computer adaptive version of the Armed Services Vocational Aptitude Battery (ASVAB) was given to NLSY97 respondents with sponsorship by the Department of Defense. Various questions in the self-administered portion of the questionnaire, including questions on health, fertility, and social relationships, have been funded by the NICHD. School surveys were undertaken in 1996 and 2000 to collect information from all high schools with a 12th grade in the 147 NLSY97 primary sampling units as well as the collection and coding of high school transcripts, and this work was funded by the Department of Education. Questions on crime and criminal activities have been sponsored by the Department of Justice, Office of Juvenile Justice and Delinquency Prevention.

The NLSY97 cohort was designed to enable research on youths' transition from school to the labor market and into adulthood for a generation born into a very different time period than youth in the '79 cohort who had transitioned into adulthood during the 1980s: NLSY79 respondents are younger baby boomers, whereas NLSY97 respondents are the oldest of the millennial generation. These two cohorts have moved into early adulthood under very different educational, employment, and family building circumstances. Current population survey time trend data (www.census.gov/hhes/socdemo/education/data/cps/historical/index.html) show that in 1990, when the youngest NLSY79 cohort member was 25, the percentages of youth ages 25 and over who had completed high school or college were 23.7% for men and 22.8% for women. In 2009 when the youngest member of the NLSY97 cohort was age 25, the percentage for males had increased only slightly to 26.6%, but for women, the rise was substantial to 34.8%. Based on figures from the March 2013 current population survey, 38% of older millennial females ages 25–32 had a bachelor's degree. The corresponding figure for their male counterparts was 31%. Higher education has become increasingly important for successful labor force participation for millennials. According to a report from the Pew Research Center (2013), women accounted for 43% of the US labor force in 1980, and this rose to 47% in 2012. Among young women (ages 25–34), 74% were in the labor force in 2012, up from 66% in 1980. Labor force participation among men on the other hand has declined over the past 30 years, from 78% in 1980 to 70% in 2012. Furthermore, each new wave of adult men younger than age 35 has been less active in the labor market than the preceding wave. Living arrangements have also changed over time. For example, in 1987 when NLSY79 respondents were ages 22–29 years old, the percentage of 25–29-year-olds who had ever cohabited was 41%. In 2009–2010 when NLSY97 cohort members were 25–30, this percentage had risen to 66% (Bumpass and Sweet 1989; Bumpass and Lu 2000; Kennedy and Bumpass 2008).

The NLSY97 cohort is also ongoing and has been surveyed every year from 1997 through 2011 and biennially since. In 2015, 16 survey rounds had been completed and respondents were ages 28–34. Up until 2015, data collection has been primarily via in-person interviewing. Beginning in round 18, set to start in late fall of 2017, there will be a shift to mostly phone interviewing. As with the NLSY79 and the NLSY79 Child and Young Adult surveys, oversamples of black and Hispanic respondents, very high retention rates, and the fact that the same people have been interviewed so frequently make the NLSY97 another remarkable panel that is highly appropriate for longitudinal and life course studies, especially during the life course stages from adolescence through early adulthood when frequent education, employment, fertility, and living arrangement transitions occur. And again, response rates have been exceedingly high: in Round 16 which was completed in 2014, 81% of respondents not known to be deceased were interviewed. Of these interviewed respondents, 69.5% had answered all 16 surveys since 1997, and a further 12% had answered 15 of them.

4 The Uniqueness of the NLSY

Many factors make the NLSY datasets a unique source of data for researchers interested in studying the life course. First, there have been many rounds of data collection at very frequent intervals: NLSY79 respondents have been interviewed up to 26 times between when they were teens in 1979 and their late forties to mid-fifties in 2015; children born to NLSY79 females have been assessed and interviewed up to 15 times, most of them from birth onward; and NLSY97 respondents have been interviewed up to 16 times from their early to mid-teens into their thirties. Such a wealth of data can seem overwhelming at times, but they also lend themselves to a better understanding of important life course trajectories and how change in one area of life can lead to both short-term and longer-term change in other realms.

The length of time that these studies have been ongoing, and the extraordinarily high response rates achieved from so many individuals who have been prepared to share of their lives round after round, means that researchers can explore potential consequences of events that happen at early stages in the life course many years later, while still being able to account for a broad array of occurrences in the intervening years. In 2004, Hayward and Gorman published a paper in *Demography* titled "The Long Arm of Childhood: The Influence of Early-Life Social Conditions on Men's Mortality" in which they drew on the NLS Older Men's cohort to study links between various childhood conditions and mortality in adulthood. Although they had to rely on retrospective reports from men in their forties and fifties about their childhood years, their results showed that men's mortality was indeed associated with an array of childhood conditions including socioeconomic status, family living arrangements, mother's work status, rural residence, and parents' nativity. With information from multiple interviews to draw from, they were then able to demonstrate how, with the exception of parental nativity, these associations were mediated by various lifestyle factors, particularly body mass and socioeconomic achievement processes in adulthood. They concluded that their findings highlighted the idea that economic and educational policies targeted at children's well-being are implicitly health policies with effects that reach far into the adult life course. As the NLSY79 cohort ages into their retirement years and beyond, it will be possible to replicate this research with prospective rather than retrospective data, and the NLSY79 Child and Young Adult data will enable researchers to go back to the earliest years of childhood and even include prenatal conditions as reported by mothers.

The United States does not have birth cohort studies as other countries, such as the United Kingdom, do. However, data on the children of the NLSY79 do provide information on children from birth. With input from child development experts, the child study was designed to gather information from their mothers during infancy and early childhood, to assess children in their elementary and middle school years and to interview them from middle school onward into adolescence and adulthood.

As illustrated in Fig. 1 below, given the wealth of data that have been collected on these children

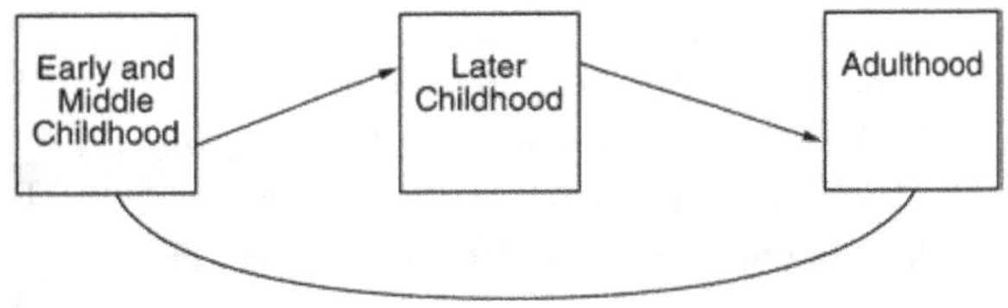

Fig. 1 Research possibilities using the NLSY79 Child and Young Adult data

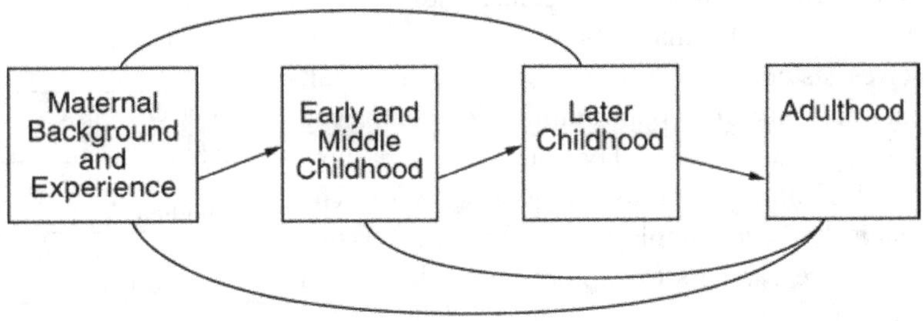

Fig. 2 Cross-generational research possibilities using the NLSY79 Maternal, Child, and Young Adult data

every other year, the NLSY79 Child and Young Adult data present researchers with enormous possibilities to link information ascertained when the child was quite young to outcomes in later childhood and beyond, plus to see how potential predictors from early or middle childhood of certain behaviors or outcomes in early adulthood or later might or might not be mediated by events and occurrences in later childhood or adolescence.

Of course, the 11,512 children of the NLSY do not constitute a birth cohort themselves as they were born between 1970 and 2011. However, they were all born to a cohort of women, and the NLSY79 Child/Young Adult files can be easily combined with information from the complete longitudinal record of their NLSY79 mothers. In addition, the Child/Young Adult dataset contains a number of created variables providing information on the mother with respect to the child's life situation. These constructed variables, drawn from the mother's record, include: family background, household composition, quarterly maternal work histories before and after each child's date of birth, educational background of members of the household, maternal health history, and information on childcare experiences during the first 3 years of life for all children of at least 1 year of age. Also available for each child are data regarding gestation and birth weight, as well as breastfeeding practices, other infant feeding practices, illnesses and injuries, and well-baby care in the first year of life. NLSY79 mothers also provide prenatal information for all births including data on their use of prenatal care, alcohol, cigarettes, marijuana, cocaine and dietary supplements and whether they had sonograms or amniocentesis during pregnancy.

As shown in Fig. 2, the availability of comprehensive child data, coupled with a wealth of longitudinal information on the background, and well-being of their NLSY79 mothers, provide researchers with a unique opportunity to undertake intergenerational research and examine linkages between maternal family behaviors and attitudes on the one hand and multiple aspects of their children's development on the other hand.

As an example, one might be interested not only in how deviancy develops from childhood into the young adult years but also in how the evolution of deviant behaviors might relate to behaviors and experiences in the prior generation—in this case among the youths' mothers. Further, as mentioned earlier, not only are similar data collected from both mothers and their children but retrospective reporting need not be relied on to link maternal reports of behaviors with those of their child, since data were collected from the NLSY79 mothers on their behaviors at, for example, ages 16 or 18 when they were 16 or 18, and then again from their children when they were 16 or 18 years old. The fact that many questions were asked of NLSY79 females and of their children when they were the same ages makes these data especially distinctive.

The information presented earlier in Table 1 provides another example of how the NLSY79 provides opportunities for life course research in ways not necessarily expected from cohort studies. Because information is collected for all children born to female respondents, and some of those NLSY79 female respondents were themselves sisters, the NLSY79 Child/Young Adult data not only offer opportunities for comparing developmental and other outcome measures between siblings but also between *cousins*. The relatively large sample of siblings and cousins permits researchers to explore both within- and cross-family effects to a greater extent than is typically possible. Over the course of the survey years, more than 3000 children in the sample have been identified as having an aunt in the NLSY79 main youth sample. Most of these children have one aunt, but there are also some child respondents with multiple aunts. The number of children who are cousins is also considerable.

More typically, researchers have tended to utilize the large number of child sibling sample cases that have been born to the female respondents. As shown in Table 3, 78.5% of NLSY79 women had at least one child, and most of them have had more than one, including a fairly large sample of women who have had three or more children by the end of their childbearing years. In addition to multiple births, there are many family units where two or more children are widely spaced in age. This enables exploring the impact of childbearing on children born to the same mother at different maternal life cycle stages.

A number of articles published in recent years have used either sibling data from the NLSY79 main youth sample or the Child and Young Adult sample or cousin data from this second generation (see, e.g., D'Onofrio et al. 2008, 2009a, b; Rodgers et al. 2008; Mendle et al. 2009; Jaffe et al. 2011; Goodnight et al. 2012 and Donahue et al. 2014).

Because there is considerable overlap in questions asked of NLSY97 and NLSY79 participants, intergenerational comparisons can be made using information from these two cohorts. Furthermore,

Table 3 NLSY79 women by number of children and race/ethnicity

Number of households				
Type of household (female)	Hispanic	Black	White	Total
Females with no children	**158**	**285**	**908**	1351
Mothers with 1 or more child	**844**	**1276**	**2812**	**4932**
Mothers with 1 child	147	278	750	1175
Mothers with 2 children	310	457	1204	1971
Mothers with 3 children	222	315	591	1128
Mothers with 4 or more children	165	226	267	658
Total	**1002**	**1561**	**3720**	**6283**

a significant number of NLSY79 Young Adults were born in the same years as NLSY97 respondents, and hence members of these two datasets can be compared with each other when overlap of questionnaire design allows. One of the drawbacks of the NLSY79 Young Adult data is that although young adults were born to women who were part of a nationally representative sample of youth living in the United States in 1979, due to immigration and fertility differentials by various background variables (e.g., race/ethnicity), the NLSY79 Young Adults are by no means nationally representative in nature. The NLSY97 respondents are, however, representative of teenagers who were living in the United States in 1997 and hence are a more generalizable sample. Although immigration since 1997 has changed the racial/ethnic makeup of the US population so that NLSY97 respondents are also no longer representative of all Young Adults in their thirties living in the US today, they are still closer than the NLSY79 Young Adults of the same ages.

On the other hand, the NLSY79 Young Adults of comparable age to the NLSY97 respondents have the strong advantage of having been followed since birth, plus in-depth information was gathered from their mothers over many years. Comparisons of research using the Young Adults with research utilizing the NLSY97 can therefore provide insights concerning the importance of non-representativeness in the Young Adult sample and potential selectivity bias in the NLSY97 due to the failure to include important prenatal or early childhood information. In other words, the strengths of one dataset can be used to evaluate potential weaknesses in the other.

Lastly, geographic residence information is available in all three datasets and the county and state of residence are provided in a separate restricted-access geocode CD that can be matched with other data sources to investigate community characteristics and contextual variables.

A number of design decisions make the NLSY97 the preferred choice of dataset to study certain behavioral choices and life events. For example, more in-depth data related to crime and delinquency are available in the NLSY97 than in the NLSY79, and a full cohabitation history also exists in the NLSY97 whereas the information available from NLSY79 respondents does not enable a complete record of living arrangements to be constructed. However, the linked NLSY79 and NLSY79 Child and Young Adult files are more ideally suited for the study of maternal and child health, since NLSY79 women have now aged through their fertile years and detailed information has been collected on all of their biological children. It is therefore the NLSY79 data that I primarily focus on in the next sections of this chapter.

5 Health Data in the NLSY Surveys

NLSY79 health sections are divided into two periods. Between 1979 and 1996, although the specific questions that were asked varied at times, most questions focused on health concerns that restricted or inhibited the respondent's ability to work. From 1998 on, as respondents reached middle age, the health section was expanded to provide a baseline profile of the respondent's overall health as they turned 40 years old. From 2008 onward, respondents have been asked another set of health questions when they turn 50.

Although the pre-1998 health questions provide a picture of the respondents' health restrictions at the time of interview, they offer little insight into chronic health problems that might affect their labor force activity in the future. For example, a serious ailment with slow development would not be picked up by the regular health questions until a respondent actually dropped out of the labor market. The extended *40-and-over health module* was therefore created to provide a baseline health profile for each respondent to facilitate research of the interrelationship of health and labor market activity in the advancement of retirement ages. Questions are not restricted to work-related health problems, and all questions are asked irrespective of the respondent's labor force status. Full information is available on www.nlsinfo.org but questions include items from the Center for Epidemiological Studies Depression Scale (CES-D), information on when respondents last saw a health care professional, and reports about the health and life status of the NLSY79 respondents' biological parents designed to improve researchers' understanding of hereditary health problems. The module also reproduces the SF-12 scale, a 12-question health survey designed by John Ware of the New England Medical Center Hospital that provides a measure of the respondents' mental and physical health irrespective of their proclivity to use formal health services (Ware et al. 1995). Finally, respondents are asked if they suffer from an extensive list of health conditions including asthma, back problems, problems with their feet and legs, kidney or bladder, stomach or intestinal ulcers, high cholesterol, chest pain, heart trouble, low blood pressure, sinus infections, joint swelling or pain, leg cramps, painful shoulders, elbows or knees, frequent headaches, severe tooth or gum trouble, skin diseases, and thyroid problems.

The *50-and-over health module* was included beginning in 2008 at which time the module was administered to respondents born in 1957–1958. In 2010, it was administered to those born in 1959–1960, and anyone who skipped the 2008 interview, and so on. This module contains many of the same questions as the 40-and-over health module. Some questions therefore provide a second decennial point of reference for general health information and many others provide updates on previously reported conditions.

Questions about diagnosis of skin cancer and other types of cancer, various heart disease-related conditions, and stroke were also asked.

50-and-over respondents are again administered the CES-D items and the SF-12 question series, as well as questions about the life and health status of their parents if they were previously reported as living. In addition, 50-and-over respondents update information on previously reported conditions such as hypertension/high blood pressure, diabetes/high blood sugar, asthma and non-asthma breathing problems, depression and other emotional/psychiatric problems, and arthritis. Questions have also been included on diagnosis of osteoporosis and the use of special equipment needed to accomplish usual activities, as well as a scale of functionality and the respondent's sleep habits.

In addition to the two health modules asked around age 40 and around age 50, other health questions have been incorporated into the NLSY79 questionnaire as mini-modules or small groups of questions to capture retrospective accounts of health in the childhood years prior to 1979, baseline measures of general health and cognition, information on the use of particular medications, and reports of head injuries. For example, in 2012 all respondents were asked a series of new questions on childhood health including overall health, major hospitalizations, or long periods of home recovery. Questions on childhood adversity that dealt with family mental health, alcohol abuse, physical abuse, and amount of parental affection were also added as researchers believe that questions such as these are predictive of adult obesity and other health-related outcomes.

Beginning in 2006, respondents ages 48 and 49 were given a battery of exercises designed to capture cognitive capabilities. Similar to the 50-and-over health module, this cognition module has also been administered to progressive 2-year birth year cohorts in the survey year during which they would turn at least age 48. This module solicits the respondent's own assessment of his/her general health, a word recall exercise using randomly assigned sets of ten words, and exercises requiring the respondent to count backward from a starting point by a specified number.

In 2004 a series of questions about asthma were added to the survey, and starting in 2008, respondents were asked if they were taking any statin drugs or heart medications. In 2012 all respondents were asked if they had experienced a serious head injury or loss of smell. Because traumatic head injury and loss of smell have been found in numerous studies to be linked to subsequent dementia, these questions were included to augment ongoing efforts to track respondents' cognitive function as they advance through middle age and beyond.

As mentioned in the section above, NLSY79 mothers have also provided a variety of information about their prenatal and postnatal activities relating to each child since 1983. Table 4 below summarizes some of the other health-related data available on *children born to NLSY79 mothers* and collected since the advent of the child survey in 1986:

Starting in 1996, mothers have additionally been asked to rate their child's health on a 4-point scale from "poor" to "excellent." Detailed information is available in the User's Guide at www.nlsinfo.org/content/cohorts/nlsy79-children/topical-guide/health.

Health questions continue as children become *Young Adults*. In some areas, questions closely parallel the health history obtained for all children of NLSY79 mothers (e.g., height and body weight, types of limitations, number of accidents and injuries in the last 12 months, hospitalizations resulting from these accidents/injuries, and insurance coverage). Young Adult respondents who do not live with their mother are also asked about illnesses and routine medical care. For younger Young Adults who do live with their mother, comparable questions are asked of the mother. Items from the CES-D depression scale are also asked of Young Adults in multiple survey rounds.

In 2004, respondents received two new series of questions. The first focused on health-related behaviors such as fruit and vegetable consumption, hours of sleep per night, and level of exercise. The second series was centered on asthma with detailed questions designed to track the onset of asthma and the persistence and severity of related symptoms. This series also includes two questions about whether anyone has smoked cigarettes in the respondent's home in the last 2 weeks and whether the respondent has routinely spent time somewhere in the last 2 weeks where they can smell cigarette smoke.

Table 4 Health-related data available on children of the NLSY79

Child health	1986	1988–1992	1994	1996–2002	2004–2012
Rating of child's health				M	M
Does health limit school or play	M	M	M	M	M
Physical, emotional, or mental condition requiring: treatment, medicine, or special equipment	M	M	M	M	M
Type/duration of limiting health conditions	M	M	M	M	M
Accidents/injuries needing medical attention in last 12 months	M	M	M	M	M
Accidents/injuries needing hospitalization since last interview/since birth		M	M	M	M
Number of illnesses requiring medical attention or treatment	M	M	M	M	M
Date of last routine health checkup	M	M	M	M	M
Date of last dental checkup/work	M	M	M	M	M
Source of health insurance, if any	M	M	M	M	M
Behavioral, emotional, or mental problems; did insurance cover doctor visit	M	M	M	M	M
Any medications or prescription drugs taken to help control activity/behavior	M	M	M	M	M
Menarche; age at first menses for female child (and mother)	M	M	M	M	M
Right-/left-handedness				M	M
Height and body weight of child	M-I	M-I	M-I	M-I	M-I
Healthcare during pregnancy leading to child's birth	M	M	M	M	M
Postnatal infant healthcare and feeding	M	M	M	M	M
Asthma					M/C

C child report, *M* mother report, *M-I* mother report or interviewer measurement

In 2006, a series of questions concerning catastrophic events that might adversely affect the health and well-being of respondents, such as death or imprisonment of a close relative, was included in the health section. These questions are a modified version of the catastrophic events series used in the NLSY97 questionnaire. Initially all respondents were asked about any such events that had occurred since they were 10 years old. Beginning in 2008, respondents who had previously answered this series are asked only about events since the date of last interview.

In 2010, several additional questions about healthy behaviors and routine checkups were included, and a *health and cognition module for respondents aged 29* and over was added. This module was modeled after the age 29 module from the NLSY97 with some adjustments and additions to also maintain comparability to the health modules in the NLSY79. For 2010 and 2012, this module was asked of all respondents ages 29 and older in order to get baseline information for all Young Adults. Thereafter, it has been asked only of respondents who are 29/30 or Young Adults who are over that age but have not yet completed the module. In 2012, a series of questions about head injuries, based on questions asked of NLSY79 respondents and described above, was incorporated into the health module.

The NLSY97 also collects information on the general health status of respondents in all rounds; for example, they report their height and weight and also describe how they would characterize their weight (very underweight, slightly underweight, etc.) and if they currently wish to lose or gain or stay at the weight they are. Information on health insurance coverage is collected in various rounds as are questions forming a five-item short version of the Mental Health Inventory (MHI-5), developed by Veit and Ware (1983). Information on various health conditions, medical treatments and visits, and out-of-the-ordinary stressors such as being a victim of a violent crime or being homeless is also collected in various survey rounds. In rounds 13–15, respondents who were 29 years of age answered a special series of health questions as a *Health-At-Age-29 health module*. These included questions about a family history of diseases (including detailed questions about diabetes), parents' mortality, respondents' health limitations (including limitations on moderate activities, climbing stairs, social activities, and productivity), energy level, and mood. Other questions were asked about whether the respondent had had a flu shot, a cholesterol test, diabetes test, pap smear, and blood pressure check at some point during the past 2 years. More information on health-related questions included in the NLSY97 can be found at https://www.nlsinfo.org/content/cohorts/nlsy97/topical-guide/health.

6 Health Research Using the NLSY Surveys

Considerable health-related research has been undertaken using the three NLSY surveys. In this section I highlight a sample of published studies and focus primarily on studies published since 2000 and those that center on child health. The NLS online bibliography (NLSinfo.org) provides a much more complete list of health focused studies. Of note, however, is the wide range of health topics studied, as well as the diversity of disciplinary backgrounds drawn upon. As the examples below illustrate, the surveys provide a great resource for examining aspects of life course health development.

Returning to Fig. 1, the first set of studies I feature use data from the NLSY79 Child and Young Adult surveys to look at health during childhood and adolescence. For example, Atkins and Matsuba (2008) use maternal ratings of childhood personality for over 1000 5- and 6-year-olds to derive resiliency, undercontrol and overcontrol prototypical profile scores. They then extend their analyses to later in childhood and examine whether childhood personality is associated with the likelihood and the timing of an unintentional injury requiring hospitalization or medical attention before the child turned age 13. Their findings suggest an inverse association between the likelihood of childhood unintentional injury and the overcontrolled prototype score. A recent paper by Cheadle and Goosby (2010) focuses on the complex interplay between childhood health and educational development over the early life course by estimating the relationship between birth weight, cognitive development, and timely high school completion. Their models therefore spanned childhood, adolescence, and early adulthood. Especially notable about this paper is the fact that they were able to adjust for fixed-family characteristics and aspects of the home environment by making use of information from siblings. Among several findings from this study, the authors noted that lower birth weight was associated with decreased cognitive skills at age 5 and marginally significantly slower growth rates into adolescence. They also showed that low birth weight increased the risk of not graduating by age 19. The authors concluded that their pattern of findings painted a multifaceted picture of disadvantage that begins in the womb and extends over the life course.

Reflecting the reality that childhood obesity is a major public health problem in the United States, many studies using the NLSY79 Child data focus on how obesity develops over the life course. For example, Huang and colleagues (Huang et al. 2013) identified developmental trajectories of obesity between ages 6 and 18 and classified four distinct categories: chronically obese, decreasing, increasing, and nonobese. They then studied associations between the various obesity trajectories and a number of risk behaviors and psychosocial health in adolescence. Although obesity trajectories were not found to be associated with greater trends in alcohol use or marijuana use, they did find that youth who became obese between childhood and adolescence had poorer psychosocial health compared to youth who followed other trajectories. Other potential effects of childhood overweight on health development have also been studied. For example, Richard Strauss (Strauss 2000) compared 9- and 10-year-old children who were obese and nonobese to see if they differed on global self-esteem scores. He found no significant difference at these ages between the two groups but by 13–14 years of age, significantly lower levels of self-esteem were observed in obese boys, obese Hispanic girls, and obese white girls compared with their nonobese counterparts. More recently, Averett and Stifel (2010) looked at the effect of obesity on cognitive development and uncovered significant effects when the relationship was examined separately by race and gender.

Other studies focusing on obesity in childhood and adolescence have incorporated maternal and family data into their analyses by merging data from NLSY79 mothers with data on their children as outlined in Fig. 2. The range of inputs varies considerably from breastfeeding versus bottle-feeding (Li et al. 2005; Salsberry and Reagan 2005; Seipel and Shafer 2013), food choices offered to young children (Faith et al. 2003), family income (Chia 2013), parental marital disruption and divorce (Arkes 2012), maternal prenatal behaviors such as smoking (Huang et al. 2014; Li et al. 2003; Salsberry and Reagan 2005, 2007; Seipel and Shafer 2013), maternal prepregnancy weight (Li et al. 2005; Salsberry and Reagan 2005, 2007), weight gain during pregnancy (Seipel and Shafer 2013), and other background factors such as parental engagement in children's daily activities, maternal age, and maternal education (Huang et al. 2014).

The relationship between various aspects of maternal employment and children's obesity has also gained attention. In a 2003 publication, Anderson, Butcher, and Levine suggest that increasing child obesity might be related to an increase in mothers working outside the home and posit that working mothers may not have time to prepare nutritious low-calorie meals and supervise their children's outdoor play that tends to expend calories. Using data on siblings to hold constant all of the family characteristics that might be correlated both with children's weight and mothers' hours worked, study results indicated that although children were more likely to be overweight if their mothers worked more hours per week over the child's life, it was higher socioeconomic status mothers whose work intensity was particularly deleterious for their children's overweight status. Others have also examined the relationship between maternal work hours and child obesity and found longer hours worked to be positively related to children's overweight (Courtemanche 2009; Liu et al. 2009). Other studies have found a more nuanced relationship, however. For example, Miller (2011) found that the timing of maternal work during a child's life mattered to the relationship and that effects of maternal work were confined to relatively low income families and to children who grew up with single mothers. Stewart et al. (2012) also found that unemployment events and the type of support that a mother received during unemployment spells were related to changes in children's weight.

Additional studies have examined various parental and family background influences on a range of child health development outcomes aside from child obesity. Some of these include how income and family structure impact routine medical and dental care provision for children (Berger 2004), the association between unwanted pregnancy and prenatal and postpartum maternal behaviors that adversely affect infant and child health (Joyce et al. 2000), the relationship between dark and cluttered home environments and the incidence of home injuries among children (Mott 1999), the distance between a child's home and a hospital and the probability of utilizing preventive care (Currie and Reagan 2003), length of maternity leave and children's immunizations (Berger et al. 2005), the effects of breastfeeding on long-term child health and well-being (Colen and Ramey 2014), various measures of economic disadvantage on intrauterine growth restriction (Reagan et al. 2007), household income histories, and changes in child depression levels (Strohschein 2005). Finally, a recent paper by Wolfe (2015) unpacked the components of socioeconomic status and found that children's health was more vulnerable to their families' wealth whereas adolescents' health was more sensitive to the current income of their families.

This brief and selected review of past studies provides a glimpse of the ways the NLSY data can be used to explore important aspects of life course health development. As the maternal and child health research community continues to explore how health develops across the life course, the NLSY can continue to be a rich source of data to answer important research questions.

7 Obtaining and Using NLSY Data

The NLSY public datasets (along with the data from the Original Cohorts) can be accessed free of charge through the NLS Investigator (www.nlsinfo.org/investigator), the data retrieval system used for obtaining public NLS data. In NLS Investigator, cohort-specific datasets can be searched by Area of Interest, Word in Title, Question Text, Question Name, Reference Number, and Survey Year. Also available at www.nlsinfo.org are cohort-specific Users Guides with an introduction to each sample, information on how to use and understand the data, topical guides, tutorials on various topics such as how to merge the NLSY79 Mother and Child data, and questionnaires for all rounds. Data can be downloaded into SAS, STATA, SPSS, and R. In addition to the public data, geocode data variables are available on a restricted basis: researchers interested in using the restricted data must complete an accessing agreement and be approved. Users with questions may also contact NLS User Services at usersvc@chrr.osu.edu for assistance with data use.

References

Anderson, P., Butcher, K., & Levine, P. (2003). Economic perspectives on childhood obesity. *Economic Perspectives, 27*(3), 30–49.

Arkes, J. (2012). Longitudinal association between marital disruption and child BMI and obesity. *Obesity, 20*(8), 1696–1702.

Atkins, R., & Matsuba, M. K. (2008). Association of personality and the likelihood of serious unintentional injury during childhood. *Journal of Pediatric Nursing, 23*(6), 451–459.

Averett, S., & Stifel, D. (2010). Race and gender differences in the cognitive effects of childhood overweight. *Applied Economics Letters, 17*(17), 1673–1679.

Berger, L. (2004). Income, family structure, and child maltreatment risk. *Children and Youth Services Review, 26*(8), 725–799.

Berger, L., Hill, J., & Waldfogel, J. (2005). Maternity leave, early maternal employment and child health and development in the US. *Economic Journal, 115*(501), F29–F47.

Bumpass, L., & Sweet, J. (1989). National estimates of cohabitation. *Demography, 26*(4), 615–625.

Bumpass, L., & Lu, H. (2000). Trends in cohabitation and implications for children's family contexts in the United States. *Population Studies, 54*, 29–41.

Caldwell, B., & Bradley, R. (1984). *Home observation for measurement of the environment*. Little Rock: University of Arkansas at Little Rock, Center for Child Development and Education.

Cheadle, J., & Goosby, B. (2010). Birth weight, cognitive development, and life chances: A comparison of siblings from childhood into early adulthood. *Social Science Research, 39*(4), 570–584.

Chia, Y. F. (2013). Dollars and pounds: The impact of family income on childhood weight. *Applied Economics, 45*(14), 1931–1941.

Colen, C., & Ramey, D. (2014). Is breast truly best? Estimating the effects of breastfeeding on long-term child health and wellbeing in the United States using sibling comparisons. *Social Science and Medicine, 109*, 55–65.

Courtemanche, C. (2009). Longer hours and larger waistlines? The relationship between work hours and obesity. *Forum for Health Economics and Policy, 12*(2). doi:10.2202/1558-9544.1123.

Currie, J., & Reagan, P. (2003). Distance to hospital and children's use of preventive care: Is being closer better, and for whom? *Economic Inquiry, 41*(3), 378–392.

D'Onofrio, B., Goodnight, J., Van Hulle, C., Rodgers, J., Rathouz, P., Waldman, I., & Lahey, B. (2009a). A quasi-experimental analysis of the association between family income and offspring conduct problems. *Journal of Abnormal Child Psychology, 37*(3), 415–429.

D'Onofrio, B., Goodnight, J., Van Hulle, C., Rodgers, J., Rathouz, P., Waldman, I., & Lahey, B. (2009b). Maternal age at childbirth and offspring disruptive behaviors: Testing the causal hypothesis. *Journal of Child Psychology and Psychiatry, 50*(8), 1018–1028.

D'Onofrio, B., Van Hulle, C., Waldman, I., Rodgers, J., Harden, K. P., Rathouz, P., & Lahey, B. (2008). Smoking during pregnancy and offspring externalizing problems: An exploration of genetic and environmental confounds. *Development and Psychopathology, 20*(1), 139–164.

Donahue, K., Van Hulle, C., Rodgers, J., & D'Onofrio, B. (2014). Psychosocial predictors of adolescent sexual risk behavior: A quasi-experimental analysis in a nationally representative sample of american youths. *Journal of Adolescent Health, 54*(2), S15–S16.

Dunn, L., & Dunn, L. (1981). *PPVT-R revised manual*. Circle Pines, Minnesota: American Guidance Service, Inc..

Faith, M., Heshka, S., Keller, K., Sherry, B., Matz, P., Pietrobelli, A., & Allison, D. (2003). Maternal-child feeding patterns and child body weight: Findings from a population-based sample. *Archives of Pediatrics and Adolescent Medicine, 157*(9), 926–932.

Goodnight, J., Lahey, B., Van Hulle, C., Rodgers, J., Rathouz, P., Waldman, I., & D'Onofrio, B. (2012). A quasi-experimental analysis of the influence of neighborhood disadvantage on child and adolescent conduct problems. *Journal of Abnormal Psychology, 121*(1), 95–108.

Harter, S. (1985). *Manual for the self-perception profile for children*. Denver, Colorado: University of Denver.

Hayward, M., & Gorman, B. (2004). The long arm of childhood: The influence of early-life social conditions on men's mortality. *Demography, 41*(1), 87–108.

Huang, D., Lanza, H. I., Wright-Volel, K., & Anglin, M. D. (2013). Developmental trajectories of childhood obesity and risk behaviors in adolescence. *Journal of Adolescence, 36*(1), 139–148.

Huang, D., Lanza, H. I., & Anglin, M. D. (2014). Trajectory of adolescent obesity: Exploring the impact of prenatal to childhood experiences. *Journal of Child and Family Studies, 23*(6), 1090–1101.

Jaffee, S., Van Hulle, C., & Rodgers, J. (2011). Effects of nonmaternal care in the first 3 years on children's academic skills and behavioral functioning in childhood and early adolescence: A sibling comparison study. *Child Development, 82*(4), 1076–1091.

Joyce, T., Kaestner, R., & Korenman, S. (2000). The effect of pregnancy intention on child development. *Demography, 37*(1), 83–94.

Kennedy, S., & Bumpass, L. (2008). Cohabitation and children's living arrangements: New estimates from the United States. *Demographic Research, 19*, 1663–1692. doi:10.4054/DemRes.2008.19.47.

Li, C., Mayo, M. S., & Ahluwalia, J. (2003). Maternal smoking during pregnancy, birth weight, and childhood overweight: A suppression effect model. *Annals of Epidemiology, 13*(8), 569.

Li, C., Kaur, H., Choi, W., Huang, T., Lee, R., & Ahluwalia, J. S. (2005). Additive interactions of maternal prepregnancy BMI and breast-feeding on childhood overweight. *Obesity Research, 13*(2), 362–371.

Liu, E., Cheng, H., Matsumoto, T., & Chou, S. (2009). Maternal full-time employment and overweight children: Parametric, semi-parametric, and non-parametric assessment. *Journal of Econometrics, 152*(1), 61–69.

Manning, W. D., & Smock, P. (2005). Measuring and modeling cohabitation: New perspectives from qualitative data. *Journal of Marriage and the Family, 67*(4), 989–1002.

Mendle, J., Harden, K. P., Turkheimer, E., Van Hulle, C., D'Onofrio, B., Brooks-Gunn, J., Rodgers, J., Emery, R., & Lahey, B. (2009). Associations between father absence and age of first sexual intercourse. *Child Development, 80*(5), 1463–1480.

Miller, D. (2011). Maternal work and child overweight and obesity: The importance of timing. *Journal of Family and Economic Issues, 32*(2), 204–218.

Mott, J. (1999). Personal and family predictors of children's medically attended injuries that occurred in the home. *Injury Prevention, 5*(3), 189–193.

Reagan, P., Salsberry, P., & Olsen, R. (2007). Does the measure of economic disadvantage matter? Exploring the effect of individual and relative deprivation on intrauterine growth restriction. *Social Science and Medicine, 64*(10), 2016–2029.

Rodgers, J., Bard, D., Johnson, A., D'Onofrio, B., & Miller, W. (2008). The cross-generational mother–daughter–aunt–niece design: Establishing validity of the MDAN design with NLSY fertility variables. *Behavior Genetics, 38*(6), 567–578.

Salsberry, P., & Reagan, P. (2005). Dynamics of early childhood overweight. *Pediatrics, 116*(6), 1329–1338.

Salsberry, P., & Reagan, P. (2007). Taking the long view: The prenatal environment and early adolescent overweight. *Research in Nursing and Health, 30*(3), 297–307.

Seipel, M., & Shafer, K. (2013). The effect of prenatal and postnatal care on childhood obesity. *Social Work, 58*(3), 241–252.

Stewart, L., Liu, Y., & Rodriguez, E. (2012). Maternal unemployment and childhood overweight: Is there a relationship? *Journal of Epidemiology and Community Health, 66*(7), 641–646.

Strauss, R. (2000). Childhood obesity and self-esteem. *Pediatrics, 105*(1), N1–N5.

Strohschein, L. (2005). Household income histories and child mental health trajectories. *Journal of Health and Social Behavior, 46*(4), 359–375.

Veit, C., & Ware, J. (1983). The structure of psychological distress and well-being in general populations. *Journal of Consulting and Clinical Psychology, 51*(5), 730–742.

Ware, J., Jr., Kosinski, M., & Keller, S. (1995). *SF-12: How to score the SF-12 physical and mental health summary scales*. New England Medical Center, Boston, MA: The Health Institute.

Wechsler, D. (1974). *Wechsler intelligence scale for children-revised*. New York: Psychological Corporation.

Wolfe, J. (2015). The effects of socioeconomic status on child and adolescent physical health: An organization and systematic comparison of measures. *Social Indicators Research, 123*(1), 39–58.

7

Life Course Health Development in Autism Spectrum Disorders

Irene E. Drmic, Peter Szatmari, and Fred Volkmar

1 Introduction

Health development results from dynamic person-environment interactions that begin before conception and continue throughout the lifespan (Halfon et al. 2014; Russ et al. 2014). Life course health development (LCHD) incorporates theories and empirical evidence from the biological, physical, and social sciences to formulate a framework that explains how health develops over the life course. The principles of life course health development (see Halfon and Forrest 2017) describe health as an emergent set of capacities that develop continuously over the lifespan in complex, nonlinear processes that result from multilevel interactions of individuals and their environments. Furthermore, health is sensitive to the timing and social structuring of environmental exposures, as well as to timing and synchronization of molecular, physiological, behavioral, social, and cultural functions. Finally, evolution enables and constrains the range of adaptive plastic responses and health developmental pathways associated with these phenotypes.

The life course health development conceptual framework can be applied to autism spectrum disorders (ASD) to help prioritize a research agenda and improve health development across the lifespan for individuals with ASD, their families, and communities. Novel approaches to understanding ASD are welcome given that ASD represents a major public health challenge. The estimated annual cost of caring for individuals with ASD in the USA is $137 billion, with a lifetime cost per individual estimated to be $2.4 million for those with co-occurring intellectual disability and $1.4 million for those without intellectual disability (Dawson and Bernier 2013). The following chapter is not an exhaustive review of the literature in ASD; rather, we highlight some issues and findings that are pertinent to an understanding of ASD using the lens of the life course health development principles.

1.1 What Is Autism Spectrum Disorder (ASD): The Clinical Phenotype

Autism spectrum disorders are a group of neuropsychiatric conditions all of which share

I.E. Drmic (✉)
Hospital for Sick Children, Toronto, ON, Canada
e-mail: Irene.drmic@sickkids.ca

P. Szatmari
Centre for Addiction and Mental Health,
Hospital for Sick Children, University of Toronto,
Toronto, ON, Canada
e-mail: Peter.Szatmari@utoronto.ca

F. Volkmar
Child Study Center, Yale University School
of Medicine, New Haven, CT, USA
e-mail: Fred.Volkmar@yale.edu

difficulties in social engagement and social interaction as their major diagnostic feature. As a result of this basic problem, difficulties arise in learning, cognitive organization, attention, and adaptive skills. Autism, the prototypic disorder, was described by Kanner in 1943 as an "inborn disturbance" of social contact. Autism was first included in a new category of pervasive developmental disorders when first recognized officially in the third edition of *Diagnostic and Statistical Manual of Mental Disorders* (DSM;APA 1980).

Autism is a condition of early onset and poses multiple problems in health development. Many parents are concerned about affected children's development by age 1 with the vast majority of parents worried by age 2 (Chawarska et al. 2008). An increasing body of work has focused on autism as it first develops in infancy (Rogers 2009). In a minority of cases (about 20%), parents report some period of normal development followed by loss of skills; the clinical significance of regression continues to be debated (Parr et al. 2011; Shattuck et al. 2009).

Problems in social interaction are a hallmark of autism and related conditions. Social difficulties are distinctive even considering any associated developmental delays. Similarly, communication problems are present and persistent even in the more cognitively able children who lack verbal and nonverbal social communication skills such as gestures, facial expression, and eye contact. Even when children do speak, they exhibit a number of difficulties including echolalia, pronoun use difficulties, abnormal prosody, and in the social use of language (Paul 2008). Kanner noted the range of unusual behaviors frequent in autism including motor mannerisms (stereotyped movement), difficulties with change, and insistence on routines. The apparent over-engagement with the nonsocial world arises in the general lack of social engagement. This suggests a potential route both as a mechanism for learning difficulties and for intervention.

The original impression that autism was not associated with cognitive problems rested, in large part, on the unusual abilities of children in some areas; in some cases, these skills are highly circumscribed and may arise even in association with overall intellectual delay (Hermelin 2001). Even for the most able individuals, scatter in abilities is often present with a relative deficit in verbal as opposed to perceptual abilities. It is also the case that there is frequently a gap between abilities in a formal testing situation and "real-world" or adaptive skills – the latter reflecting the significant difficulties individuals have in generalization and in tasks that involved fast-paced decision making, executive functioning, and social interaction (Robinson et al. 2009). In more classical autism, nonverbal skills tend to be much stronger than verbal abilities; the opposite profile may hold true for Asperger's disorder although this has been debated (Klin et al. 1996; Meyer and Minshew 2002; Noterdaeme et al. 2010).

As noted above in addition to classic autism of the type described by Kanner, a number of other conditions with some apparent similarity to autism have been recognized, although their validity apart from autism continues to be hotly debated. Asperger's disorder was described (Asperger 1944) the year after Kanner's report first appeared. Although the children (all boys) had major problems in social interaction, in contrast to Kanner's (1943) cases, they demonstrated good language abilities and were more likely to exhibit motor difficulties, unusual and all-consuming esoteric special interests, and their problems seemed to come to clinical attention rather later (Woodbury-Smith and Volkmar 2009). Although included in DSM-IV and *International Statistical Classification of Diseases and Related Health Problems* (ICD)-10 as a distinctive disorder, Asperger's disorder has been the focus of much debate and is not considered a diagnosable disorder in DSM-V.

A subthreshold pervasive developmental disorder category was included in DSM since 1980 to encompass individuals whose difficulties appear to fall close to autism but do not achieve thresholds for diagnosis of that, or related, conditions. Interestingly this concept also was described in the 1940s although not with great precision. It has as always been recognized to significantly outnumber more classical autism (Fombonne 2005a, b) by probably four or five times although research in this area has, paradoxically, been limited. In recent years, the tendency to equate pervasive developmental disorder not otherwise specified with more classic autism has led to a broader autism spectrum concept although it must be emphasized that the DSM-5 autism spectrum disorder concept would likely exclude many cases that in the past had been said to have pervasive developmental disorder not otherwise specified (Volkmar and McPartland 2014).

1.2 Epidemiology

It is clear that ASD has a strong genetic component and is likely related to the interaction of multiple genes (Devlin and Scherer 2012); ASD invariably originates in the first years of life. Poverty and lack of access to adequate resources and intervention clearly impact identification, service provision, and likely outcome (Liptak et al. 2008; Thomas et al. 2007), but this area of work remains one that is relatively little studied. Various factors complicate the study of prevalence rates in ASD. There has been a concern that rates have risen over time although in his review of the topic Fombonne (2005a, b) suggests that a median rate of strictly defined autism would be about 1 per 800 to 1000 people with the much broader pervasive developmental disorder category being much more common. Several recent studies have reported higher rates (e.g., Brugha et al. 2011; Elsabbagh et al. 2012), but studies of adults in community settings report similar rates to those estimated by Fombonne and others (Brugha et al. 2011; Elsabbagh et al. 2012; Rutter 1973) and various factors which might account for apparent increases in rates have been identified (King and Bearman 2009; Rutter 1982) with potential overestimation due to methodology (i.e., case-confirmation strategies) and small sample sizes resulting in high estimates (Levy et al. 2009). Such factors include increased public awareness and increased recognition of more cognitively able individuals, applying the diagnosis to individuals with specific syndromes such as Down syndrome and widening of diagnostic criteria, sundry methodological problems, and "diagnostic substitution" – the latter referring to an issue, particularly in the USA, where an educational label of autism may be used to obtain services in preference to other labels such as mental retardation (Fombonne 2005a, b).

Most studies have reported significantly higher rates of ASD in boys than in girls although girls with more strictly defined autism are also more likely to have intellectual disability (Fombonne 2005a, b). The three- to fivefold increase in boys is similar to other neurodevelopmental disorders such as language disorders and attention deficit hyperactivity disorder (ADHD). It is possible that milder expression in some girls is underdiagnosed (Landa et al. 2007). There has been speculation that greater severity sometimes observed in girls is a function of a greater genetic risk for the condition (Fombonne 2005a, b) and that observed sex differences might relate to fundamental cognitive mechanisms (Baron-Cohen 2011). In reality, sex differences have been remarkably little studied and our understanding of this phenomenon remains very limited.

Potential social class correlates of autism first noted by Kanner (1943) in his original sample have not generally held up in subsequent research, presumably reflecting a referral bias in Kanner's original cases (Fombonne 2005a, b; Wing 1980). However, disparities in diagnosis rates are observed with children from backgrounds of poverty or minority status often going undiagnosed (LaFramboise et al. 2009). Although diagnostic presentation is rather similar around the world, cultural factors may impact both diagnosis and treatment (Brown and Rogers 2003).

1.3 Classification and Diagnosis

Several approaches were undertaken in the late 1970s to provide more operational definitions of autism. Rutter's approach (1978) emphasized difficulties in social interaction, communication, and unusual behaviors of early onset that were not solely attributable to mental retardation. Both family genetic and longitudinal studies provided important information on the stability and validity of the diagnosis apart from other conditions and led to the inclusion of autism in DSM-III (APA 1980). The DSM-III approach was modified in 1987 when DSM-III-R appeared and yet again with DSM-IV which appeared in 1994. The DSM-IV definition was based on results of a large international field trial and became consistent with the tenth revision of the ICD leading to two decades of diagnostic stability (Volkmar and McPartland 2014). For DSM-5, a number of changes were made and have proven controversial. The adoption of the term autism spectrum disorder seems well justified; however, the criteria proposed appear to really be more relevant to classic "Kanner's autism," and many individuals, particularly the more cognitively able, would likely lose their diagnosis (Volkmar and McPartland 2014). As a result, cases with "well-established" diagnosis of Asperger's or pervasive developmental disorder not otherwise specified (PDD-NOS; in DSM-IV terms) could retain an ASD diagnosis – thus effectively creating two diagnostic systems in current use; the advent of ICD-11 and the Research Domain Criteria (RDoC) approach suggest that for some time there may be considerable controversy about definitional issues (see Baker et al. 2012; Brand et al. 2012; Mattilla et al. 2011; McGrew et al. 2012; Watts 2012; Huerta et al. 2012).

2 Pathogenesis

2.1 Hereditability

ASD is now considered a disorder caused at least in part by genetic factors (Szatmari et al. 1998). The evidence for this comes from studies showing that ASD runs within families, from twin studies that show that this familial aggregation is due to genetic and possibly to shared environmental risk factors (Sullivan et al. 2012) and to the recent identification of several different networks of genes responsible for synaptic and axonal development and neuronal migration (Malhotra and Sebat 2012).

Early family studies looked at the recurrence risk to a sibling if one child in the family had ASD. Those sibling risks were around 2% which were considered to be very much higher than the general population rate estimated at that time to be 4 per 10,000 (Szatmari et al. 1998). With better study designs and with a better appreciation of the breadth of the ASD phenotype, these family studies now suggest that the risk to sibling is closer to 9% (Ritvo et al. 1989). This needs to be seen in the context thought of more recent prevalence estimates of ASD of around 1%. Thus, it seems the sibling recurrence risk is roughly ten times the population base rate (Constantino et al. 2010).

The baby sibs paradigm provides a more valid estimate of sibling recurrence risk. In these studies, the infant sibling of an older child with ASD is followed from birth to 3 years of age. In this context, the emergence of autistic signs and symptoms can be carefully documented prospectively, and the presence or absence of an ASD diagnosis is determined by 3 years of age. These studies have shown that signs and symptoms of the ASD phenotype begin to emerge around 6–12 months of age, and upward of 20% of siblings will have a diagnosis of ASD at 3 years of age (Chawarska et al. 2008; Zwaigenbaum et al. 2012). Interestingly, despite the fact that these studies have demonstrated that ASD can be diagnosed as early as 3 years and that best practice in ASD, such as the 2007 American Academy of Pediatrics guideline that all children should be screened for ASD at 18 and 24 months, the average age of diagnosis in the USA is still close to 5 years and higher in those with milder forms of ASD (CDC 2014).

Twin studies are used to determine the mechanism of familial aggregation. Earlier studies suggested very sharp discrepancies between monozygous and dizygous concordance rates suggesting not only that the mechanism of heritability was genetic but that there was little room for environmental risk factors in playing an important role in causation. The twin study with the largest sample size and the one carried out with the most methodological rigor was recently published (Hallmayer et al. 2011). In that study, monozygous concordance rates were closer to 60%, and dizygous rates were 20% rate seen in the recent infant sibling studies. While the Hallmayer et al. twin study also provides support for the importance of genetic factors in the etiology of the disorder, the higher than expected dizygous concordance rate also suggests a significant role for shared environmental risk factors.

2.2 Genetic Contribution

Hundreds of different genes have been described in ASD that have been disrupted by either deletions or duplications of copy number. These genes all appear to be related to different aspects of neuronal development (largely synaptic functioning) or neuronal migration (Li et al. 2012). This is an important finding as it steers mechanisms of etiology away from neurotransmitters and monoamines, a theory which had dominated the field for several decades (McDougle et al. 2005).

With the discovery of copy number variants as important structural genomic risk factors for a variety of human diseases has come the realization that these variants might play an important role in the etiology of ASD (Marshall et al. 2008). Copy number variants represent deletions or duplications covering more than 1000 kbs of DNA. In general, copy number variants can be common or rare, and they can be either de novo or inherited from parents. The first copy number variant identified in ASD in a genome-wide study was a rare deletion in the neurexin gene (Szatmari et al. 2007), and this has been followed up with many reports of other copy number variants affecting important brain-expressed genes (for a review see Malhotra and Sebat 2012). These copy number variants tend to be extremely rare, found in less than 1% of the ASD samples, and tend to rise de novo. This would explain the frequent lack of family history in ASD families and would provide a mechanism whereby the prevalence of the disorder remains stable in the context of a condition associated with reduced fertility (Power et al. 2012). Common genetic variants (either polymorphisms or copy number variants) have not been reliably identified in ASD, although such variants likely do exist and will require very large sample sizes for their identification (Devlin et al. 2011). If they do exist, their effect size must be very small or else they operate as modifying factors as opposed to susceptibility genes. Currently, copy number variants explain less than 10% of cases in ASD, and the population attributable risk is less than 5% (Pinto et al. 2010). The etiology of the vast majority of cases of ASD remains to be explained. The next generation of genetic studies will focus on much smaller copy number variants or DNA sequence variants identified either in exomes or in whole genome sequencing.

2.3 Nongenetic Contributions

The search for environmental risk factors has been underway for many decades. There seems reasonably good evidence that certain maternal anticonvulsants such as carbamazepine, valproic acid, and perhaps other anticonvulsants increase risk for ASD (Palac and Meador 2011). Other putative environmental risk factors that may have been more common in earlier decades such as congenital rubella have now virtually disappeared. A complication in all this work is disentangling the sometimes complex issues of severe mental handicap and "autistic-like" behaviors, particularly since stereotyped mannerisms become much more common with severe intellectual deficiency, but characteristic social-communicative features may be either difficult to judge or not clearly present (Volkmar et al. 2005). Pregnancy and birth complications have been studied extensively, and other than low birth weight or being small for gestational age, it is difficult to identify a risk factor (see Gardener et al. 2009 for a recent meta-analysis). It should be noted, however, that low birth weight may in fact represent a *consequence* of genetic vulnerability rather than an environmental risk factor interacting with genetic susceptibility (Rutter 2005). Other potential environmental markers signaled by inflammatory indices are of interest but remain highly speculative at this point (Muller et al. 2015). Perhaps the most convincing evidence for an environmental risk factor is that of advanced parental age (Shelton et al. 2010). Since paternal and maternal age is so highly correlated, it is difficult to determine if both are risk factors or if only one. This is important as the mechanism by which the risk factor might operate will be quite different based on the maternal/paternal risk factor (Veltman and Brunner 2012). De novo copy number variants are more common with advanced paternal age, while chromosomal abnormalities (like trisomies) are more common with advanced maternal age.

2.4 Epigenetic Contributions

Epigenetic studies of non-syndromic ASD are in their infancy but do hold promise once technological and methodical issues associated with this area of study are resolved. Genes that regulate DNA methylation have been implicated in the etiology of ASD, and single gene disorders associated with ASD have implicated epigenetic mechanisms (Loke et al. 2015). It is anticipated that this will be an active field in the future and will yield novel insights in how person-environment interactions lead to the development of ASD.

2.5 Physical Biomarkers

Magnetic resonance imaging and diffusion tensor imaging studies have provided some insight into brain structure, circuitry, and connectivity in ASD. Courchesne and colleagues followed toddlers from 12 months to 48 months and found an abnormal brain growth trajectory in autism (Schumann et al. 2010). Toddlers, who were ultimately diagnosed with ASD, showed enlargement of cerebral gray and white matter, which was most pronounced in the frontal, temporal, and cingulate cortices, and some gray matter regions showed an abnormal growth rate. In addition, in those infants who later developed ASD, there was a difference in the development of white matter tracks between 6 and 12 months of age (i.e., increases in fractional anisotropy), with a slowing in development by 24 months (Wolff et al. 2012). Thus, abnormal neurodevelopmental connectivity early in life could potentially serve as an important biomarker for ASD.

2.6 Genotype-Phenotype Contributions

In addition, genotype-phenotype correlations have been virtually impossible to establish, and the fact that the genetic variants identified in ASD also appear to be playing a role in intellectual disability, epilepsy, schizophrenia, and ADHD has emphasized the nonspecificity of these susceptibility risk factors (State 2010). These genetic findings in ASD have influenced healthcare recommendation and practice, such that microarray testing is part of the standard of care for diagnosis of ASD (McGrew et al. 2012). It is likely that in the future, whole exome sequencing will also become standard clinical practice. However, to date, no studies have directly assessed the impact of genetic testing on health outcomes such as earlier age of diagnosis or reduced use of other diagnostic tools such as MRI (Sun et al. 2015). In the future, we anticipate that there will be an increased application of genetics and neuroimaging to the early identification of ASD (Dawson and Bernier 2013). It is also likely that the discovery of genetic variants that impact the development of the synapse will lead to clinical trials of new (or "repurposed") drugs targeting those mechanisms. Such trials are already underway in fragile X and tuberous sclerosis but so far with disappointing results (Geschwind and State 2015).

3 Outcome Studies

3.1 An Overview of Developmental Course

Before reviewing approaches to assessing outcome, an overview of what is known, and what is not known, about the course of autism spectrum disorders may be helpful. It must be emphasized that outcome is usually very specifically defined as adult independence and that little information is available on health-related outcomes and vanishingly little relates to older individuals with ASD. Variations in life course are, in part, one of the rationales used to support previous diagnostic distinctions between subtypes. In more "classical" autism, it is clear that diagnosis in infancy is of great interest but also somewhat problematic until about age 3 when reasonable stability in clinical manifestations occurs. Before that time, the issue usually is between change from (or to) a more classic picture to a more "subthreshold" condition (an issue that may be mitigated by the broad approach adopted in DSM-5). Often the difficulty, using the DSM-IV, was that social and communication problems are present but the "restricted interests" criteria were not fully met (even though some likely precursor behaviors are present). Rarely a child moves off the autism spectrum entirely. There is good evidence (NRC 2001) that treatments are most effective when started early in life; although for reasons not well understood, some children do not improve as dramatically as others. It is important to emphasize that apart from a reasonably robust literature on adult outcome (i.e., early in adult life), the literature on adults with autism is very limited both in terms of actual numbers of studies and individuals studied and an absence of literature on the topic of aging in autism (Howlin 2013; Perkins and Berkman 2012). For example, few studies address the issue of rates of employment among adults with autism/ASD and rates of suicide or suicide attempts (even though depression is thought to be a frequent co-occurring condition), and no studies are available on the life course changes for individuals with autism/ASD. Put another way (and viewed in the starkest possible light), it is as if adults with autism/ASD vanish from the scene once they've become adult and "had their outcome," such as capacities in young adulthood for personal independence and self-sufficiency.

School-age children with more "classic" autism often become more sociable as they get older, and gains in cognitive and communication skills also typically are made – sometimes dramatic ones and other times not. Social language use and peer relationships often remain areas of difficulties, and problems with agitation and self-stimulatory behavior may require behavioral or pharmacologic intervention. As first observed by Leo Kanner (Kanner 1971), in adolescence, some children make major gains, while another group unfortunately exhibits some degree of deterioration in functioning. A number of outcome studies now suggest a gradual change in overall prognosis presumably reflecting both earlier and better intervention as well as some changes in diagnostic practice over the time (i.e., including recognizing autism in more cognitively able individuals) (Howlin 2005). An increasing number of individuals are able to live independently and self-sufficiently as adults, and many now go to college or pursue technical/vocational training. Major predictors of adult outcome include level of intellectual functioning and communication competence. Some adults require intermediate levels of support, and in many cases, affected individuals never attain independence and must live in highly structured residential settings. Age-related vulnerabilities have been noted, e.g., the risk of seizure disorder is substantially increased both in early childhood and again in adolescence and possibly well into adulthood. More able adults with autism and related conditions also are apparently more vulnerable to anxiety and depression which can require specific treatments (Howlin 2013; Skokauskas and Gallagher 2010; Szatmari and McConnell 2011; White et al. 2009).

Data on outcome in Asperger's disorder are, expectedly, less extensive but suggest (also as might be expected) overall better outcomes in terms of independence, educational attainment, employment, and social independence. However, comorbid conditions, such as anxiety and depression, can be a complicating factors and negatively impact outcomes (Skokauskas and Gallagher 2010; Szatmari and McConnell 2011; White et al. 2009; Volkmar et al. 2014). There is some suggestion of increased risk for both psychosis and legal difficulties in adolescence and adulthood, but the evidence for this consists largely of case reports (Skokauskas and Gallagher 2010; Szatmari and McConnell 2011; White et al. 2009).

Studies of children with "subthreshold" pervasive developmental disorder are very uncommon although, on balance, these individuals appear to have a better outcome than those with more classical autism (Towbin 2005). The outcome in childhood disintegrative disorder and Rett's does appear, unfortunately, to be poor (Volkmar et al. 2005; Van Acker et al. 2005). In childhood disintegrative disorder, children lose skills but then plateau and make relatively minimal gains. In Rett's, the course is well known with children becoming somewhat more sociable over time but also more incapacitated due to neurological and movement problems.

3.2 Adult Independence

Information on long-term prognosis is limited and difficult to interpret. This review will focus primarily on long-term follow-up outcome studies that have been published over the past decade (for reviews of earlier outcome studies see Gillberg 1991; Henninger and Taylor 2012; Howlin 2000; Howlin and Moss 2012; Levy and Perry 2011; Nordin and Gillberg 1998). The majority of studies that report on "outcomes" for people with ASD have focused on a few domains (e.g., work status, residential situation, friendships; see more detailed discussion below). Predicting outcome has been difficult due to the wide variability in cognitive, linguistic, social, and behavioral abilities in this group of individuals. Consistent interpretation of different findings has also been difficult due to varied sample size (generally small), sampling procedures (clinical versus population based), differences in diagnostic criteria over time, wide range of age at diagnosis, differences in amount of time between initial and follow-up assessments, differences in measures used, imprecise and/or poor quality data on early intellectual functioning, and the lack of information about early intervention services. These factors may account, in part, for the substantial variability reported in adult outcomes for people with ASD.

As noted previously, although psychosocial outcomes have generally been poor, there is a trend over time for higher rates of improvement (see Table 1 – description of how the outcome categories were defined is provided below; Beadle-Brown et al. 2002; Billstedt et al. 2005, 2007, 2011; Eaves and Ho 2008; Farley et al. 2009; Gillberg 1991; Hofvander et al. 2009; Howlin 1998; Howlin et al. 2004; Kobayashi et al. 1992; Lockyer and Rutter 1969, 1970; Lotter 1978; Lovaas 1987; Nordin and Gillberg 1998; Rutter et al. 1967; Rutter and Lockyer 1967; Szatmari et al. 1989). Studies conducted from the 1950s to 1970s reported that less than 15% of individuals had good/very good outcomes and the majority had poor/very poor outcomes (Eisenberg 1956; Rutter et al. 1967; Lotter 1974). Over the past three decades, outcomes have improved but remain variable; the proportion of good to very good outcomes ranges from 4% to 62% and poor to very poor outcome ranges from 3% to 78% (see Table 1). Outcomes have been classified into different outcome categories ranging from "very poor to very good" by various studies over the years. Of note, these ratings were more subjective in earlier studies (pre-2000), whereas more objective criteria have been used in recent studies (for a detailed discussion, see Henniger and Taylor 2012).

The group of studies published within the last decade used quantifiable outcome criteria to classify individuals with ASD into these different outcome categories ranging from very poor to very good (see Howlin et al. 2004, Appendix 2, for detailed criteria). In general, the criteria used to determine outcome were based on a 5-point composite rating of overall social and independent living functioning that was derived by summing individual scores for work status (ranging from 0 = employed or self-employed to 3 = no occupation), residential situation (ranging from 0 = living independently to 5 = being in hospital care or at home because nowhere else would accept the individual), and number and quality of meaningful friendships (ranging from 0 = more than one friendship to 3 = no friendships or joint activities) . Based on the 5-point composite rating, a score of 0 indicated a "very good" outcome (i.e., total for all three areas between 0 and 2); 1 = "good" outcome (total 3–4); 2 = "fair" outcome (total 5–7); 3 = "poor" outcome (total 8–10); and 4 = "very poor" outcome (total 11). Thus, the concept of "outcome" is related to practical independence and autonomy achieved in adult life.

Howlin and her colleagues (2004) surveyed 68 adults (average age of 29 years) with autism who had a performance IQ of 50 or above in childhood and found that the majority (58%) had

Table 1 Review of adult outcome studies

Authors	*N*	Mean age at intake (IN) and follow-up (FU) (years)	Functioning level at intake (IN) and follow-up (FU)	Mean follow-up time (years)	Method of initial assessment	*Dx*	Very poor to poor	Restricted to fair	Good to very good
Gillespie-Lynch et al. (2012)	AUT = 20	IN: 3.9 FU: 26.6	IN: 54.7[a] FU: n/a	–	DSM-III	AUT	50	20	30
Billstedt et al. (2011)[b]	TOT = 108 (AUT = 73 ATY = 35)	IN: <10 years FU: 25.5 (17–40)	AUT IN: 21% IQ > 70 FU: 7% IQ > 70 ATY IN: 14% IQ > 70 FU: 3% IQ > 70	17.8	DSM-III-R	AUT& ATY	12	26	62
Farley et al. (2009)	AUT = 48	IN: 7.2 (3–25) FU: 32.5 (22–46)	IN: IQ > 70 (IQ Estimate = 86.66) FU: FSIQ = 88.93	24.4	DSM-III	AUT	17	34	48
Eaves and Ho (2008)	AUT = 48 ASD = 40	IN: 6.8 (3–12) FU: 24.0 (19–31)	IN: 17% IQ ≥ 70 FU: n/a	–	DSM I–III; Rutter	AUT	46	32	21
Cederlund et al. (2008)	ASP = 70 AUT = 70 (includes AUT & ATY)	ASP IN: 11.3 (5–24) FU: 21.5 (16–33) AUT IN: <10.0 FU: 24.5 (16–36)	ASP: IN: 100% IQ ≥ 70 (FSIQ =101.4) FU: 98% IQ ≥ 70 (FSIQ = 103.0) AUT: IN: 19% IQ ≥ 70 FU: 7% IQ ≥ 70	–	Gillberg's criteria, DSM-III, DSM-III-R	ASP AUT	3 76	70 24	27 0
Billstedt et al. (2005)	TOT = 108 (AUT = 73 ATY = 35)	IN: <10.0 FU: 25.5 (17–40)	AUT: IN: 21% IQ > 70 FU: 7% IQ > 70 ATY IN: 14% IQ > 70 FU: 3% IQ > 70	17.8	Rutter, DSM-III	AUT& ATY	78	21	0
Howlin et al. 2004	AUT = 68	IN 7.24 (3–15) FU 29.3 (21–48)	IN: PIQ = 80.21 VIQ = 61.49 FU: PIQ = 75.00 VIQ = 79.78	–	Criteria applicable at time of diagnosis (1950–1979)	AUT	58	19	22

(continued)

Table 1 (continued)

Authors	*N*	Mean age at intake (IN) and follow-up (FU) (years)	Functioning level at intake (IN) and follow-up (FU)	Mean follow-up time (years)	Method of initial assessment	*Dx*	Very poor to poor	Restricted to fair	Good to very good
Engstrom et al. (2003)	ASP = 32 HFA = 10	IN: HFA 13.5 (4–20); ASP 28.0 (15–41) FU: 30.8 (18–49)	IN: n/a FU: 100% IQ > 70	–	DSM-IV	ASP& HFA	12	75	12
Howlin (2000) and Mawhood et al. (2000)	AUT = 19	IN: (7–8) FU: 23.8 (21–26)	IN: NVIQ ≥ 70 NVIQ = 94.28 VIQ = 66.56 FU: NVIQ = 82.78 VIQ = 82.33	–	Rutter	AUT	74	10	16
Larsen and Mouridsen (1997)	AUT = 9 ASP = 9	IN: ASP = 9.2; AUT = 5.9 FU: ASP 39.1 (33–44); AUT 36.5 (32–39)	IN: ASP: 100% IQ > 70 AUT: 56% IQ > 70 FU: N/A	30	ICD-10	ASP AUT	22 67	44 11	33 22
Ruble and Dalrymple (1996)	AUT = 46	IN: 5.2 FU: 17.1	IN: 26.7% IQ >70 FU: 15.2% IQ > 70	8.6	DSM-III-R	AUT	100	0	0
Kobayashi et al. (1992)	AUT = 201	IN: 6.4 FU: 21.5	IN: 23.4% IQ ≥ 70 FU: n/a	15.4	DSM-III-R	AUT	46	27	27
Gillberg and Steffenburg (1987)	AUT = 23	IN: <6 FU: (16–23)	IN: 26% IQ > 70 FU: n/a	6–11	DSM-III; Kanner & Eisenberg; Rutter	AUT	44	48	4
Lotter 1974	AUT = 32	IN: (8–10) FU: (16–18)	IN: 66.7% IQ < 55 FU: n/a	8	Creak (1961)	AUT	63	24	13
Rutter et al. (1967) and Rutter and Lockyer (1967)	IP = 57	IN: 5.9 (2–10) FU: 15.6	IN: 29% IQ > 70 (mean IQ 62) FU: n/a	9.7	Agreement among psychiatrists	IP	61	25	14
Eisenberg (1956)	AUT = 63	IN: 6 FU: 15	n/a	9	Unclear	AUT	73	22	5

ASP Asperger syndrome, *ATY* atypical autism, *AUT* autism, *HFA* high-functioning autism, *IP* infantile psychosis
[a]Developmental quotient (mental age divided by chronological age)
[b]QOL scale

poor or very poor outcomes, 19% had fair outcome, and 22% had good or very good outcome. Those individuals with a performance IQ of at least 70 in childhood had significantly better outcome than those with an IQ below 70. More specifically, of those individuals with a performance IQ between 50 and 69 (n = 23), only one individual had very good outcome, three were rated as fair, and the remaining had poor or very poor outcome. Individuals in this IQ category had much poorer prognosis with few having jobs, friends, or achieving independence as adults. In the group of individuals with near average to average IQ, outcome was generally better, although still quite variable. Of those individuals with an IQ of 70 or above (n = 45; parental data missing on one individual), 14 individuals were rated as good or very good, 10 as fair, and 20 as poor or very poor. Furthermore, there was no difference in outcome in those individuals with an IQ over 100 and those with and initial IQ between 70 and 99. Interestingly, many individuals with an IQ between 70 and 99 made better progress in terms of academics, jobs, and general level of functioning, than those with an IQ above 100. Thus, having an IQ of about 70 seemed to be a critical cutoff point for better outcome (e.g., level of independence); however, outcome in these individuals was still quite variable.

Other studies found a similar pattern of results. Billstedt et al. (2005) examined a group of low- to middle-functioning individuals (82% had an IQ below 70) with autism or atypical autism and found that 91% had poor or very poor outcome and none were reported to have good outcome. Eaves and Ho (2008) reported somewhat better outcomes in a group of low- to middle-functioning individuals (majority had IQ < 70) with approximately half having fair to good outcome and half poor (but none very poor). Similar outcomes were reported by Gillespie-Lynch et al. (2012), with 50% reporting poor outcome and 50% fair to very good outcome. Engstrom, Ekstrom, and Emilsson (2003) reported on the psychosocial functioning of a systematically selected sample of patients with Asperger syndrome (AS) and high-functioning autism (HFA) all of whom had an IQ above 70. The majority were rated as having a fair outcome (75%), with few being rated as good or poor (12% each) and none being rated as very poor. Farley et al. (2009) also examined adult outcomes for 41 individuals with average or near average cognitive abilities and found better outcomes compared to the other studies with 48% showing good or very good outcome, 34% with fair outcome, and only 17% with poor outcome (none with very poor outcome). Taken together, these studies suggest that outcomes for adults may be improving and that this is likely related to availability of services for individuals with ASD (Gillespie-Lynch et al. 2012; Kobayashi et al. 1992). However, it is important to also take into consideration the pattern of attrition in longitudinal studies. For instance, selective attrition of lower functioning individuals may account for the more positive outcomes in some studies (Eaves and Ho 2008; Gillespie-Lynch et al. 2012).

3.3 Quality of Life

Although the vast majority of studies have based outcomes on level of independence achieved in adulthood and IQ, symptom severity and language development are thought to be important factors in these outcomes; there is increasing interest in examining outcomes based on quality of life (QOL) indictors. QOL is a more comprehensive and multidimensional concept that also encompasses one's subjective evaluations of their experiences (Burgess and Gutstein 2007). According to the World Health Organization (WHO), the concept of QOL not only includes level of independence and social relationships but also is composed of the person's health, personal beliefs, and their relationship to salient features of their environment (Saxena and Orley 1997).

Generally, studies show that overall QOL and health-related QOL is relatively low for people with ASD (Kamp-Becker et al. 2011; van Heijst and Geurts 2015; Potvin et al. 2015). van Heijst and Geurts (2015) conducted a meta-analysis on QOL studies that included children, adolescents, and adults with ASD and found that QOL is lower in people with ASD compared to people without ASD and age did not have an effect. The lack of association with age has previously been reported (Kamino et al. 2012; Kamp-Becker et al. 2011), although it had also been reported that increasing age is associated with decreasing quality of life (Bennett et al. 2005). Characteristics that were relevant predictors in the traditional adult outcome studies, including symptom severity, IQ, and early language, were not examined because information was too sparse. Given the dearth of information about the elderly, the authors also conducted an empirical study examining QOL in intellectually able elderly individuals with ASD and again found large difference in QOL in people with versus without ASD with lower QOL in individuals with ASD. Interestingly, age, IQ, and symptom severity did not predict QOL in the elderly.

Billstedt et al. (2011) examined aspects of quality of life (QOL) in adults diagnosed with autism or atypical autism in childhood and found that the majority of the ASD group remained dependent on parents for support in education, recreation, and occupational situations in late adolescents and early adulthood, but QOL was quite positive (independent of intellectual functioning). The QOL scale used in this study measured both objective and subjective (although by proxy) indicators of well-being. The authors who evaluated the participants completed a QOL scale assessing "autism-friendly environment" using a five-item scale (QOL-1). The item categories were (1) staff and caregivers have specific "autism knowledge," (2) applied structured education implemented, (3) individual specific treatment/training plan for the person with autism implemented, (4) occupation or everyday life activity corresponding to his/her level of capacity, and (5) overall quality of life. Each item was rated on a 1 (very good) to 5 (very poor). A second QOL scale assessing "parent/care rating of individual's well-being" was obtained to estimate how the individual with autism enjoyed or liked his/her residential conditions (QOL-2). Sixty-two percent of individuals were rated as having a very good or good QOL by the authors (QOL-1), and 91% of families reported high or very high residential well-being (QOL-2). This is consistent with reports among young adults with intellectual disabilities who reported satisfaction with their lives even though they remained quite dependent on caregivers (Keogh et al. 2004) and a greater sense of empowerment than those individuals who were still in the school system (Kraemer et al. 2003). Howlin (2013) emphasized that traditional definitions of "good outcome" or "independent living" may not be the most suitable goal to strive for individuals with ASD, because it may lead to a life with little support that is isolated and lacking in stimulation. More research examining QOL is needed in ASD. Raphael et al. (1996) conceptualize a QOL model, which is relevant to persons with developmental disabilities, as containing three domains that include "being, belonging, and becoming" (p. 28). The "being" domain includes being who one is or wants to become, "belonging" includes how one fits within their environment, and "becoming" involves pursuit of personal goals and wants. They also noted that within each domain, it is important to consider the perceived importance, enjoyment experienced, perceived control, and opportunities for change and enhancement. Thus, it is important to also examine and understand the subjective experience of the individuals with ASD and their families when assessing outcome. As with any chronic disability, having a condition like ASD may predispose to other problems – particularly difficulties with depression and anxiety disorder; the relative dearth of work on adult outcome and complexities of the problems of comorbidity and diagnosis limit our understanding of the developmental pathways that result in these outcomes. Similarly, even for the most cognitively able adults (e.g., those who attend college), challenges remain in various areas including adaptive (real-world) skills and generalization, social interaction, organization abilities, and so forth (Farley et al. 2009). As noted previously, the significant limitations of the available literature must be emphasized – issues of QOL have not frequently been assessed, even more cognitively able individuals may lead lives of social isolation with comorbid mental health conditions, medication use is quite high, limitations in daily life can result from poor adaptive skills, and essentially no information is available on aging (Howlin 2013). Thus, given the large differences between quality of life in people with and without ASD, a great deal of work needs to be done to understand how to support optimal health development in individuals with ASD and provide their families with the kinds of interventions that will enable them to achieve a higher QOL and promote well-being. A shift in research focus is needed to understand factors that lead to a better QOL across the life course. There is some evidence indicating that a higher QOL is related to earlier diagnosis (Kamino et al. 2012), greater perceived support (Renty and Roeyers 2006), and supported employment, residential, and leisure programs (Garcia-Villamisar et al. 2002, García-Villamisar and Dattilo 2010; Gerber et al. 2011). Thus, considerable work is needed to improve QOL in people with ASD, and a better understanding of the developmental trajectory across the lifespan may help to better understand the need and interventions required to support these individuals.

3.4 Predictors of Adult Independence

Intellectual functioning (IQ) and language have been most consistently identified as the best predictor of adult personal independence as outcome in ASD (Billstedt et al. 2005, 2007; Gillberg and Steffenburg 1987; Gillespie-Lynch et al. 2012; Howlin et al. 2004; Kobayashi et al. 1992; Lotter 1974; Nordin and Gillberg 1998; Rumsey et al. 1985), although reports have been variable (Farley et al. 2009; Gillespie-Lynch et al. 2012). Farley et al. (2009) reported that early childhood variables were weakly associated with adult outcomes, but the participants in their study all had communicative phrase speech or better language by age 6 and near average to average IQ. Gillespie-Lynch et al. (2012) also found that early intellectual functioning did not predict adult outcomes but suggested that this may be because the average age of the first assessment was quite young (mean age of 3.9 years). Cognitive testing of children with autism older than 4–5 years of age is reported to give more stable measures than in those children who are tested at younger ages (Lord and Schopler 1989; Howlin et al. 2004). In general, however, the presence of an intellectual disability (ID) is associated with poorer outcome in people with ASD in adult life (Cederlund et al. 2008; Gillberg and Steffenberg 1987; Howlin et al. 2004; Rumsey et al. 1985; Shattuck et al. 2007), with the poorest outcomes for those individuals with an IQ below 50 (Lord and Bailey 2002). Few people with this level of cognitive impairment (IQ < 50), regardless of an ASD diagnosis, achieve a high level of independence as adults (Keogh et al. 2004; Kraemer and Blacher 2001). Conversely, higher levels of intellectual functioning (IQ > 70) are associated with better outcome (Billstedt et al. 2007; Eaves and Ho 2008; Gillberg and Steffenberg 1987; Howlin et al. 2004; Rumsey et al. 1985; Szatmari et al. 1989), but outcome can still be quite variable in these individuals (Billstedt et al. 2005; Howlin et al. 2004). These data further underscore the importance of focusing on early language development and learning (IQ) in early intervention programs for children with ASD.

With regard to verbal and performance (nonverbal) IQ, the results are more inconsistent. Some have reported that childhood verbal IQ is a better predictor of later functioning than performance IQ (Billstedt et al. 2005; Lord and Bailey 2002), whereas another study found neither to be a consistent prognostic indicator (Howlin et al. 2004). In addition, the presence of good early language skills before age 5–6 is crucial for positive outcome in ASD (Billstedt et al. 2007; Gillberg and Steffenberg 1987; Gillespie-Lynch et al. 2012; Lockyer and Rutter 1969; Lotter 1978; Szatmari et al. 2003). Mawhood et al. (2000) have shown that individuals who tended to have better linguistic outcome in adulthood were functioning at a higher cognitive level more generally.

Other factors have also been suggested to be related to outcome, including symptom severity, repetitive/stereotyped behaviors in childhood, adaptive behavior, education, gender, the presence of a diagnosed medical disorder, onset of epilepsy before age 5 years, and joint attention skills (Billstedt et al. 2007; De Meyer et al. 1973; Farley et al. 2009; Gillespie-Lynch et al. 2012; Howlin and Goode 1998; Totsika et al. 2010; Venter et al. 1992). For instance, Farley et al. (2009) reported that adaptive behavior measures (in particular the Daily Living Skills domain) evaluated at follow-up were most closely correlated to better outcomes. They described a group of individuals with a high IQ but poor practical living skills who felt frustrated by these limitations. Furthermore, they also described individuals who had a low IQ but who were able to manage with little assistance and obtained good or very good outcome rating despite poor cognitive skills. These results have important implications for intervention programs that foster these practical living skills in adulthood.

The development of joint attention skills may be another important area to target in early intervention programs because of the relationship of this developmental skill set with later health development outcomes. Joint attention skills typically develop between 6 and 18 months of age and refer to ability of the infant to coordinate their attention with another individual during a social interaction. Joint attention skills are important because they are considered early markers of social cognitive development; that is, they reflect the early development of the infant's ability to think about the perspective of another individual (Tomasello 1995). These skills are critical to social learning and social information processing (Mundy and Jarrold 2010), language development (Sigman and Kasari 1995), and the emergence of social and behavioral competence in childhood (Vaughan Van Hecke et al. 2007). Children with ASD present with deficits in joint attention regardless of their developmental or intellectual level, and these deficits are neither absolute nor uniform (Mundy et al. 2009).

In a recent longitudinal study into adult outcomes, responsiveness to joint attention, but not initiation of joint attention (IJA), was found to predict later outcomes. Responsiveness to joint attention was found to predict gains in IQ from early childhood (M = 3.9 years) to later childhood (M = 11.7 years) and receptive language in late adolescents/early adulthood (M = 18.3 years) (Sigman and McGovern 2005; Sigman and Ruskin 1999). In terms of adult outcomes, responsiveness to joint attention predicted adult nonverbal communication, social skills, and symptoms (Gillespie-Lynch et al. 2012). In addition, responsiveness to joint attention and early language both predicted a composite measure of adult social functioning and independence. Taken together, responsiveness to joint attention measured in early childhood may reflect early emerging social cognition, and preliminary evidence suggests that it may be a good predictor of social behaviors in adulthood. Gillespie-Lynch and colleagues also suggested examining the relationship with responsiveness to joint attention and early executive functioning in childhood on later outcomes given that executive functioning is related to adaptive functioning in children with autism (Gilotty et al. 2012).

Gulsrud et al. (2014) examined the developmental trajectories of specific joint attention gestures (i.e., pointing, showing, coordinated joint looking) and expressive language over a 6-year period and found that coordinated joint looking and showing increased over time and pointing to share interest increased over the preschool years (3–5 years of age) and then decreased. They also reported a causal relationship between early pointing and later language development; that is, those children with high rates of pointing in the preschool years had better expressive language skills later. Hence, an understanding of the developmental course of joint attention skills allows for better consideration deciding "when" to intervene. Based on the data, the authors suggested that it may be useful to focus on pointing in early childhood when the child is preverbal and less useful when the child begins to use spoken language. Thus, the interval when early joint attention skills develop may represent a critical or sensitive period to intervene and potentially impact the developmental trajectory and outcomes for individuals with ASD. In addition, the children who received the joint attention intervention showed the fastest improvement compared to the control condition or child who received a different intervention. Participation in the joint attention treatment placed these children on a different developmental trajectory. This highlights that "what" you target and "when" you intervene are important (Gulsrud et al. 2014).

3.5 Diagnostic Stability and Symptom Severity

There is considerable debate in the literature regarding the stability of a diagnosis of autism and other forms of ASD over time. Some studies report that individuals diagnosed in childhood continue to meet criteria for the disorder at follow-up (Billstedt et al. 2005; Cederlund et al. 2008; Howlin et al. 2004; Lotter 1978); whereas others report a change in diagnosis or movement "off" the spectrum in some individuals (Daniels et al. 2011; Kleinman et al. 2008; Turner and Stone 2007). Two recent studies reported that a diagnosis of autism was reasonably stable, whereas for other forms of ASD such as pervasive developmental disorder, the results were more variable (Rondeau et al. 2011; Woolfenden et al. 2012). Rondeau et al. (2011) did a meta-analysis on eight longitudinal studies, published between 1996 and 2009, examining autism and pervasive developmental disorder. All diagnoses were made before 36 months of age, and the interval between the initial and follow-up assessment was short, ranging from 12 to 84 months. They reported that an autism diagnosis tended to be a more stable than pervasive developmental disorder. Of those with pervasive developmental disorder, only 35% retained the same diagnosis (versus the 76% reported for autism), 39% moved to autism, and 25% moved off the spectrum. The authors concluded that those children diagnosed with pervasive developmental disorder at a young age should be reassessed at an older age.

The diagnosis of autism is relatively reliable and stable over time. Issues arise for very young children (the full syndrome picture sufficient for diagnosis may not be observed until age 3 years) and for individuals with "autistic-like" or "spectrum" conditions not so clearly satisfying strict diagnostic criteria. For example, Woolfenden et al. (2012) conducted a systematic review of 23 longitudinal studies (many overlapping with Rondeau et al. 2011) examining the stability of the diagnosis of children initially diagnosed with autism and other forms of ASD. The mean age of children at baseline ranged from 1.8 to 11.3 years, and mean duration at follow-up ranged from 2.1 to 32.5 years. Overall, autism was found to be a stable diagnosis although lower estimates (as low as 53%) were reported for children diagnosed in the preschool years (below 3 years of age). A small percentage of individuals diagnosed with autism, between 12% and 15%, move off the spectrum altogether. For other ASD's (including pervasive developmental disorder, Asperger's disorder, but not autism), based on the highest quality studies, the pattern of stability was more variable with 14–61% retaining their initial diagnosis at follow-up. A few studies reported on optimal outcome in autism (Fein group), and while these adults are indeed quite independent and functional, it appears that some autistic traits remain.

Taken together, a diagnosis of autism is more stable than the other ASD subtypes such as pervasive developmental disorder (Rondeau et al. 2011; Woolfenden et al. 2012), which is consistent with the rationale for the DSM-5 (Szatmari 2011). Given that the ASD category is less stable due to the inclusion of pervasive developmental disorder individuals, this presents challenges to clinicians when sharing a diagnosis of ASD with parents in terms of making appropriate intervention recommendations (Woolfenden et al. 2012).

Impairments in the core ASD symptoms (impairment in communication, reciprocal social interaction, and repetitive or stereotyped behaviors and interests) also tend to persist into adulthood (Billstedt et al. 2007; Howlin 2003; Matson et al. 2008), although symptom severity is reported to decrease in some individuals over time (Seltzer et al. 2003; Shattuck et al. 2007). Totsika et al. (2010) found that an older (50 years or older) group of adults with ASD and ID presented with fewer behavioral problems than the younger (<50 years) group, which is consistent with reports of decreases in behavior problems in the general adult intellectual disability population (Holden and Gitlesen 2006). Billstedt et al.

(2007) found that social interaction problems were still present in the vast majority of adults with ASD, but the occurrence of behavioral impairments (maladaptive and stereotyped behaviors) was much more variable with only a few symptoms in each category affecting half or more of the study sample. Others have reported that behavioral problems continue into the adult years (Ballaban-Gil et al. 1996) and that unusual responses to sensory (e.g., touch, pain, auditory, and visual) stimuli also remain common in adulthood (Billstedt et al. 2007; Leekam et al. 2006).

3.6 Cognitive Stability

There is considerable variability in measures of cognitive ability over time. Some have reported that IQ is relatively stable in ASD (e.g., Ballaban-Gil et al. 1996; Begovac et al. 2009; Howlin et al. 2004; Lockyer and Rutter 1970; Venter et al. 1992), whereas others have reported gains and/or losses over time (Billstedt et al. 2005; Farley et al. 2009; Mawhood et al. 2000). Howlin and colleagues reported that IQ remained remarkably stable over the life course; however, stability tended to be greatest among individuals with an initial IQ of at least 70. On the other hand, Billstedt et al. (2005) found that many individuals who initially had near average intelligence (IQ between 71 and 85) were later diagnosed with a mild (IQ 50–70) or severe (IQ < 50) intellectual disability, and those individuals with a severe intellectual disability (IQ < 50) in the original diagnostic study were all still in this category at follow-up. Overall, they found a downward shift of IQ level from the diagnostic study to the follow-up evaluation. A decrease in IQ may be an important biological marker in a subset of individuals with ASD (Farley et al. 2009). Farley et al. (2009) reported that over half of the sample had either large gains or losses in cognitive ability of greater than 1 standard deviation. Cognitive gain was associated with better outcome, as was better adaptive functioning. Some of the variability in results may be, in part, accounted for by the way IQ was measured or assessed, the age of initial assessment (IQ less stable in young children), and level of functioning of the participant, and the sometimes highly varied cognitive profiles of individuals which may evolve over time. This variability in IQ trajectory may also be due to the cumulative or time-specific impact of other risk or protective factors on the plasticity of IQ development.

4 Transitions Over the Life Course

4.1 Childhood

Children with ASD, like all other children, undergo several transitions throughout their school years. For instance, this may include the transition from early intervention to preschool, changing grades each year and moving into adolescence and then into adult life. Individuals with ASD also struggle with smaller transitions that are required on a daily basis, such as transitioning from one context to another. For example, this may include a transition between classes or transitions to unfamiliar settings (e.g., doctor's office). It is important to plan for these transitions because ineffective transition planning can have a negative impact on social and academic progress (Adreon and Stella 2001). Thus, numerous studies have emphasized the importance of transition planning for all children with special needs (Polloway et al. 2001), and this is particularly significant for children with ASD who frequently struggle with transitions. The ease with which a child transitions depends on the strategies adopted by educators when working with the child with ASD and their family (Harris and Handelman 2000). Parents of young children with ASD identified a number of factors that support successful and effective transitions, such as good communication between the school and home, transition plans that are child-centered, and inclusion of parents (Stoner et al. 2007).

Longitudinal studies of ASD have emphasized documenting the prevalence of certain outcomes (such as the stability of the diagnosis) rather than a more detailed look at developmentally related changes over time. Some studies are now taking a life course health development perspective by focusing on trajectories (Kim et al. 2015). The Pathways in ASD study, for example, followed roughly 400 children from the point of diagnosis at 2–4 years of age to the transition into primary school at 6 years of age allowing for the possibility of heterogeneous trajectories of autism symptoms and adaptive functioning. The results suggested (Szatmari et al. 2015) that heterogeneity in the rate of change of both phenotypes occurred, with some children doing remarkably well in adaptive function, but autism symptom severity remained more stable. There was little overlap of the autistic symptom severity and adaptive functioning developmental trajectories so that the course of the two seemed relatively independent, thereby highlighting the importance of close surveillance and treatment of these two domains independently over time because improvement in one area does not ensure improvement in the other area. These data also suggested that at least for the transition into primary school, continued improvement is possible for the majority of children with ASD.

A growing evidence base suggests that behavioral interventions can be associated with positive outcomes for children with ASD, with little evidence and generally poor quality studies available in adolescents and adults (Lounds Taylor et al. 2012; Weitlauf et al. 2014; National ASD Center National Standards Project 2009, 2015). Early interventions that were based on high-intensity applied behavior analysis over extended periods of time were associated with improvements in cognitive functioning and language skills, although the magnitude of effects varied across studies (Weitlauf et al. 2014). This variability may be related to the scarcity of information about modifying factors related to subgroups (Weitlauf et al. 2014). For instance, the majority of evidence supports the efficacy of comprehensive early intensive behavioral interventions (EIBI), which is currently the standard of care in many clinics and schools (Peters-Scheffer et al. 2011; Reichow 2012). Meaningful gains have been shown in IQ, language skills, and adaptive outcomes with medium to large effects (Reichow 2012; Strauss et al. 2013) and a decrease in autism severity over time (Zachor and Itzchak 2010). Gains are not universal, some making rapid progress and others only modest or no progress (Peters-Scheffer et al. 2011; Reichow and Wolery 2009). Inclusion of parents in skill generalization has led to overall higher effect sizes (Strauss et al. 2013). Early intensive parent programs have been shown to modify parent behavior during interactions, but there is less data about their ability to improve developmental skills beyond language gains for some children (Weitlauf et al. 2014). Predictors of positive outcome and/or changes in trajectory include younger age at entry into EIBI programs (between 18 months and 5 years), higher IQ or adaptive functioning or language (mild to moderate range of functioning), and less severe autism symptoms (Strauss et al. 2013). With regard to program characteristics, intensity of EIBI programs was related to gains in IQ, adaptive functioning, and language ability, whereas duration of the program was generally not related to gains with the exception of some evidence that it was related to language and adaptive behavior gains (Strauss et al. 2013). Contemporary early intervention ABA approaches are more naturalistic, child-directed, and guided by developmental theory and are currently referred to as naturalistic developmental behavioral interventions (NDBI's) (for detailed discussion see Schreibman et al. 2015). Other behavioral interventions that have shown some positive effects include, but are not limited to, social skills, treatment targeting joint attention, and cognitive behavior therapy (Weitlauf et al. 2014). Research is beginning to show that behaviorally based interventions have an effect on patterns of brain activity, particularly in regions involved in social processing (Dawson et al. 2012), and that neural plasticity in response to intervention may exist throughout the lifespan (Faja et al. 2012).

Thus, the evidence supports that early interventions are effective in ASD; however, less is known about how sustainable these intervention effects are after transitions from early intervention into preschool and elementary school. There is emerging evidence that young children with ASD who received early intervention sustained social, language, and/or nonverbal cognitive gains through a 6–37-month follow-up period (e.g., Kasari et al. 2010; Landa et al. 2011; Landa and Kalb 2012). For instance, Landa and Kalb (2012) examined outcomes in 2-year-old toddlers enrolled in a 6-month nursery school-based intervention immediately following intervention (M age = 35 months), at short-term (M age = 41 months) and long-term follow-up (M age = 72 months; 37 months after children completed intervention). At long-term follow-up, they found gains in IQ and communication; however, increases were not evenly distributed across the different time points. Gains in IQ and communication were robust initially from pre- to post-intervention, followed by a period of stabilization, which was then followed by another developmental burst. In contrast, the trajectory of autism severity was different with an initial decrease in severity form pre- to post-intervention, followed by an increase in severity to pre-intervention levels by the final time point. Magiati et al. (2011) reassessed outcomes even later at 5 years after departing preschool and found that children maintained standardized IQ scores, but adaptive functioning scores decreased. Longer-term outcome studies are needed to determine the sustainability of gains, as well as to determine whether there are sensitive periods in development as well as the developmental scaffolding that is necessary, especially during key life course transitions that are likely to promote optimal health development outcomes (e.g., age, type of intervention, duration, intensity, content, etc.) (Landa and Kalb 2012).

4.2 Transition from Adolescence into Adulthood

For youth with ASD and their families, the transition into adulthood is a time of uncertainty and loss of entitlement to many services that were available while in the school system. In comparison to early childhood, there often is a dearth of appropriate supports and opportunities for adults with ASD. Leaving high school can have a disruptive effect on youth and young adults with ASD in a number of areas, including ASD symptom presentation, maladaptive behaviors, and family functioning (Taylor and Seltzer 2010, 2011a, b). Taylor and Seltzer (2010) examined the impact of exiting high school and observed that in general, autism symptoms and maladaptive behaviors continued to improve while adolescents were part of the secondary school system, but improvement significantly slowed (by over half) after exiting high school for internalizing behavior and all but one of the autism symptom domains (i.e., verbal communication impairments). The authors suggested that this change was likely related to the lack of disability-related services or that occupational or day program services were less stimulating than those in the school system. Interestingly, youth without comorbid intellectual disability improved more in both autism symptoms and maladaptive behaviors while in high school compared to those with intellectual disability (Shattuck et al. 2007), but after exiting high school, improvement slowed more for those individuals without an ID (Taylor and Seltzer 2010). Indeed, only 6% of individuals with ASD without comorbid ID were receiving day services immediately after high school, compared to 74% with ASD and ID, and over one-quarter had no occupational, educational, or day activities. In addition, the improvement in the mother-youth relationship seen in high school slowed or stopped after high school (i.e., decreasing maternal warmth), with the greatest impact on relationships for youth with ASD and no ID (Taylor and Seltzer 2011a). Thus, leaving high school had a negative impact on individuals with ASD, with the most pronounced effect on those youth with ASD without an ID, suggesting a particular lack of adequate educational and occupational activities for this group of individuals in adulthood. It also highlights that individuals with ASD and no ID are often impaired in their adaptive skills and encounter difficulty generalizing these skills in daily life. When services are inadequate, parents will often take on this responsibility, leading some families to experience this transition period as a time of stress and anxiety (Howlin 2005). Other families view this period as an opportunity for new and more positive possibilities, such as finding more appropriate occupational placements and leaving high school, which for some youth, was a negative experience (Taylor 2009).

Access to autism-related services is also related to family income. Families with lower incomes and less parental education may have less access to autism-related services in childhood compared to families with higher incomes (Liptak et al. 2008; Thomas et al. 2007). Improvement in maladaptive behaviors slows after high school more so for those families with a lower income (Taylor and Seltzer 2011b). Thus, it is important to better understand the factors that promote optimal transition for individuals with ASD, as well as the impact on families. Taylor (2009) underscores the importance of examining contextual and environmental factors that are amenable to change or can be targeted in intervention in order to improve success with transition and suggests that exclusively focusing on characteristics such as IQ and early language that although are predictive of later outcome is more difficult to intervene once the individual with ASD becomes an adolescent or adult. For instance, the implementation of transition planning has been associated with more successful achievement of adult milestones (Frank and Siltington 2000). Indeed, factors such as the post-high school goals for the student and parental expectations were predictive of participation in postsecondary education (Chiang et al. 2012). In addition, the development of appropriate educational, occupational, and day programs for individuals with ASD of all ability levels is important as is a lifelong emphasis on generalization of skills.

4.2.1 Educational Attainment

With regard to education, many individuals in the follow-up studies published in the last decade attended specialized schools or classrooms (Billstedt et al. 2011; Farley et al. 2009, Howlin et al. 2004). Only a few individuals with ASD obtained formal qualifications (Eaves and Ho 2008; Howlin et al. 2004), although results of recent studies have been more promising (Hofvander et al. 2009; Farley 2009). For example, Farley and colleagues reported that 44% completed high school at grade 12 with a diploma, and 39% went on to postsecondary education. With regard to those students who are capable of entry into college or university, many do not seek or gain entry or drop out prematurely (Glennon 2001; VanBergeijk et al. 2008) due to a number of factors including social isolation and loneliness, difficulty managing changing routines and schedules, difficulty with independent living, and the absence of monitoring and guidance (Howlin et al. 2004; Jobe and White 2007; White et al. 2011).

Students with ASD are able to succeed both academically and socially in postsecondary education when the transition is carefully planned, appropriate accommodations are obtained, and supports are available (for detailed discussion, see VanBergeijk et al. 2008). Preparing students for the transition to postsecondary education is important for many adolescents but is particularly important for individuals with ASD, most of whom have difficulty with transitions. VanBergeijk and colleagues stress the importance of a good fit between the student and the prospective academic institution. For instance, this may include careful consideration of the size of the school and classes, level of supports, and receptiveness to serving students with disabilities – specifically ASD, access to mental health services, and availability of supports to address both academic concerns (e.g., organizational help, accommodations related to evaluation and test taking, support with complex assignments, etc.), as well as nonacademic concerns including life skills, issues of daily living (e.g., laundry, budgeting), organizational difficulties, communication limitations, and social skills (e.g., socializing with peers, getting along with roommates, romantic relationships). Indeed, adolescents with ASD reported greater concern about social acceptance and being able to function independently than about accessing academic accommodations and resources in postsecondary educational settings, and thereby identified a need for built in social supports and access to trained staff members as a resource (Camarena and Sarigiani 2009). Many individuals with ASD also have difficulty with issues related to sexuality and may require support or direct instruction (see Volkmar 2004). Furthermore, postsecondary educational programs must also include planning and preparation for the transition to work and independent living that includes vocational training and life coaching (VanBergeijk et al. 2008). Families and educators are also encouraged to support the development of self-advocacy skills which are important to the transition process so that adolescent and young adults are able to navigate the journey through higher education, work, and independent living (Camarena and Sarigiani 2009). Thus, for students with aspirations for postsecondary education, careful planning and supports are required to help students with ASD achieve academic success.

4.2.2 Employment, Independent Living, and Social Life

The research on transition into adulthood in individuals with ASD has primarily focused on the traditional view of transition which describes the degree of independence in living arrangements, ability to gain and maintain employment, and the presence of intimate relationships outside of the family unit (Fussell and Furstenberg 2005). The majority of individuals with ASD have difficulty achieving the developmental tasks of adulthood and remain dependent on parents/caregivers for support in employment and accommodation, and most do not have intimate relationships (friendship or romantic).

Many persons with ASD are able to work successfully within the community (Garcia-Villamisar et al. 2000; Mawhood and Howlin 1999); however, the majority experience difficulty securing meaningful employment (Billstedt et al. 2011; Eaves and Ho 2008; Howlin et al. 2004; Newman et al. 2011). Findings from the National Longitudinal Transition Study-2 (NLTS2) examined a nationally representative sample of youth and young adults with disabilities in the USA and found that up to 8 years post-high school, only 63% of adults with autism had worked at some point after high school and only 37% were employed at the time of the survey (Newman et al. 2011). In a group of individuals with near average to average intelligence, the outcomes were somewhat more promising with 54% in full-time or part-time independent paid jobs, 12% in supported employment or part-time volunteer positions, 24% in day programs, and 10% unemployed (Farley et al. 2009). Even among those who are employed, many worked few hours, and most jobs tended to be low level, were found by parental contacts (versus open job market), and were poorly paid such that individuals did not have adequate financial support to live independently (Cimera and Cowan 2009; Eaves and Ho 2008; Howlin et al. 2004). Furthermore, many individuals were in part-time, volunteer, supported, or sheltered employment; few worked independently with little or no support, and some had no daytime occupation at all. Jobs often ended prematurely because of social or behavioral difficulties or other work-related difficulties (Mawhood and Howlin 1999). Cimera and Cowan (2009) examined cost of services and employment outcomes achieved by adults with ASD in the vocational rehabilitation system. The study found that adults with autism were employed at higher rates than other disability groups; however, the rate of employment was only 41% (60% do not obtain employment), and as noted earlier, they worked fewer hours and earned lower wages. Adults with autism were also the most costly group of individual to serve, and services were difficult to implement. Howlin (2013) underscores that generic employment services do not meet the needs of individuals with ASD, and there is a need for more programs and research specific to individuals with ASD. Although limited, research is beginning to emerge showing that supported employment models for individuals with ASD are effective (Howlin et al. 2005; Keel et al. 1997; Shattuck et al. 2012; Taylor et al. 2012).

Critical factors in finding and maintaining a long-term placement include a thorough assessment to appropriately match the skills and abilities of the person with ASD to the requirements of the job, as well as having the appropriate level and type of employment support (Mawhood and Howlin 1999; Smith and Paulippen 1999).

Hagner and Cooney (2005) found that a set of supervisory accommodation strategies were commonly associated with successful supervision, including maintaining a consistent schedule and set of job responsibilities, using organizers to structure the job, minimizing unstructured or idle time, being direct with communication, and providing reminders and reassurances. Longer job retention has been correlated with higher levels of social inclusion and acceptance on the job (Belcher and Smith 1994). Furthermore, engaging in work is often related to other meaningful outcomes, such as contributing to one's self-worth and confidence, providing opportunities to shares one's strengths that are valued by others, opportunities to develop friendships or other supportive relationships, as well as engagement in the larger community (Lee and Carter 2012). On the other hand, failure to find suitable work resulted in frustration and in some serious problems with depression and/or anxiety (Mawhood and Howlin 1999). With supported employment, individuals with ASD are able to find and maintain suitable employment (Mawhood and Howlin 1999).

Most individuals with ASD live with their parents or in other supported arrangements (e.g., community-based group home), and few live independently either with or without some level of support (Billstedt et al. 2011; Farley et al. 2009). Eaves and Ho (2008) reported that 56% lived with their parents, 35% were in supported arrangements such as group homes or foster care, and the remainder lived more or less independently. With regard to friendship, it has been reported that up to approximately 30% of individuals have one or more friends (Eaves and Ho 2008; Howlin et al. 2004). Social contacts often result from special interests and skills rather than close friendships (Howlin 2000). Some individuals have been reported to want friendships but were unable to form these relationships, whereas others had no interest or did not understand the concept of friendship (Billstedt et al. 2011). Few individuals had close intimate relationships or were married at some point (Eaves and Ho 2008; Farley et al. 2009; Hofvander et al. 2009; Howlin et al. 2004). In a group of higher functioning individuals with ASD, Farley and colleagues reported that 7% were married, 5% divorced, 7% were in long-term relationships, 44% never dated, 32% dated in both group and couple situations, and 22% dated only in group settings. When parents were asked whether they felt their adult child wished to have a romantic relationship, of those participants not already in relationships, 44% felt their son or daughter would like to be in a relationship. On the other hand, 41% did not want a romantic partner because parents thought their children were concerned about passing on autism to a child or themselves being too difficult for a partner to manage.

4.2.3 Summary

Taken together, the research to date focuses primarily on the attainment of traditional skills that are indicative of successful transition into adulthood and less on more subjective or quality of life indicators. Although outcomes are quite variable, in general, outcomes related to level of independence, employment status, and intimate relationships are poor, suggesting that the transition to adulthood is fraught with many challenges. Evidence suggests that better outcomes are related to better cognitive abilities and earlier language skills, although even these individuals struggle with attaining the developmental tasks of adulthood. Furthermore, availability of appropriate resources, services, and supports for the individuals with ASD and their families are key ingredients for successful transition into adulthood and better outcomes throughout adult life. Lee and Carter (2012) identified seven elements that are important for high-quality transition services, which include individualized services that reflect the strengths of the individual, positive career development and early work experiences, collaboration and interagency involvement, family supports and expectations, fostering self-determination and independence, social- and employment-related skill instruction, and establishment of job-related supports. Thus, the impetus of future research is to examine factors that will support successful transition (e.g., environmental and contextual factors) and find other ways to define transition such as from a psychosocial or attachment perspective (for review, see Taylor 2009), especially as the epidemiology of ASD changes from autism with ID to a preponderance of ASD without ID.

4.3 Aging and ASD

Autism is a lifelong condition; however, little is known about older adults with ASD. Indeed, much of the research to date has examined the aging ASD population but not the aged (65 plus) (Perkins and Berkman 2012). Although information is quite limited, research suggests that life expectancy is shortened compared to the general population and causes of death include high rates of seizures and accidental deaths (e.g., drowning) (Mouridsen et al. 2008; Piven and Rabins 2011). It is unclear whether deaths that are related to diseases (e.g., nervous and sensory disease) in ASD are due to a predisposition to certain health concerns or due to poor health surveillance leading to poor diagnosis and management (Perkins and Berkman 2012). A number of medical and psychiatric concerns have been reported in children and adolescents with ASD, such as sleep disorders, psychiatric symptoms, gastrointestinal disorders, feeding selectivity and aversions, metabolic conditions, and epilepsy; however, there is little information about these concerns as individuals age (Piven and Rabins 2011). Similarly, it is unclear whether treatments that are effective in children and adolescents would also benefit adults. Given the dearth of information of older adults with ASD, a group of experts were convened to characterize the gaps in knowledge and define a research agenda to bridge this gap (see Piven and Rabins 2011). Research priorities included developing diagnostic criteria and tools to diagnose older adults, conducting cross-sectional descriptive studies in adults of phenomenology and associated features, longitudinal studies of lifespan trajectories, neurobiological studies examining underlying changes over time, intervention studies, and mechanism to support clinical and research training in aging. This research is needed to improve the lives of individuals with ASD and to inform clinical practice and policies that can address these healthcare disparities (Piven and Rabins 2011).

5 Mental Health Issues in ASD

5.1 Prevalence Rates

In terms of quality of adult life, there is increasing evidence suggesting that comorbid psychiatric symptoms and disorders are common in individuals with ASD, with estimated rates ranging from 30% to 70% (e.g., Bradley et al. 2004; Gjevik et al. 2011; Leyfer et al. 2006; Moseley et al. 2011; Simonoff et al. 2008; Skokauskas and Gallagher 2010). Understanding comorbid mental health problems is important not only because of the high prevalence but also because of the impact on daily functioning, long-term prognosis, and the added burden and challenges faced by individuals and their families. Individuals with ASD have higher rates of comorbidity compared to the general population (Ghaziuddin et al. 1998; Moseley et al. 2011), a psychiatrically referred population of youth without ASD (Joshi et al. 2010), as well as individuals with ID alone (Bradley et al. 2004; Brereton et al. 2006; LoVullo and Matson 2009), although the latter has not been consistently found (Tsakanikos et al. 2006). The most commonly reported psychiatric disorders include anxiety and depression (MacNeil et al. 2009; Sterling et al. 2008; White et al. 2009). ASD has also been found to co-occur with obsessive compulsive disorder (OCD), disruptive behavioral disorders, attention deficit hyperactivity disorder (ADHD), bipolar disorder, Tourette's disorder, tic disorder, and eating disorders (Drmic amd Szatmari 2014; Skokauskas and Gallagher 2010; Szatmari and McConnell 2011; Volkmar et al. 2014; White et al. 2009). Studies examining schizophrenia have been mixed; some studies report high rates (Chang et al. 2003), whereas others have not found an increased rate (Seltzer et al. 2004; Volkmar and Cohen 1991). Although the two disorders are quite different, misclassification of ASD as schizophrenia may also contribute to the variability in reported rates (Perlman 2000;

Palucka, Bradley, Lunsky 2008). Furthermore, ASD often co-occurs with multiple psychiatric disorders (Leyfer et al. 2006; Simonoff et al. 2008). For instance, Simonoff et al. (2008), using a population-based cohort, conducted a structured psychiatric interview (not modified for ASD) with 112 10–14-year olds and found that 70% of ASD participants had at least one comorbid disorder and 41% had two or more. It is important to better understand this comorbidity given that many individuals with ASD are likely to struggle with mental health concerns, and more importantly, psychiatric problems may cause considerable distress and interference with daily functioning and significantly impact long-term prognosis and outcome (Kim et al. 2000; Mattila et al. 2010; Muris et al. 1998; Russell and Sofronoff 2005; White et al. 2009).

To date, the majority of research on psychiatric comorbidity has been conducted in children and adolescents (Amr et al. 2012; Gjevik et al. 2011; Leyfer et al. 2006; Mattila et al. 2010; Skokauskas and Gallagher 2010). In a review conducted by Skokauskas and Gallagher (2010) examining comorbid disorders in children with autism and Asperger syndrome, wide ranges in rates of co-occurring symptoms or diagnoses were found: 0–6% for schizophrenia, 5–35% for generalized anxiety, 10–64% for simple phobias, 1–37% for OCD, and 0–50% for affective disorders or symptoms. Fewer studies have examined this issue in adults, although research in this area is beginning to emerge (Cederlund et al. 2010; Ghaziuddin and Zafar 2008; Hofvander et al. 2009; La Malfa et al. 2007; Lugnegard et al. 2011; Moseley et al. 2011), and a number of follow-up studies have reported on psychiatric outcomes (Billstedt et al. 2005; Eaves and Ho 2008; Farley et al. 2009). A study that examined young adults with Asperger syndrome found high rates of depression and anxiety, consistent with the literature in children and adolescents with ASD, whereas psychotic and substance-induced disorders were uncommon (Lugnegard et al. 2011). Hofvander et al. (2009) assessed 122 consecutively referred adults with ASD and normal intelligence ranging in age from 16 to 60 years. Lifetime axis I comorbidity was common, and they also found that mood (53%) and anxiety disorders (50%) were most common, followed by ADHD (43%), OCD (34%), and chronic tic disorders (20%). With regard to the rate of lifetime axis II disorders, 62% met criteria for at least one personality disorder. Other studies have reported somewhat lower rates of anxiety (Farley et al. 2009; Moseley et al. 2011) and depression (Billstedt et al. 2005; Eaves and Ho 2008; Farley et al. 2009; Moseley et al. 2011). A study examining adolescents and young adults with autism (over three-quarters had an intellectual disability) found that 42% had an additional mental health disorder, a rate that is two to four times seen in typically developing young people (Moseley et al. 2011). There is some evidence that the rates of mood and anxiety disorders in parents of children with autism is higher than that in the general population and when compared to Down syndrome (Bolton et al. 1998; Mazefsky et al. 2008). This may reflect an effect of stress on family members. A more thorough examination of genetic variable expressivity would involve a study of mood disorders in second- and third-degree relatives.

5.2 Mental Health Services

Given the high rate of psychiatric comorbidity, there is a need for appropriate mental health services for individuals with ASD of all ages. This includes preventive interventions designed to optimize mental functioning and life course trajectories. In a study investigating the healthcare experiences of children with ASD and their families, it was found that 15% of families reported unmet mental health services, and provider lack of skills was a barrier to obtaining these services (Chiri and Warfield 2012). With regard to the utilization of mental health services by individuals with ASD, the reports are mixed, with some reporting underutilization of services (Bryson et al. 2008) and others reporting relatively high rates of service use (Narendorf et al. 2011). Narendorf et al. (2011) reported that of those youth who received mental health services (i.e., 46%), 49% received it through the school.

African-American youth and youth from lower-income families were more likely to use school-based services than accessing community-based services, underscoring the importance of schools in providing these services for underserved group and the importance of ensuring the continuation of services after high school. For students with ASD, there is emerging research examining the delivery of mental health services in schools for anxiety (Drmic, Aljunied, Reaven 2017; Luxford, Hadwin, Kovshoff 2016). Bryson et al. (2008) found that short-term crisis-oriented mental health services were effective at stabilizing children with ASD but that many remained highly symptomatic at discharge, suggesting that changes are needed to the current system in order to serve those individuals with chronic and long-term needs.

Many individuals with ASD may be at risk for psychiatric hospitalization. Indeed, approximately 11% of children and youth aged 5–21 years experienced at least one psychiatric hospital inpatient admission (Mandell 2008), and 48% used psychiatric hospital services by age 40 (Mouridsen et al. 2008). Children with a diagnosis of Asperger's disorder and pervasive developmental disorder, compared to children with autism, were more likely to experience inpatient hospitalization (Bryson et al. 2008). Lunsky et al. (2009) compared patients with ASD and ID to other individuals accessing tertiary level mental healthcare in Ontario and found that individuals with ASD and ID were younger, spent more days in hospitals, and were less likely to have a psychotic disorder diagnosis than both patients with and without ID. Interestingly, fewer than half of the individuals with ASD and ID had an additional psychiatric diagnosis, although almost all (91%) were prescribed psychotropic medication, which is consistent with previous studies (Tsakanikos et al. 2006, 2007a). Tsakanikos et al. (2007b) reported that behavioral management problems predicted psychotropic medication and use of psychiatric services in adults with pervasive developmental disorder and ID. A study examining referral trends to specialist mental health services in south London from 1983 to 2000 for individuals with ASD and ID reported an increase in diagnosable psychiatric disorders over time and a significant reduction of medication at time of referral, but no change in the use of other therapeutic interventions, which is in contrast to services received by younger children with ASD. Thus, there continues to be a need for specialized inpatient and outpatient mental health services for individuals with ASD, as well as more training for service providers.

6 Summary

ASD is a neurodevelopmental disorder that represents a chronic, lifelong condition based on atypicalities in brain development. While there are changes in syndrome expression over time, new challenges often emerge. Much of the current research has focused on static or crosssectional outcomes as opposed to developmental trajectories and changes in those trajectories. This can include looking at the developmental course of the disorder, the developmental course of specific skills that are important to later outcomes such as joint attention skills, as well as trajectories, related to the effects of early intervention. Longer-term studies are critical to treatment research in order to determine the sustainability of early intervention treatment gains, to explore whether there are sensitive periods of child development when treatments are most effective, and to determine factors that promote treatment outcome. Research needs to include enough information about factors that might be important to outcome so that predictors can be better elucidated, as well as a shift to focus on mediators and moderators of outcome. There is a need for more longitudinal studies and some consensus about the type of information that should be gathered by all research groups so that findings are comparable among different studies and can be combined into meta-analyses. For instance, standardized IQ measures could be used to document intellectual abilities. It may be beneficial to convene a group of experts as well as parents and individuals with ASD to determine what basic set of factors are important.

The current review highlights that outcomes for people with ASD have been improving over time; although relative to typically developing children and adolescents, outcomes are still generally poor. Much of the work to date has focused on achieving the traditional developmental tasks of adulthood, including independence in living arrangements, gaining and maintaining employment, and developing intimate relationships outside of the family unit. Research examining quality of life is beginning to emerge, which is an important next step to further our understanding of how to help improve the lived experiences of individuals with ASD. QOL studies need to shift focus and include information about factors and developmental processes that are thought to be important to achieving better life course health development outcomes, such as IQ, symptom severity, and language development. In addition, examining other factors that promote thriving in individuals with ASD is needed. Understanding what those factors are is critical so that better programs and interventions can be developed, which include the developmental scaffolding that children and families need to optimize long-term health development outcomes. It is also important to understand what impact access to adequate resources and intervention has on the identification, service provision, and likely outcomes on people with ASD. Another key theme is the development and emergence of mental health comorbidities which often represent an enormous challenge for young adults with ASD and their families. Research needs to include information about the developmental pathways that lead to these outcomes so that risk and protective factors can be targeted early, with the intent of optimizing the trajectory of mental health outcomes. There is also a need for more basic research such as epigenetic studies of non-syndromic ASD, genetic studies that focus on much smaller copy number variants or DNA sequence variants identified either in exomes or in whole genome sequencing, and continued research examining environmental risk factors.

A number of recommendations to facilitate the transition periods and support individual with ASD and their families can be gleaned from the existing literature. Implementation of a transition plan is crucial since it is associated with more successful transition from early intervention into preschool (Stoner et al. 2007) and attainment of adult milestones (Frank and Siltington 2000) and may help temper the disruptive effect of leaving high school (Taylor and Seltzer 2010, 2011a, b). Parents, clinicians, and educators are encouraged to begin the transition planning process for the transition to adulthood early and include planning for treatment, independence (i.e., daily living skills, skills for independent living), education, employment, living arrangements, mental health, and medical care. For instance, good practical living skills, even in those individuals who have a cognitive disability, led to better outcomes and quality of life (Farley et al. 2009). Therefore, focusing on developing independence in daily living skills starting from a young age is an important target for intervention programs and transition planning. This highlights the importance of planning early so that skills can be integrated into treatment and educational programs at younger ages, allowing for ample practice and supervision of these skills well before the individual is expected to be able to manage on their own.

For many individuals and families, the transition to adulthood is a time of worry and uncertainty because many services that were available through the educational system are no longer available and there are few appropriate supports or services for adults with ASD. Taylor and Seltzer (2010) showed that the improvement slowed significantly after exiting high school, particularly for those youth with ASD and no ID. This change was likely related to a lack of services or that available services were less stimulating than those provided in the educational system. Thus, the development of new models of care that incorporate appropriate educational, occupational and day programs for adults with ASD of all ability levels is essential. However, simply having a program is not enough; it is also important to ensure that the appropriate training and support is provided on an ongoing basis to the individual with ASD and that service providers are adequately trained to work with this group of individuals. For instance, given the prevalence and impact of mental health issues in individuals with ASD and their families, there is a need for ongoing mental health services and staff who are trained in this area and able to support families. A worrying trend is the increased use of psychopharmacology in adults with ASD often as a result of lack of psychosocial services that might better meet those needs in a way that improves life course outcomes and promotes thriving. Another example relates to successfully obtaining and maintaining long-term employment, which may involve supportive employment programs that include training related to general job skills (e.g., resume writing, interviewing skills, proper social behavior), specific skills needed for a particular job (e.g., learning job requirements and skills, learning about the culture and expectations for that job), and ongoing support (e.g., job coach). Training and support should also be provided to the employers in order to educate them about ASD in general, help them understand the needs of a particular individual, as well as highlight their unique skills and abilities that can positively contribute to workplace. Indeed, parents, educators, employers, and other professionals are encouraged to appreciate the many strengths, skills, and unique talents of individuals with ASD and approach current programs and future planning from a strength-based approach, leveraging each individual's unique set of assets, versus a deficits-based approach that focuses on what needs to be fixed.

There is a stark lack of information about ASD in the aging and elderly population. Given this gap in knowledge, a group of experts were convened to identify and describe these gaps and define a research agenda (see Piven and Rabins 2011). The research proprieties included developing diagnostic criteria and tools to diagnose older adults, conducting cross-sectional descriptive studies in adults of phenomenology and associated features, longitudinal studies of lifespan trajectories, neurobiological studies examining underlying changes over time, and intervention studies and mechanism to support clinical and research training in aging.

This change in perspective might be part of a shift from treatment of deficits to accommodation of unique characteristics of the adult with ASD. There comes a time when the relentless pursuit of treatment to "make things better" will have a negative impact on the person with ASD and their family. People with ASD should not always be considered "disabled," and taking a lifespan perspective to developmental trajectories should be part of this switch for service providers as well as parents.

7 Research Priorities

There has been a marked increase in ASD-related research over the past decades. Considerable advances have been made in key areas, including: the genetic basis of ASD and its diagnosis; studies of the social brain; the connections between timing of diagnosis and long-term outcomes; new treatment models, some pharmacological and behavioral treatments can now be viewed as evidence based; psychiatric co-morbidities with particular emphasis on anxiety and depression; and, research on basic issues like employment, living arrangements, medical survelillance, etc. Thus, a number of gaps remain that need to be addressed. The following summarizes a number of recommendations for research, some of which were noted earlier in the paper, to better understand life course health development in ASD.

7.1 Research Priorities

(i) Basic mechanism research:
   (a) Better understanding of epigenetic mechanisms in non-syndromic ASD.
   (b) Continued research in the area of genetics and neuroimaging. For example, this could include:
   - Genetic studies that focus on much smaller copy number variants or DNA sequence variants identified either in exomes or in whole genome sequencing
   - Studies that assess the impact of genetic testing (e.g., microarrays) on health outcomes
   - Studies combining genetics and neuroimaging work

- Neuroimaging studies examining the trajectories of brain development
- Neuroimaging studies examining the impact of behavioral treatments on the brain

(c) Continued research examining environmental risk factors, as well as gene-environment interactions.

(d) Identification of biomarkers (e.g., genetics, neural circuitry) is a high priority. For instance, the National Institutes of Health Interagency Coordinating Committee Strategic Plan called for the identification of biological markers, which separately or in combination with behavioral markers accurately identified ASD before age 2 (Dawson and Bernier 2013).

(e) Development of novel therapeutics, e.g., creating medicine that can target core ASD symptoms.

(f) Focus on early developmental skills or early markers of development that may impact the developmental trajectory. For instance, there is evidence that early joint attention skills are important for social cognitive development and later language and adaptive skills. Further, interventions targeting joint attention have been shown to be effective. Thus, research further examining the role of joint attention skills in ASD would be beneficial. It is also important to identify other potential early developing skills that may provide early targets for intervention.

(ii) Clinical Research:

(a) Early diagnosis remains a treatment priority. The recent advances in technology (e.g., neuroimaging) and genetics suggest the next wave of advances in our ability to detect autism through the use of biomarkers and new screening tools. Thus, research examining the utility of these biomarkers in clinical contexts will be needed. The availability of predictive biomarkers could index risk for ASD before or at the onset of symptoms, thereby preventing the symptoms from developing or alleviating symptoms and improving the trajectory of outcomes.

(b) Development of more evidence-based treatment research throughout the lifespan is needed.

- A growing body of literature has shown that interventions can be associated with positive outcomes in children; however, there is still a need for studies across setting and improvements in methodological rigor.
- Little evidence is available about treatment in adolescents and adults. There is a need to develop treatment across the lifespan and determine "which" treatments are most needed and effective at the different life stages and "when" these treatments are most effective.
- Substantial scientific advances are needed to improve our understanding of which interventions are most effective for specific children with ASD and to elucidate the factors or components of interventions most associated with positive outcomes.
- Exciting potential to bring together basic science and treatment in development of new metrics/measures (e.g., predicting response to treatments – recent work on EEG/fMRI and treatment change).

(c) Very little evidence is available for specific treatment approaches in adolescents and adults; this is especially the case for evidence-based approaches to support the transition of youth with autism to adulthood. (Lounds et al. 2012). Thus, more research is needed to focus transition period.

(d) Little information exists about the aging population in ASD with virtually no information about the aged (65+). More research is needed in various areas from basic and clinical research to data/method development and translational research. A research agenda spanning all these areas for the aging population was described in Piven and Rabins (2011). As noted earlier, the research

priorities included developing diagnostic criteria and tools to diagnose older adults, conducting cross-sectional descriptive studies in adults of phenomenology and associated features, longitudinal studies of lifespan trajectories, neurobiological studies examining underlying changes over time, and intervention studies and mechanism to support clinical and research training in aging.
   (e) Studies examining quality of life and the person, environmental, and person-environmental interactions that lead to a thriving life.
(iii) Translational research:
   (a) Need innovative solutions for training physicians, clinicians, and other professionals working with individuals with ASD throughout the lifespan. In particular, there is a serious lack of well-trained healthcare professional to serve the large number of adults with ASD. This includes multiple areas, including diagnosis and assessment of adult, mental health and medical supports, and supports for daily life.
   (b) Research related to transition planning as it relates to treatment, independence, education, employment, living arrangements, mental health, and medical care.

7.2 Data/Method Development Priorities

(a) A shift toward longitudinal studies to better understand developmental trajectories (with attention to child and family characteristics – e.g., SES, parental education)
(b) Inclusion of characteristics that might be important to outcome (e.g., IQ, language ability, etc.) so that predictors of outcome can be better elucidated, as well as a shift to focus on mediators and moderators of outcome.
(c) A shift in focus examining not only risk factors but also on factors that are protective and promote thriving.
(d) Better metrics throughout the lifespan. There is an exciting potential to bring together basic science and treatment in development of new metrics/measures (e.g., predicting response to treatments as was seen in recent work on fMRI and treatment change).
(e) Development of better measures to look at outcome determination and more focus on quality of life (QOL) measures for the individual and family.
(f) Greater focus in critical or sensitive periods of development when environemntal exposures can have long-lasting effects on outcomes.

7.3 Translational Priorities

(a) Early diagnosis. A wide gap remains between our knowledge about best practices in ASD (e.g., screening for ASD at 18 and 24 months) and Centers for Disease Control and Prevention (CDC) data showing that the average age of diagnosis in the USA is 5 years and higher for individuals with milder forms of ASD. This is a problem given that much of the literature on early intervention shows best outcomes when intervention is initiated early (between 18 months and 5 years). This is a major challenge and will require innovative solutions and a focus on dissemination and implementation science.
(b) Better coordination of different systems related to children's health development (e.g., school and health systems).
(c) Development of physician guidelines for healthcare.
(d) Challenge in providing access to behavioral, mental health, and medical healthcare and, thus, the need for improved and expanded healthcare services with care providers who are well trained in working with individuals with ASD and their families.
(e) Innovative solutions to better serve those in remote regions or underserved population (e.g., individuals living in poverty).

(f) Incorporating independent living skills into treatment/educational programs starting at a young age.
(g) Although our understanding of autism has increased, there is a major gap in translating this to public school settings.
(h) Development of new models/systems of care that incorporate appropriate educational, occupational and day programs for adults with ASD of all ability levels is essential.
(i) Vocational system for adults.
(j) Generic employment services do not meet the needs of individuals with ASD, therefore the need for more programs and research specific to individuals with ASD (e.g., supported employment models). Supportive employment programs – training related to general job skills, specific skills needed for a particular job, and ongoing support (e.g., job coach).
(k) Training and support for employers.

8 Conclusions

Taken together, there has been a tremendous growth in research in the ASD field. However, there remain a number of gaps that need to be addressed, with a particular focus on optimizing life course trajectories for individuals and populations with ASD. The principles of the life course health development framework describe health as an emergent set of developmental capacities that develop continuously over the lifespan in a complex, nonlinear process occurring in multiple dimensions, levels, and phases and are sensitive to timing. This is a valuable framework to direct the research agenda to continue to move the field forward and to improve the lives of individuals with ASD, their families, and their communities.

References

Adreon, D., & Stella, J. (2001). Transition to middle and high school: Increasing the success of students with Asperger syndrome. *Intervention in School and Clinic, 36*, 266–271.

American Psychiatric Association. (1980). *Diagnostic and statistical manual*. Washington, DC: APA Press.

Amr, M., Raddad, D., El-Mehesh, F., Bakr, A., Sallam, K., & Amin, T. (2012). Comorbid psychiatric disorders in Arab children with autism spectrum disorders. *Research in Autism Spectrum Disorders, 6*, 240–248.

Asperger, H. (1944). Die "autistichen Psychopathen" im Kindersalter. *Archive fur psychiatrie und Nervenkrankheiten, 117*, 76–136.

Baker, T. B., Breslau, N., Covey, L., & Shiffman, S. (2012). DSM criteria for tobacco use disorder and tobacco withdrawal: A critique and proposed revisions for DSM-5. *Addiction, 107*(2), 263–275. doi:10.1111/j.1360-0443.2011.03657.x.

Ballaban-Gil, K., Rapin, I., Tuchman, R., & Shinner, S. (1996). Longitudinal examination of the behavioral, language and social changes in a population of adolescents and young adults with autistic disorder. *Pediatric Neurology, 15*, 217–223.

Baron-Cohen, S. (2011). *The science of evil: On empathy and the origins of cruelty*. New York: Basic Books.

Beadle-Brown, J., Murphy, G., Wing, L., Gould, J., Shah, A., & Holmes, N. (2002). Changes in social impairment for people with intellectual disabilities: A follow-up of the Camberwell cohort. *Journal of Autism and Developmental Disorders, 32*, 195–206.

Begovac, I., Begovac, B., Majic, G., & Vidovic, V. (2009). Longitudinal studies of IQ stability with childhood autism-literature survey. *Psychiatria Danubina, 21*(3), 310–319.

Belcher, R., & Smith, M. D. (1994). Coworker attitudes towards employees with autism. *Journal of Vocational Rehabilitation, 4*, 29–36.

Bennet, H. E., Wood, C. L., & Hare, D. J. (2005). Providing care for adults with autistic spectrum disorders in learning disability services: Needs-based or diagnosis-driven? *Journal of Applied Research in Intellectual Disabilities, 18*, 57–64.

Billstedt, E., Gillberg, C., & Gillberg, C. (2005). Autism after adolescents: Population-based 13- to 22-year follow-up study of 120 individuals with autism diagnosed in childhood. *Journal of Autism and Developmental Disorders, 35*(3), 351–360.

Billstedt, E., Gillberg, C., & Gillberg, C. (2007). Autism in adults: Symptom patterns and early childhood predictors. Use of the DISCO in a community sample followed from childhood. *Journal of Child Psychology and Psychiatry, 48*(11), 1102–1110.

Billstedt, E., Gillberg, I. C., & Gillberg, C. (2011). Aspects of quality of life in adults diagnosed with autism in childhood: A population-based study. *Autism, 15*(1), 7–20.

Bolton, P. F., Pickles, A., Murphy, M., & Rutter, M. (1998). Autism, affective, and other psychiatric disorders: Patterns of familial aggregation. *Psychological Medicine, 28*, 385–395.

Bradley, E. A., Summers, J. A., Wood, H. L., & Bryson, S. E. (2004). Comparing rates of psychiatric and behavior disorders in adolescents and young adults with severe intellectual disability with and without autism. *Journal of Autism and Developmental Disorders, 34*, 151–161.

Brand, B. L., Lanius, R., Vermetten, E., Loewenstein, R. J., & Spiegel, D. (2012). Where are we going? An update on assessment, treatment, and neurobiological research in dissociative disorders as we move toward the DSM-5. *Journal of Trauma & Dissociation, 13*(1), 9–31.

Brereton, A. V., Tonge, B. J., & Einfeld, S. L. (2006). Psychopathology in children and adolescents with autism compared to young people with intellectual disability. *Journal of Autism and Developmental Disorders, 36*, 862–870.

Brown, J. R., & Rogers, S. J. (2003). Cultural issues in autism. In R. L. Hendren, S. Ozonoff, & S. Rogers (Eds.), *Autism spectrum disorders* (pp. 209–226). Washington, DC: American Psychiatric Press.

Brugha, T. S., McManus, S., Bankart, J., Scott, F., Purdon, S., Smith, J., et al. (2011). Epidemiology of autism spectrum disorders in adults in the community in England. *Archives of General Psychiatry, 68*(5), 459–466.

Bryson, S. A., Corrigan, S. K., McDonald, T. P., & Holmes, C. (2008). Characteristics of children with autism spectrum disorders who received services through community mental health centers. *Autism, 12*, 65–82.

Burgess, A. F., & Gutstein, S. E. (2007). Quality of life for people with autism: Raising the standard for evaluating successful outcomes. *Child and Adolescent Mental Health, 12*, 80–86.

Camarena, P. M., & Sarigiani, P. A. (2009). Postsecondary educational aspirations of high-functioning adolescents with autism spectrum disorders and their parents. *Focus on Autism and Other Developmental Disabilities, 24*(2), 115–128.

Cederlund, M., Hagberg, B., Billstedt, E., Gillberg, I. C., & Gillberg, C. (2008). Asperger syndrome and autism: A comparative longitudinal follow-up study more than 5 years after original diagnosis. *Journal of Autism and Developmental Disorders, 38*, 72–85.

Cederlund, M., Hagberg, B., & Gillberg, C. (2010). Asperger syndrome in adolescent and young adult males. Interview, self – And parent assessment of social, emotional, and cognitive problems. *Research in Developmental Disabilities, 31*, 287–298.

Centers for Disease Control and Prevention (CDC). (2014). Prevalence of Autism Spectrum disorder among children aged 8 years — Autism and Developmental disabilities monitoring network, 11 sites, United States, 2010. *Morbidity and Mortality Weekly Report, 63*(SS02), 1–21.

Chang, H. L., Juang, Y. Y., Wang, W. T., Huang, C. I., Chen, C. Y., & Hwang, Y. S. (2003). Screening for autism spectrum disorder in adult psychiatric outpatients in a clinic in Taiwan. *General Hospital Psychiatry, 25*, 284–288.

Chawarska, K., Klin, A., & Volkmar, F. R. (2008). Autism spectrum disorders in infants and toddlers: diagnosis, assessment, and treatment. *Autism spectrum disorders in infants and toddlers: Diagnosis, assessment, and treatment* (pp. 327–336, 348). New York: Guilford Press.

Chiang, H.-M., Cheung, Y. K., Hickson, L., Xiang, R., & Tsai, L. Y. (2012). Predictive factors of participation in postsecondary education for high school leavers with autism. *Journal of Autism and Developmental Disorders, 42*, 685–696. doi:10.1007/s10803-011-1297-7.

Chiri, G., & Warfield, M. E. (2012). Unmet needs and problems accessing core health care services for children with autism spectrum disorders. *Journal of Child and Maternal Health, 16*, 1081–1091.

Cimera, R. E., & Cowan, R. J. (2009). The costs of services and employment outcomes achieved by adults with autism in the US. *Autism, 13*(3), 285–302.

Constantino, J. N., Zhang, Y., Frazier, T., Abbacchi, A. M., & Law, P. (2010). Sibling recurrence and the genetic epidemiology of autism. *The American Journal of Psychiatry, 167*(11), 1349–1356.

Creak, M. (1961). Schizophrenic syndrome in childhood. *Developmental Medicine and Child Neurology, 3*, 501–504.

Daniels, A. M., Rosenberg, R. E., Law, J. K., Lord, C., Kaufmann, W. E., & Law, P. A. (2011). Stability of initial disorder diagnoses in community settings. *Journal of Autism and Developmental Disorders, 41*(1), 110–121.

Dawson, G., & Bernier, R. (2013). A quarter century of progress on early detection and treatment of autism spectrum disorder. *Development and Psychopathology, 25*, 1455–1472.

Dawson, G., Jones, E. J., Merkle, K., Venema, K., Lowy, R., Faja, S., et al. (2012). Early behavioral intervention is associated with normalized brain activity in young children with autism. *Journal of the American Academy of Child & Adolescent Psychiatry, 51*, 1150–1159.

DeMyer, M. K., Barton, S., DeMyer, W. E., Norton, J. S., Allen, J., & Steele, R. (1973). Prognosis in autism: A follow-up study. *Journal of Autism and Childhood Schizophrenia, 3*, 199–246.

Devlin, B., & Scherer, S. W. (2012). Genetic architecture in autism spectrum disorder. *Current Opinion in Genetics and Development, 22*, 229–237.

Devlin, B., Melhem, N., & Roeder, K. (2011). Do common variants play a role in risk for autism? Evidence and theoretical musings. *Brain Research, 1380*, 78–84.

Drmic, I., Aljunied, M., & Reaven, J. (2017). Facing your fears in schools: Implementing CBT for teens with ASD and anxiety in Singapore. *Journal of Autism and Developmental Disabilities*. doi:10.1007/s10803-016-3007-y.

Drmic, I., & Szatmari, P. (2014). Emotional dysregulation and comorbidity in Autism Spectrum Disorder. *Invited review for Cutting Edge Psychiatry in Practice – Autism Issue, 1*, 119–131.

Eaves, L. C., & Ho, H. H. (2008). Young adult outcomes of autism spectrum disorders. *Journal of Autism and Developmental Disorders, 38*, 739–747.

Eisenberg, L. (1956). The autistic child in adolescence. *The American Journal of Psychiatry, 112*, 607–612.

Elsabbagh, M., Divan, G., Koh, Y.-J., Kim, Y. S., Kauchali, S., Marcin, C., et al. (2012). Global prevalence of autism and other pervasive developmental disorders. *Autism Research, 5*(3), 160–179. doi: http://dx.doi.org/10.1002/aur.239.

Engstrom, I., Ekstrom, L., & Emilsson, B. (2003). Psychosocial functioning in a group of Swedish adults with Asperger syndrome or high-functioning autism. *Autism, 7*(1), 99–110.

Faja, S., Webb, S. J., Jones, E., Merkle, K., Kamara, D., Bavaro, J., et al. (2012). The effects of face expertise training on the behavioral performance and brain activity of adults with high functioning autism spectrum disorders. *Journal of Autism and Developmental Disorders, 42*, 278–293.

Farley, M. A., McMahon, W. M., Fombonne, E., Jenson, W. R., Miller, J., Gardner, M., et al. (2009). Twenty-year outcome for individuals with autism and average or near-average cognitive abilities. *Autism Research, 2*, 109–118.

Fombonne, E. (2005a). Epidemiology of autistic disorder and other pervasive developmental disorders. *Journal of Clinical Psychiatry, 66*(Suppl 10), 3–8.

Fombonne, E. (2005b). The changing epidemiology of autism. *Journal of Applied Research in Intellectual Disabilities, 18*(4), 281–294. doi: http://dx.doi.org/10.1111/j.1468-3148.2005.00266.x.

Frank, A. R., & Siltington, P. L. (2000). Young adults with mental disbailities – Does transition planning make a difference? *Education and Training in Mental Retardation and Developmental Disabilities, 35*, 119–134.

Fussell, E., & Furstenberg, F. F. (2005). The transition to adulthood during the twentieth century. In R. A. Settersten, F. F. Furstenberg, & R. G. Rumbaut (Eds.), *On the frontier of adulthood: Theory, research and public policy* (pp. 29–75). Chicago: University of Chicago Press.

García-Villamisar, D. A., & Dattilo, J. (2010). Effects of a leisure pro-gramme on quality of life and stress of individuals with ASD. *Journal of Intellectual Disability Research, 54*, 611–619.

Garcia-Villamisar, D., Ross, D., & Wehman, P. (2000). Clinical differential analysis of persons with autism in a work setting: A follow-up study. *Journal of Vocational Rehabilitation, 14*, 183–185.

García-Villamisar, D., Wehman, P., & Navarro, M. D. (2002). Changes in the quality of autistic people's life that work in supported and sheltered employment: A 5-year follow-up study. *Journal of Vocational Rehabilitation, 17*, 309–312.

Gardener, H., Spiegelman, D., & Buka, S. L. (2009). Prenatal risk factors for autism: Comprehensive meta-analysis. *British Journal of Psychiatry, 195*(1), 7–14.

Gerber, F., Bessero, S., Robbiani, B., et al. (2011). Comparing residential programmes for adults with autism spectrum disorders and intellectual disability: Outcomes of challenging behaviour and quality of life. *Journal of Intellectual Disability Research, 55*, 918–932.

Geschwind, D.H., & State, M.W. (2015). Gene hunting in autism spectrum disorder: on the path to precision medicine. *Lancet Neurology*, Published online http://dx.doi.org/10.1016/S1474-4422(15)00044-7.

Ghaziuddin, M., & Zafar, S. (2008). Psychiatric comorbidity in adults with autism spectrum disorders. *Clincial Neuropsychiatry, 5*, 9–12.

Ghaziuddin, M., Weidmer-Mikhail, E., & Ghaziuddin, N. (1998). Comorbidity of Asperger syndrome: A preliminary report. *Journal of Intellectual Disability Research, 42*, 278–283.

Gillberg, C. (1991). Outcome in autism and autistic-like conditions. *Journal of the American Academy of Child and Adolescent Psychiatry, 30*, 375–382.

Gillberg, C., & Steffenburg, S. (1987). Outcomes and prognostic factors in infantile autism and similar conditions: A population-based study of 46 cases followed through puberty. *Journal of Autism and Developmental Disorders, 17*, 272–288.

Gillespie-Lynch, K., Sepeta, L., Wang, Y., Marshall, S., Gomez, L., Sigman, M., & Hutman, T. (2012). Early childhood predictors of the social competence of adults with autism. *Journal of Autism and Developmental disorder, 42*, 161–174.

Gilotty, L., Kenworthy, L., Sirian, L., Black, D. O., & Wagner, A. E. (2012). Adaptive skills and executive function in autism spectrum disorders. *Child Neuropsychology, 8*(4), 241–248.

Gjevik, E., Eldevik, S., Fjaeran-Granum, T., & Sponheim, E. (2011). Kiddie-SADS reveals high rates of DSM-IV disorders in children and adolescents with autism spectrum disorders. *Journal of Autism and Developmental Disorders, 41*, 761–769.

Glennon, T. J. (2001). The stress of the university experience for students with Asperger syndrome. *Work: Journal of Prevention, Assessment & Rehabilitation, 17*(3), 183–190.

Gulsrud, A. C., Hellemann, G. S., Freeman, F. N., & Kasari, C. (2014). Two to ten years: Developmental trajectories of joint attention with ASD who received targeted social communication interventions. *Autism Research, 7*, 207–215.

Hagner, D., & Cooney, B. F. (2005). "I do that for everybody": Supervising employees with autism. *Focus on Autism and Developmental Disabilities, 20*(2), 91–97.

Halfon, N., & Forrest, C. B. (2017). The emerging theoretical framework of life course health development. In N. Halfon, C. B. Forrest, R. M. Lerner, & E. Faustman (Eds.), *Handbook of life course health-development science*. Cham: Springer.

Halfon, N., Larson, K., Lu, M., Tullis, E., & Russ, S. (2014). Lifecourse health development: Past, present and future. *Journal of Maternal Child Health, 18*, 344–365.

Hallmayer, J., Cleveland, S., Torres, A., Phillips, J., Cohen, B., Torigoe, T., et al. (2011). Genetic heritability and shared environmental factors among twin pairs with autism. *Archives of General Psychiatry, 68*(11), 1095–1102. doi:10.1001/archgenpsychiatry.2011.76.

Harris, L. J., & Handelman, J. S. (Eds.). (2000). *Preschool education programs for children with autism* (2nd ed.). Austin: PRO-ED.

Henninger, N. A., & Taylor, J. L. (2012). Outcomes in adults with autism spectrum disorders: A historical perspective. *Autism, 0*(0), 1–14. doi:10.1177/1362361312441266.

Hermelin, B. (2001). *Bright Splinters of the mind: A personal story of research with Autistic savants*. London: Jessica Kingsley.

Hofvander, B., Delorme, R., Chaste, P., Nyden, A., Wentz, E., Stahlberg, O., et al. (2009). Psychiatric and psychosocial problems in adults with normal-intelligence autism spectrum disorders. *BMC Psychiatry, 9*, 35. doi:10.1186/1471-244X-9-35.

Holden, B., & Gitlesen, J. P. (2006). A total population study of challenging behavior in the country of Hedmark, Norway: Prevalence, and risk markers. *Research in Developmental Disabilities, 27*(4), 456–465.

Howlin, P. (1998). *Children with autism and Asperger syndrome. A guide for practitioners and carers*. Chichester: John Wiley & Sons.

Howlin, P. (2000). Outcome in adult life for more able individuals with Autism or Asperger Syndrome. *Autism, 4*(1), 63–83.

Howlin, P. (2003). Outcome in high-functioning adults with autism with and without early language delays: Implications for the differentiation between autism and Asperger syndrome. *Journal of Autism and Developmental Disorders, 33*, 3–13.

Howlin, P. (2005). Outcomes in autism spectrum disorders. In P. Howlin (Ed.), *Handbook od autism and pervasive developmental disorder, volume 1: Diagnosis, development, neurobiology, and behavior* (3rd ed.). Hoboken: John Wiley & Sons.

Howlin, P. (2013). Outcomes in adults with autism spectrum disorders. In F. Volkmar, S. Rogers, R. Paul, & K. Pelphrey (Eds.), *Handbook of autism* (4th ed.). Hoboken: Wiley.

Howlin, P., & Goode, S. (1998). Outcomes in adult life for individuals with autism. In F. Volkmar (Ed.), *Autism and developmental disorders*. New York: Cambridge University Press.

Howlin, P., & Moss, P. (2012). Adults with autism spectrum disorders. *Canadian Journal of Psychiatry, 57*(5), 275–283.

Howlin, P., Alcock, J., & Burkin, C. (2005). An 8 year follow-up of a specialist supported employment service for high-ability adults with autism or Asperger syndrome. *Autism, 9*(5), 533–549.

Howlin, P., Goode, J., Hutton, J., & Rutter, M. (2004). Adult outcomes for children with autism. *Journal of Child Psychology and Psychiatry, 45*, 212–229.

Huerta, M., Bishop, S. L., Duncan, A., Hus, V., & Lord, C. (2012). Application of the DSM-5 criteria for autism spectrum disorder to three samples of children with DSM-IV diagnoses of pervasive developmental disorders. *American Journal of Psychiatry, 169*(10), 1056–1064.

Jobe, L., & White, S. W. (2007). Loneliness, social relationships, and a broader autism phenotype in college students. *Personality and Individual Differences, 42*, 1479–1489.

Joshi, G., Petty, C., Wozniak, J., Henin, A., Fried, R., Galdo, M., et al. (2010). The heavy burden of psychiatric comorbidity in youth with autism spectrum disorders: A large comparative study of psychiatrically referred population. *Journal of Autism and Developmental Disorders, 40*, 1361–1370.

Kamio, Y., Inada, N., & Koyama, T. (2012). A nationwide survey on quality of life and associated factors of adults with high-functioning autism spectrum disorders. *Autism, 17*, 15–26.

Kamp-Becker, I., Schröder, J., Muehlan Remschmidt, H., et al. (2011). Health-related quality of life in children and adolescents with autism spectrum disorder. *Zeitschrift für Kinder - und Jugendpsychiatrie und Psychotherapie, 39*(2), 123–131.

Kanner, L. (1943). Autistic disturbances of affective contact. *Nervous Child, 2*, 217–250.

Kanner, L. (1971). Follow-up study of eleven autistic children originally reported in. *Journal of Autism & Childhood Schizophrenia, 1*(2), 119–145.

Kasari, C., Gulsrud, A. C., Wong, C., Kwon, S., & Locke, J. (2010). Randomized controlled caregiver mediated joint engagement intervention for toddlers with autism. *Journal of Autism Developmental Disorders, 40*(9), 1045–1056.

Keel, J. H., Mesibov, G. B., & Woods, A. V. (1997). TEACCH-supported employment program. *Journal of Autism and Developmental Disabilities, 27*(1), 3–9.

Keogh, B. K., Bernheimer, L. P., & Guthrie, D. (2004). Children with developmental delays twenty years later: Where are they? How are they? *American Journal on Mental Retardation, 109*(3), 219–230.

Kim, S.H., Macari, S., Koller, J., & Chawarska, K. (2015). Examining the phenotypic heterogeneity of early autism spectrum disorder: Subtypes and short-term outcomes. *Journal of Child Psychology and Psychiatry*. doi:10.1111/jcpp.12448.

King, M., & Bearman, P. (2009). Diagnostic change and the increased prevalence of autism. *International Journal of Epidemiology, 38*(5), 1224–1234. Epub 2009 Sep 7. PubMed PMID: 19737791.

Kleinman, J., Ventola, P., Pandey, J., Verbalis, A., Barton, M., Hodgson, S., et al. (2008). Diagnostic stability in very young children with autism spectrum disorder. *Journal of Autism and Developmental Disorders, 38*(4), 606–615. doi:10.1007/s10803-007-0427-8.

Klin, A., Volkmar, F. R., Sparrow, S. S., Cicchetti, D. V., & et al. (1996). Validity and neuropsychological characterization of Asperger syndrome: Convergence with nonverbal learning disabilities syndrome. *Annual Progress in Child Psychiatry & Child Development*, 241–259.

Kobayashi, R., Murata, T., & Yoshinaga, K. (1992). A follow-up study of 201 children with autism in Kyushu and Yamaguchi areas, Japan. *Journal of Autism and Developmental Disorders, 22*, 395–411.

Kraemer, B. R., & Blacher, J. (2001). Transition for young adults with severe mental retardation: School preparation, parent expectations, and family involvement. *Mental Retardation, 39*, 432–455.

Kraemer, B. R., McIntyre, L. L., & Blacher, J. (2003). Quality of life for young adults with mental retardation during transition. *Mental Retardation, 41*, 250–262.

Kim, J., Szatmari, P., Bryson, S. E., & Wilson, F. J. (2000). Prevalence of anxiety and mood problems among children with autism and Asperger syndrome. *Autism, 4*, 117–132.

LaFramboise, T., Winckler, W., & Thomas, R. K. (2009). A flexible rank-based framework for detecting copy number aberrations from array data. *Bioinformatics, 25*(6), 722–728.

La Malfa, G., Lassi, S., Salvini, R., Giganti, C., Bertelli, M., & Albertini, G. (2007). The relationship between autism and psychiatric disorders in intellectually disabled adults. *Research in Autism Spectrum Disorders, 1*, 218–228.

Landa, R. J., & Kalb, L. G. (2012). Long-term outcomes of toddlers with autism spectrum disorders exposed o short-term intervention. *Pediatrics, 130*(2), S186–S190. doi:10.1542/peds.2012-0900Q.

Landa, R. J., Holman, K. C., & Garrett-Mayer, E. (2007). Social and communication development in toddlers with early and later diagnosis of autism spectrum disorders. *Archives of General Psychiatry, 64*(7), 853–864.

Landa, R. J., Holman, K. C., O'Neill, A. H., & Stuart, E. A. (2011). Intervention targeting development of socially synchronous engagement in toddlers with autism spectrum disorder: A randomized controlled trial. *Journal of Child Psychology and Psychiatry, 52*(1), 13–21.

Larsen, F. W., & Mouridsen, S. E. (1997). The outcome in children with childhood autism and Asperger syndrome originally diagnosed as psychotic. A 30-year follow-up study of subjects hospitalized as children. *European Child and Adolescent Psychiatry, 6*(4), 181–190.

Lee, G. K., & Carter, E. W. (2012). Preparing transition-age students with high-functioning autism spectrum disorders for meaningful work. *Psychology in the Schools, 49*(10), 988–1000. doi:10.1002/pits.21651.

Leekam, S. R., Nieto, C., Libby, S. J., Wing, L., & Gould, J. (2006). Describing the sensory abnormalities of children and adults with autism. *Journal of Autism and Developmental Disorders, 37*, 894–910. doi:10.1007/s10803-006-0218-7.

Levy, A., & Perry, A. (2011). Outcome in adolescents and adults with autism: A review of the literature. *Research in Autism Spectrum Disorders, 5*, 1271–1282.

Levy, S. E., Mandell, D. S., & Schultz, R. T. (2009). Autism. *Lancet, 374*, 1627–1638.

Leyfer, O. T., Folstein, S. E., Bacalman, S., Davis, N. O., Dinh, E., Morgan, J., et al. (2006). Comorbid psychiatric disorders in children with autism: Interview development and rates of disorders. *Journal of Autism and Developmental Disorders, 36*, 849–861.

Li, X., Zou, H., & Brown, W. T. (2012). Genes associated with autism spectrum disorder. *Brain Research Bulletin, 88*(6), 543–552.

Liptak, G. S., Benzoni, L. B., Mruzek, D. W., Nolan, K. W., Thingvoll, M. A., Wade, C. M., & Fryer, G. E. (2008). Disparities in diagnosis and access to health services for children with autism: Data from the national survey of children's health. *Journal of Developmental & Behavioral Pediatrics, 29*(3), 152–160.

Lockyer, L., & Rutter, M. (1969). A five- to fifteen-year follow-up study of infantile psychosis: III. *Psychological aspects. The British Journal of Psychiatry, 115*, 865–882.

Lockyer, L., & Rutter, M. (1970). A five- to fifteen-year follow-up study of infantile psychosis: IV. Patterns of cognitive ability. *British Journal of Social and Clinical Psychology, 9*(2), 152–163.

Loke, Y. J., Hannan, A. J., & Craig, J. M. (2015). The role of epigenetic change in autism spectrum disorders. *Frontiers in Neurology, 6*, 107. doi:10.3389/fneur.2015.00107.

Lord, C., & Bailey, A. (2002). Autism spectrum disorders. In M. Rutter & E. Taylor (Eds.), *Child and adolescent psychiatry* (4th ed., pp. 664–681). Oxford, MA: Blackwell Scientific.

Lord, C., & Schopler, E. (1989). The role of age at assessment, developmental level, and test in the stability of intelligence scores in young autistic children. *Journal of Autism and Developmental Disorders, 19*(4), 483–499.

Lotter, V. (1974). Social adjustment and placement of autistic children in Middlesex: A follow-up study. *Journal of Autism and Childhood Schizophrenia, 4*, 11–32.

Lotter, V. (1978). Follow-up studies. In M. Rutter & E. Schopler (Eds.), *Autism: A reappraisal of concepts and treatment* (pp. 475–495). New York: Plenum Press.

Lounds Taylor, J., Dove, D., Veenstra-VanderWeele, J., Sathe, N.A., McPheeters, M.L., Jerome, R.N., Warren, Z.. (2012). *Interventions for adolescents and young Adults with Autism Spectrum disorders.* Comparative effectiveness review no. 65. (Prepared by the Vanderbilt evidence-based practice Center under contract no. 290–2007-10065-I.) AHRQ publication no. 12-EHC063-EF. Rockville, MD: Agency for Healthcare Research and Quality. www.effectivehealthcare.ahrq.gov/reports/final.cfm

Lovaas, I. (1987). Behavioral treatment and normal educational and intellectual functioning in young autistic children. *Journal of Consulting and Clinical Psychology, 55*(1), 3–9.

LoVullo, S. V., & Matson, J. L. (2009). Comorbid psychopathology in adults with autism spectrum disorders and intellectual disabilities. *Research in Developmental Disabilities, 30*, 1288–1296. doi:10.1016/j.ridd.2009.05.004.

Lugnegard, T., Hallerback, M. U., & Gillberg, C. (2011). Psychiatric comorbidity in young adults with a clinical diagnosis of Asperger syndrome. *Research in Developmental Disabilities, 32*, 1910–1917.

Lunsky, Y., Gracey, C., & Bradley, E. (2009). Adults with autism spectrum disorders using psychiatric hospitals in Ontario: Clinical profile and service needs. *Research in Autism Spectrum Disorders, 3*, 1006–1013.

Luxford, S., Hadwin, J. A., & Kovshoff, H. (2016). Evaluating the effectiveness of a school-based cognitive behavioural therapy intervention for anxiety in adolescents diagnosed with autism spectrum disorder. *Journal of Autism and Developmental Disorders*, doi:http://dx.doi.org/10.1007/s10803-016-2857-7

Magiati, I., Moss, J., Charman, T., & Howlin, P. (2011). Patterns of change in children with autism spectrum disorders who received community based comprehensive interventions in their pre-school years: A seven year follow-up study. *Research in Autism Spectrum Disorders, 5*(3), 1016–1027.

Malhotra, D., & Sebat, J. (2012). Copy number variants: Harbingers of a rare variant revolution in psychiatric genetics. *Cell, 148*(6), 1223–1241.

Mattila, M.-L., Hurtig, T., Haapsamo, H., Jussila, K., Kuusikko-Gauffin, S., Kielinen, M., et al. (2010). Comorbid psychiatric disorders associated with Asperger syndrome/high functioning autism: A community and clinic-based study. *Journal of Autism and Developmental Disorders, 40*, 1080–1093.

Mattilla, M.-L., Kielinen, M., Linna, S.-L., Jussilla, K., Ebeling, H., Bloigu, R., et al. (2011). Autism Spectrum disorders According to DSM-IV-TR and comparison with DSM-5 draft criteria an epidemiological study. *Journal of the American Academy of Child & Adolescent Psychiatry, 50*(6), 583–592.

MacNeil, B. M., Lopes, V. A., & Minnes, P. M. (2009). Anxiety in children and adolescents with autism spectrum disorders. *Research in Autism Spectrum Disorders, 3*, 1–21. doi:10.1016/j.rasd.2008.06.001.

Mandell, D. (2008). Psychiatric hospitalization among children with autism spectrum disorders. *Journal of Autism and Developmental Disorders, 38*, 1059–1065.

Marshall, C. R., Noor, A., Vincent, J. B., Lionel, A. C., Feuk, L., Skaug, J., et al. (2008). Structural variation of chromosomes in autism spectrum disorder. *American Journal of Human Genetics, 82*(2), 477–488.

Matson, J. L., Wilkins, J., & Ancona, M. (2008). Autism in adults with severe intellectual disability: An empirical study of symptom presentation. *Journal of Intellectual & Developmental Disability, 33*, 36–42. doi:10.1080/13668250701829837.

Mawhood, L., & Howlin, P. (1999). The outcome of a supported employment scheme for high functioning adults with autism or Asperger syndrome. *Autism, 3*, 229–254.

Mawhood, L., Howlin, P., & Rutter, M. (2000). Autism and developmental receptive language disorder-a comparative follow-up in early adult life I: Cognitive and language outcomes. *Journal of Child Psychology and Psychiatry, 41*, 547–559.

Mazefsky, C. A., Folstein, S. E., & Lainhart, J. E. (2008). Overrepresentation of mood and anxiety disorders in adults with autism and their first degree relatives: What does it mean? *Autism Research, 1*, 193–197.

McGrew, S. G., Peters, B. R., Crittendon, J. A., & Veenstra-VaderWeele, J. (2012). Diagnostic yield of chromosomal microarray analysis in autism primary care practice: Which guidelines to implement? *Journal of Autism and Developmental Disorders, 42*(8), 1582–1591.

McDougle, C. J., Erickson, C. A., Stigler, K. A., & Posey, D. J. (2005). Neurochemistry in the pathophysiology of autism. *Journal of Clinical Psychiatry, 66*(Suppl 10), 9–18.

Meyer, J. A., & Minshew, N. J. (2002). An update on neurocognitive profiles in Asperger syndrome and high-functioning autism. *Focus on Autism and Other Developmental Disabilities, 17*(3), 152–160. http://dx.doi.org/10.1177/10883576020170030501.

Moseley, D. S., Tonge, B. J., Brereton, A. V., & Einfeld, S. L. (2011). Psychiatric comorbidity in adolescents and young adults with autism. *Journal of Mental Health Research in Intellectual Disabilities, 4*, 229–243.

Mouridsen, S. E., Rich, B., Isager, T., & Nedergaard, N. J. (2008). Psychiatric disorders in individuals diagnosed with infantile autism as children: A case control study. *Journal of Psychiatric Practice, 14*, 5–12.

Muller, N., Myint, A., & Schwarz, M. J. (2015). *Immunology and psychiatry: From basic research to therapeutic interventions*. Cham: Springer International Publishing.

Mundy, P., & Jarrold, W. (2010). Infant joint attention, neural networks and social cognition. *Neural Networks, 23*, 985–997. doi:10.1016/j.neunet.2010.08.009.

Mundy, P., Sullivan, L., & Mastergeorge, A. M. (2009). A parallel and distributed processing model of joint attention, social cognition, and autism. *Autism Research, 2*, 2–21.

Muris, P., Steerneman, P., Merckelbach, H., Holdrinet, I., & Meesters, C. (1998). Comorbid anxiety symptoms in children with pervasive developmental disorders. *Journal of Anxiety Disorders, 12*, 387–393.

Narendorf, S. C., Shattuck, P. T., & Sterzing, P. R. (2011). Mental health services among adolescents with an autism spectrum disorder. *Psychiatric Services, 62*, 975–978.

National Autism Center. (2015). *Findings and conclusions: National standards project, phase 2*. Randolph, MA: Author.

National Autism Center. (2009). *National Standards Report – Addressing the need for evidence-based practice guidelines for Autism Spectrum Disorders*. Massachusetts: National Autism Center.

National Research Council. (2001). *Educating young children with autism*. Washington, DC: National Academy Press.

Newman, L., Wagner, M., Knokey, A. M., Marder, C., Nagle, K., Shaver, D., & Wei, X. (2011). *The posy-high school outcomes of young adults with disabilities up to 8 years after high school*. Menlo Park: SRI International.

Nordin, V., & Gillberg, C. (1998). The long-term course of autistic disorders: Update on follow-up studies. *Acta Psychiatrica Scandinavica, 97*, 99–108.

Noterdaeme, M., Wriedt, E., & Höhne, C. (2010). Asperger's syndrome and high-functioning autism: Language, motor and cognitive profiles. *European Child & Adolescent Psychiatry, 19*(6), 475–481.

Palac, S., & Meador, K. J. (2011). Antiepileptic drugs and neurodevelopment: An update. *Current Neurology and Neuroscience Reports, 11*(4), 423–427.

Palucka, A. M., Bradley, E., & Lunsky, Y. (2008). A case of unrecognized intellectual disability and autism misdiagnosed as schizophrenia: Are there lessons to be learned? *Mental Health Aspects of Developmental Disabilities, 11*(2), 55–60.

Parr, J. R., Le Couteur, A., Baird, G., Rutter, M., Pickles, A., Fombonne, E., Bailey, A. J., & International Molecular Genetic Study of Autism Consortium. (2011). Early developmental regression in autism spectrum disorder: Evidence from an international multiplex sample. *Journal of Autism & Developmental Disorders, 41*(3), 332–340.

Paul, R. (2008). Communication development and assessment. In K. Chawarska, A. Klin, & F. Volkmar (Eds.), *Autism Spectrum disorders in infants and toddlers: Diagnosis, Assessment, and treatment* (pp. 76–103). New York: Guilford Press.

Pinto, D., Pagnamenta, A. T., Klei, L., Anney, R., Merico, D., Regan, R., et al. (2010). Functional impact of global rare copy number variation in autism spectrum disorders. *Nature, 466*(7304), 368–372.

Piven, J., & Rabins, P. (2011). Autism spectrum disorders in older adults: Toward defining a research agenda. *Journal of the American Geriatrics Society, 59*(11), 2151–2155.

Perkins, E. A., & Berkman, K. A. (2012). Into the unknown: Aging with autism spectrum disorders. *American Journal on Intellectual and Developmental Disabilities, 117*(6), 478–496.

Perlman, L. (2000). Adults with Asperger disorder misdiagnosed as schizophrenic. *Professional Psychology: research & Practice, 31*(2), 221–225. False.

Peters-Scheffer, N., Didden, R., Hubert, K., & Sturmey, P. (2011). A meta-analytic study on the effectiveness of comprehensive ABA-based early intervention programs for children with Autism Spectrum disorders. *Research in Autism Spectrum Disorders, 5*(1), 60–69.

Polloway, E. A., Patton, J. R., & Serna, L. (2001). *Strategies for teaching learners with special needs.* Upper Saddle River: Merrill Prentice Hall.

Potvin, M. C., Snider, L., Prelock, P. A., Wood-Dauphinee, S., & Kehayia, E. (2015). Health-related quality of life in children with high-functioning autism. *Autism, 19*(1), 14–19.

Power, R. A., Kyaga, S., Uher, R., Maccabe, J. H., Långström, N., Landen, M., et al. (2012). Fecundity of patients with schizophrenia, Autism, bipolar disorder, depression, anorexia nervosa, or substance abuse vs their unaffected siblings. *Archives of General Psychiatry, 12*, 1–8.

Raphael, D., Brown, I., Renwick, R., & Rootman, I. (1996). Assessing the quality of life of persons with developmental disabilities: Description of a new model, measuring instruments, and initial findings. *International Journal of Diability, 43*(1), 25–42.

Reichow, B. (2012). Overview of meta-analyses on early intensive behavioral intervention for young children with autism spectrum disorders. *Journal of Autism and Developmental Disorders, 42*, 512–520.

Reichow, B., & Wolery, M. (2009). Comprehensive synthesis of early intensive behavioral interventions for young children with autism based on the UCLA young Autism Project model. *Journal of Autism and Developmental Disorders, 39*(1), 23–41.

Renty, J., & Roeyers, H. (2006). Quality of life in high-functioning adults with autism spectrum disorder: The predictive value of disability and support characteristics. *Autism, 10*, 511–524.

Ritvo, E. R., Jorde, L. B., Mason-Brothers, A., Freeman, B. J., Pingree, C., Jones, M. B., et al. (1989). The UCLA-University of Utah epidemiologic survey of autism: Recurrence risk estimates and genetic counseling. *American Journal of Psychiatry, 146*(8), 1032–1036.

Robinson, S., Goddard, L., Dritschel, B., Wisley, M., & Howlin, P. (2009). Executive functions in children with autism spectrum disorders. *Brain and Cognition, 71*(3), 362–368. http://dx.doi.org/10.1016/j.bandc.2009.06.007

Rogers, S. J. (2009). What are infant siblings teaching us about autism in infancy? *Autism research : Official Journal of the International Society for Autism Research, 2*(3), 125–137.

Rondeau, E., Klein, L. S., Masse, A., Bodeau, N., Cohen, D., & Guile, J.-M. (2011). Is pervasive developmental disorder not otherwise specified less stable than autistic disorder? A meta-analysis. *Journal of Autism and Developmental Disorders, 41*, 1267–1276.

Ruble, L. A., & Dalrymple, N. J. (1996). An alternative view of outcome in autism. *Focus on Autism and Other Developmental Disabilities, 11*(1), 3–14.

Rumsey, J. M., Rapoport, J. L., & Sceert, W. R. (1985). Autistic children as adults: Psychiatric, social, and behavioral outcomes. *Journal of the American Academy of Child Psychiatry, 24*(4), 465–473.

Russ, S. A., Larson, K., Tullis, E., & Halfon, N. (2014). A lifecourse approach to health development: Implications for the maternal and child health research agenda. *Maternal and Child Health Journal, 18*(2), 497–510.

Russell, E., & Sofronoff, K. (2005). Anxiety and social worries in children with Asperger syndrome. *Australian and New Zealand Journal of Psychiatry, 39*, 633–638.

Rutter, M. (1967). The autistic child. *Royal Institute of Public Health & Hygiene Journal, 30*(4), 130–132.

Rutter, M. (1973). Why are London children so disturbed? *Proceedings of the Royal Society of Medicine, 66*(12), 1221–1225.

Rutter, M. (1978). Diagnosis and definition of childhood autism. *Journal of Autism & Childhood Schizophrenia, 8*(2), 139–161.

Rutter, M. (1982). Prevention of children's psychosocial disorders: Myth and substance. *Pediatrics, 70*(6), 883–894.

Rutter, M. (2005). Environmentally mediated risks for psychopathology: Research strategies and findings. *Journal of the American Academy of Child & Adolescent Psychiatry, 44*(1), 3–18.

Rutter, M., & Lockyer, L. (1967). A five to fifteen year follow-up study of infantile psychosis I. Description of sample. *British Journal of Psychiatry, 113*(504), 1169–1182.

Rutter, M., Greenfield, D., & Lockyer, L. (1967). A five to fifteen year follow-up of infantile psychosis II social and behavioral outcome. *The British Journal of Psychiatry, 113*, 1183–1199.

Schreibman, L., Dawson, G., Stahmer, A. C., Landa, R., Rogers, S., et al. (2015). Naturalistic developmental behavioral interventions: Empirically validated treatments for autism spectrum disorder. *Journal of Autism and Developmental Disorders, 45*(8), 2411–2428.

Saxena, S., & Orley, J. (1997). Quality of life assessment: The world health organization perspective. *European Psychiatry, 12*, 263s–266s.

Schumann, C. M., Bloss, C. S., Barnes, C. C., Wideman, G. M., Carper, R. A., Akshoomoff, N., et al. (2010). Longitudinal magnetic resonance imaging study of cortical development through early childhood in autism. *Journal of Neuroscience, 30*, 4419–4427.

Seltzer, M. M., Krauss, M. W., Shattuck, P. T., Orsmond, G., Swe, A., & Lord, C. (2003). The stmptoms of autism spectrum disorders in adolescents and adulthood. *Journal of Autism and Developmental Disorders, 33*, 565–581.

Seltzer, M. M., Shattuck, P., Abbeduto, L., & Greenberg, J. S. (2004). Trajectory of development in adolescents and adults with autism. *Mental Retardation and Developmental Disabilities, 10*, 234–247.

Shattuck, P. T., Durkin, M., Maenner, M., Newschaffer, C., Mandell, D. S., Wiggins, L., et al. (2009). Timing of identification among children with an autism spectrum disorder: Findings from a population-based surveillance study. *Journal of the American Academy of Child & Adolescent Psychiatry, 48*(5), 474–483.

Shattuck, P. T., Roux, A. M., Hudson, L. E., Taylor, J. L., Maenner, M. J., & Trani, J.-F. (2012). Services for adults with autism spectrum disorder. *Canadian Journal of Psychiatry, 57*(5), 284–291.

Shattuck, P. T., Seltzer, M. M., Greenberg, J. S., Orsmond, G. I., Bolt, D., Kring, S., et al. (2007). Change in autism symptoms and maladaptive behaviors in adolescents with an autism spectrum disorder. *Journal of Autism and Developmental Disorders, 37*, 1735–1747.

Shelton, J. F., Tancredi, D. J., & Hertz-Picciotto, I. (2010). Independent and dependent contributions of advanced maternal and paternal ages to autism risk. *Autism Research, 3*(1), 30–39.

Sigman, M., & Kasari, C. (1995). *Joint attention across contexts in normal and autistic children.* (pp. 189–203). Hillsdale: Lawrence Erlbaum Associates, Inc. Retrieved from http://search.proquest.com/docview/618769168?accountid=14771

Sigman, M., & McGovern, C. W. (2005). Improvement in cognitive and language skills from preschool to adolescence in autism. *Journal of Autism and Developmental Disorders, 35*(1), 15–23.

Sigman, M., & Ruskin, E. (1999). Continuity and change in the social competence of children with autism, down syndrome, and developmental delays. *Monographs of the Society for Research in Child Development, 64*(1), 1–139.

Simonoff, E., Pickles, A., Charman, T., Chandler, S., Loucas, T., & Baird, G. (2008). Psychiatric disorders in children with autism spectrum disorders: Prevalence, comorbidity, and associated factors in a population-derived sample. *Journal of the American Academy of Child and Adolescent Psychiatry, 47*, 921–929.

Skokauskas, N., & Gallagher, L. (2010). Psychosis, affective disorders, and anxiety in autistic spectrum disorder: Prevalence and nosological considerations. *Psychopathology, 43*, 8–16.

Smith, M., & Paulippen, L. (1999). Community integration and supported employment. In D. Zager (Ed.), *Autism: Identification, education, treatment* (pp. 301–319). Mahwah: Erlbaum.

State, M. W. (2010). The genetics of child psychiatric disorders: Focus on autism and Tourette syndrome. *Neuron, 68*(2), 254–269.

Sterling, L., Dawson, G., Estes, A., & Greenson, J. (2008). Characteristics associated with presence of depressive symptoms in adults with autism spectrum disorder. *Journal of Autism and Developmental Disorders, 38*, 1011–1018.

Stoner, J. B., Angell, M. E., House, J. J., & Bock, S. J. (2007). Transitions: Perspectives from parents of young children with autism spectrum disorders (ASD). *Journal of Developmental Disabilities, 19*, 23–39.

Strauss, K., Mancini, F., & Fava, L. (2013). Parent inclusion in early intensive behavior interventions for young children with ASD: A synthesis of meta-analyses from 220 to 2011. *Reseach in Developmental Disabilities, 34*(9), 2967–2985.

Sullivan, P. F., Daly, M. J., & O'Donovan, M. (2012). Genetic architectures of psychiatric disorders: The emerging picture and its implications. *Nature Reviews Genetics, 13*(8), 537–551.

Sun F, Oristaglio J, Levy SE, Hakonarson H, Sullivan N, Fontanarosa J, Schoelles KM. 2015. Genetic testing for developmental disabilities, intellectual disability, and Autism Spectrum disorder. Technical brief no. 23. (prepared by the ECRI institute–Penn medicine evidence-based practice Center under contract no. 290–2012-00011-I.) AHRQ publication no.15-EHC024-EF. Rockville, MD: Agency for Healthcare Research and Quality. www.effectivehealthcare.ahrq.gov/reports/final.cfm.

Szatmari, P. (2011). New recommendations on autism spectrum disorder shifting the focus from subtypes to dimensions carriers potential costs and benefits. *BMJ, 342*. doi:10.1136/bmj.d2456.

Szatmari, P., & McConnell, B. (2011). Anxiety and mood disorders in individuals with autism spectrum disorder. In D. G. Amaral, G. Dawson, & D. H. Geschwind

(Eds.), *Autism spectrum disorders* (pp. 330–338). New York: Oxford University Press, Inc.

Szatmari, P., Bartolucci, G., Brenner, R., Bond, S., & Rich, S. (1989). A follow-up study of high-functioning autistic children. *Journal of Autism and Developmental Disorders, 19*, 213–225.

Szatmari, P., Bryson, S. E., Boyle, M. H., Streiner, D. L., & Duku, E. (2003). Predictors of outcome among high functioning children with autism and Asperger syndrome. *Journal of Child Psychology and Psychiatry, 44*(4), 529–528.

Szatmari, P., Georgiades, S., Duku, E., Bennett, T. A., Bryson, S., et al. (2015). Developmental trajectories of symptom severity and adaptive functioning in an inception cohort of preschool children with autism spectrum disorder. *JAMA Psychiatry, 72*(3), 276–283.

Szatmari, P., Jones, M. B., Zwaigenbaum, L., & MacLean, J. E. (1998). Genetics of autism: Overview and new directions. *Journal of Autism and Developmental Disorders, 28*(5), 351–368.

Szatmari, P., Paterson, A. D., Zwaigenbaum, L., Roberts, W., Brian, J., Autism Genome Project Consortium, et al. (2007). Mapping autism risk loci using genetic linkage and chromosomal rearrangements. *Nature Genetics, 39*(3), 319–328.

Taylor, J. L. (2009). The transition out of high school and into adulthood for individuals with autism and for their families. *International Review of Research in Mental Retardation, 38*, 1–32. doi:10.1016/S0074-7750(08)38001-X.

Taylor, J. L., & Seltzer, M. M. (2010). Changes in the autism behavioral phenotype during the transition to adulthood. *Journal of Autism and Developmental Disorders, 40*, 1431–1446.

Taylor, J. L., & Seltzer, M. M. (2011a). Changes in the mother-child relationship during the transition to adulthood for youth with autism spectrum disorders. *Journal of Autism and Developmental Disorders, 41*, 1397–1410. doi:10.1007/s10803-010-1166-9.

Taylor, J. L., & Seltzer, M. M. (2011b). Employment and post-secondary educational activities for young adults with autism spectrum disorders during the transition to adulthood. *Journal of Autism and Developmental Disorders, 41*, 566–574.

Taylor, J. L., McPheeters, M. L., Sathe, N. A., Dove, D., Veenstra-VanderWeele, J., & Warren, Z. (2012). A systematic review of vocational interventions for young adults with autism spectrum disorders. *Pediatrics, 130*(3), 531–538. doi:10.1542/peds.2012-0682.

Thomas, K. C., Ellis, A. R., McLaurin, C., Daniels, J., & Morrissey, J. P. (2007). Access to care for autism-related services. *Journal of Autism and Developmental Disorders, 37*, 1902–1912.

Totsika, V., Flece, D., Kerr, M., & Hastings, R. P. (2010). Behavior problems, psychiatric symptoms, and quality of life for older adults with intellectual disability with and without autism. *Journal of Autism and Developmental Disorders, 40*, 1171–1178.

Tomasello, M. (1995). Joint attention as social cognition. In C. Moore, & P. J. Dunham (Eds.), *Joint attention: Its origins and role in development; joint attention: Its origins and role in development* (pp. 103-130, Chapter vii, 286 Pages). Hillsdale: Lawrence Erlbaum Associates, Inc.

Towbin, K. E. (2005). Pervasive developmental disorder not otherwise specified. In F. R. Volkmar, A. Klin, R. Paul, & D. J. Cohen (Eds.), *Handbook of autism and pervasive developmental disorders* (Vol. 1, 3rd ed., pp. 165–200). Hoboken: Wiley.

Tsakanikos, E., Costello, H., Holt, G., Bouras, N., Sturmey, P., & Newton, T. (2006). Psychopathology in adults with autism and intellectual disability. *Journal of Autism and Developmental Disorders, 36*, 1123–1129.

Tsakanikos, E., Costello, H., Holt, G., Sturmey, P., & Bouras, N. (2007a). Behavior management problems as predictors of psychotropic medication and use of psychiatric services in adults with autism. *Journal of Autism and Developmental Disorders, 37*, 1080–1085.

Tsakanikos, E., Sturmey, P., Costello, H., Holt, G., & Bouras, N. (2007b). Referral trends in mental health services for adults with intellectual disability and autism spectrum disorders. *Autism, 11*, 9–17.

Turner, L. M., & Stone, W. L. (2007). Variability in outcome for children with an ASD diagnosis at age 2. *The Journal of Child Psychology and Psychiatry, 48*(8), 793–802.

Van Acker, R., Loncola, J. A., & Van Acker, E. Y. (2005). Rett syndrome: A pervasive developmental disorder. In F. R. Volkmar, R. Paul, A. Klin & D. Cohen (Eds.), Handbook of autism and pervasive developmental disorders: Diagnosis, development, neurobiology, and behavior (vol. 1) (3rd ed) (pp. 126–164, Chapter xxv, 703 Pages). Hoboken: John Wiley & Sons Inc.

VanBergeik, E., Klin, A., & Volkmar, F. (2008). Supporting more able students on the autism spectrum: College and beyond. *Journal of Autism and Developmental Disorders, 38*, 1359–1370. doi:10.1007/s10803-007-0524-8.

van Heijst, B. F. C., & Geurts, H. M. (2015). Quality of life in autism across the lifespan: A meta-analysis. *Autism, 19*(2), 158–167. doi:10.1177/1362361313517053.

Vaughan Van Hecke, A., Mundy, P., Acra, C. F., Block, J. J., Delgado, C. E. F., Parlade, M. V., et al. (2007). Infant joint attention, temperament, and social competence in preschool children. *Child Development, 78*(1), 53–69.

Veltman, J. A., & Brunner, H. G. (2012). De novo mutations in human genetic disease. *Nature Reviews Genetics, 13*(8), 565–575.

Venter, A., Lord, C., & Schopler, E. (1992). A follow-up study of high-functioning autistic children. *Journal of Child Psychology and Psychiatry, 33*(3), 489–507.

Volkmar, F. R. (2004). Adolescence and sexuality. In F. R. Volkmar & L. A. Wiesner (Eds.), *Healthcare for children on the autism spectrum* (pp. 245–260). New York: Harbour House.

Volkmar, F. R., & McPartland, J. (2014). From Kanner to DSM-5: Autism as an evolving diagnostic concept. *Annual Review of Clinical Psychology, 10*, 193–212.

Volkmar, F. R., & Cohen, D. J. (1991). Comorbid association of autism and schizophrenia. *The American Journal of Psychiatry, 148*(12), 1705–1707.

Volkmar, F. R., Koenig, K., & State, M. (2005). Childhood disintegrative disorder. In F. R. Volkmar, A. Klin, R. Paul, & D. J. Cohen (Eds.), *Handbook of autism and pervasive developmental disorders* (Vol. 1, 3rd ed., pp. 70–78). Hoboken: Wiley.

Volkmar, F. R., Klin, A., & McPartland, J. (2014). Asperger's syndrome: An overview. In J. McPartland, A. Klin, & F. Volkmar (Eds.), *Asperger syndrome: Assessing and treating high-functioning autism spectrum disorders* (pp. 1–42). New York: Guilford Press.

Watts, G. (2012). More psychiatrists attack plans for DSM-5. *BMJ, 344*, e3357. http://dx.doi.org/10.1136/bmj.e3357

Weitlauf, A.S., McPheeters, M.L., Peters, B., Sathe, N., Travis, R., Aiello, R., Williamson, E., Veenstra-VanderWeele, J., Krishnaswami, S., Jerome, R., Warren, Z. (2014). Therapies for Children With Autism Spectrum Disorder: Behavioral Interventions Update. Comparative Effectiveness Review No. 137. (Prepared by the Vanderbilt Evidence-based Practice Center under Contract No. 290–2012-00009-I.) AHRQ Publication No. 14-EHC036-EF. Rockville, MD: Agency for Healthcare Research and Quality. www.effectivehealthcare.ahrq.gov/reports/final.cfm

Wing, L. (1980). Childhood autism and social class: a question of selection? *British Journal of Psychiatry, 137*, 410–417.

White, S., Oswald, D., Ollendick, T., & Scahill, L. (2009). Anxiety in children and adolescents with ASD. *Clinical Psychology Review, 29*, 216–229.

Wolff, J. J., Gu, H., Elison, J. T., Styner, M., Gouttard, S., et al. (2012). Differences in white matter fiber tract development present from 6 to 24 months in infants with autism. *The American Journal of Psychiatry, 169*, 589–600.

Woodbury-Smith, M. R., & Volkmar, F. R. (2009). Asperger syndrome. *European Child & Adolescent Psychiatry, 18*(1), 2–11.

Woolfenden, S., Sarkozy, V., Ridley, G., & Williams, K. (2012). A systematic review of the diagnostic stability of autism spectrum disorder. *Research in Autism Spectrum Disorders, 6*, 345–354. doi:10.1016/j.rasd.2011.06.008.

Zachor, D. A., & Itzchak, E. B. (2010). Treatment approach, autism severity and intervention outcomes in young children. *Research in Autism Spectrum Dosorders, 4*(3), 425–432.

Zwaigenbaum, L., Bryson, S. E., Szatmari, P., Brian, J., Smith, I. M., Roberts, W., et al. (2012). Sex differences in children with autism spectrum disorder identified within a high-risk infant cohort. *Journal of Autism and Developmental Disorders, 42*(12), 2585–2596.

8

Life Course Research Agenda (LCRA), Version 1.0

Neal Halfon, Christopher B. Forrest, Richard M. Lerner, Elaine M. Faustman, Ericka Tullis, and John Son

1 Introduction

A rapidly growing number of research studies show that experiences and exposures in the early years can influence health development throughout life. This research also shows that suboptimal experiences and higher rates of early risk exposures can result in a cascading array of poor health outcomes, with compounding effects across subsequent life stages. This emerging life course health science has fundamentally challenged older models of how health develops and how diseases manifest over the lifecourse. It has also challenged thought leaders, researchers, policymakers, and service providers to redefine the role of health programs and policies as a platform to organize strategies that improve immediate health outcomes for children and their mothers, while also enhancing the health development of the adults those children will become (Wise 2016).

Authors' note: In 2010, the Maternal and Child Health Bureau of the Health Resources and Services Administration created the Maternal and Child Health Life Course Research Network (LCRN) and charged it with creating a new infrastructure for catalyzing progress and enhancing funding to support basic, theoretical, applied, and translational life course health development research of relevance to practice and policy. In addition to undertaking a variety of other activities and projects aimed at advancing the emerging field, the LCRN initiated an inclusive agenda-setting process that resulted in the Handbook of Life Course Health Development, including this chapter and the research agenda it contains. For a more detailed description of the development and history of the LCRN, the Handbook, and the research agenda, please see the Preface and Introduction to this volume.

N. Halfon (✉)
Department of Pediatrics, David Geffen School of Medicine, UCLA, Los Angeles, CA, USA

Department of Health Policy and Management, Fielding School of Public Health, UCLA, Los Angeles, CA, USA

Department of Public Policy, Luskin School of Public Affairs, UCLA, Los Angeles, CA, USA

Center for Healthier Children, Families, and Communities, UCLA, Los Angeles, CA, USA
e-mail: nhalfon@ucla.edu

C.B. Forrest
Applied Clinical Research Center, Children's Hospital of Philadelphia, Philadelphia, PA, USA

R.M. Lerner
Tufts University, Medford, MA, USA

E.M. Faustman
Institute for Risk Analysis and Risk Communication, Department of Environmental and Occupational Health Sciences, School of Public Health, University of Washington, Seattle, WA 98105, USA

E. Tullis • J. Son
Center for Healthier Children, Families and Communities, UCLA, Los Angeles, CA, USA

Life course health science research is "connecting the dots" between child health development, adult patterns of premature morbidity and mortality, and more integrated notions of healthy aging. It is also starting to inform new ways of controlling costs by limiting the prevalence of chronic health conditions. One indication of how fertile, important, and interconnected this research is becoming is the growing number of research studies that are spawning in this nascent field. There are not only many outstanding questions about the relationship between early experiences and lifelong health and well-being, but a growing need to understand how emerging knowledge can be applied to the development of evidence-based practice and policy that can reduce risks, minimize exposures, and optimize lifelong health. As major national research initiatives advance clinical translational research and precision medicine, the life course health sciences can play an important role in informing research questions, leveraging life course informed health development focused strategies, and advancing translational activities from laboratories to patients to communities. Life course health science can play an important role in pinpointing key molecular leverage points, linking those processes to higher-level (body system, organism, family, or social) influences, and illuminating the often overlooked relationship between the individual and population manifestations of underlying health development processes. The findings from life course health science research will also shape the organization, design, and financing of emerging and future healthcare systems (Halfon et al. 2014a, b).

Although this Handbook is far from comprehensive, in that there are numerous health conditions and issues it does not address, it does offer state-of-the-art reviews and analyses of life course health development research focused on key life stages and a variety of specific health conditions. Based on their analysis of existing research, the authors of each chapter have suggested how life course health development research can be supported and advanced. In developing this concluding chapter, we synthesized their findings and recommendations in order to propose an integrated set of research priorities and strategies that can advance the entire field of life course health development research.

The resulting transdisciplinary research agenda focuses on foundational research types and topics, including research that addresses life course epidemiology, research that elucidates life course health development (LCHD) processes (e.g., sensitive periods, epigenetics), and research that identifies effective interventions, with a special emphasis on health disparities research and research on high priority conditions (e.g., obesity and mental health conditions) and specific vulnerable populations (e.g., children in foster care, premature infants, and children with medical complexity). Next, we consider essential research capacity-building activities focused on data, data systems, and methods, as well as strategies for building the human, technical, cultural, and financial capacity required to carry out this challenging work. Lastly, we discuss the importance of translational and intervention research that can speed the application of concepts and findings to the practice and policy arenas. We conclude with a discussion of advancing the overall life course health development research paradigm, including the framework and principles that have emerged from the research thus far, and that are helping to define a robust explanatory and theoretical LCHD framework.

2 Rationale: Why a Life Course Research Agenda?

Until recently, a strong US-based life course focused research and data infrastructure has been lacking. There have also been limits on funding currently available in the US to support the development of new methodologies and collaborative approaches to life course health development research. This has hampered the production of the transformative research that is needed to advance the emerging field of life course health development. The recently aborted National Children's Study is a major example of an unsuccessful attempt to launch a cohort study and research infrastructure that would have allowed the US to start catching up with the many other nations that have launched one or more national cohorts in the past, are in the process of conducting millennium cohort studies, or already have well developed national data systems that permit exploration into life course specific health development questions. Nonetheless, the move toward multidisciplinary LCHD research is advancing in the U.S. as research continues to break out of discipline-specific silos that have often constrained rapid transdicsiplinary progress. Over time, we believe that life course health development will become an increasingly productive and impactful transdisciplinary field.

Current and future production, dissemination, and application of life course health development research can improve our understanding of the origins, development, and manifestation of health and disease. This research must also be strategically aligned with and responsive to ongoing and emerging trends that are important influences on health development research. Because the epidemiology of human health and the capacity of the health system to respond to challenges are constantly changing, a robust LCHD research strategy must be informed by and responsive to emerging trends and shifts. These include but are not limited to:

- The ongoing epidemiologic shift in diseases and disease burdens, from infectious diseases of the past to chronic, preventable, noncommunicable diseases.
- The recognition that health is not the absence of disease, and that health as an outcome is a key target for healthcare systems.
- The "new" epidemics of obesity, several mental health conditions, and multi-morbidity, particularly in older adults.
- The growing recognition that contributing to the US's dubious distinction as the sickest of rich nations is the fact that it spends more on healthcare late in life, compared to nations with better health outcomes that invest in social and education services early in the life course.
- The World Economic Forum's recent focus on what they have termed as "inflection points" across the life course that serve as strategic targets for intervention and present opportunities to leverage population health improvement goals. These inflection points of health development suggest that life course health development research can be translated into effective policy frameworks.
- The transition in how healthcare services are organized and paid for, including the focus on preventing disease and designing payment methodologies that pay for health instead of services. These major system-level changes can use the new science of health development to define the value of healthcare, align payments with health development time frames, and establish overall health system goals.
- A range of different research organizing strategies—from those focused on translating research into action at a patient, community, or health system level to the Clinical Translation Science Institutes, to the National Institutes of Health's new efforts focused on precision medicine—can potentially benefit from new insights from the life course health sciences and can also help advance this type of basic, clinical, applied, and translational research.

The research revolution that gave birth to the life course health sciences is now about four decades old. Several disciplines, fields, and seminal research studies have contributed to the emergence of the field. These converging, interacting, and interdependent empirical and analytic trends are important to recognize and to strategically leverage as we advance the life course health sciences through a robust research agenda.

Longitudinal cohort studies that have allowed for direct empirical interrogation of the role of early life factors on adult health behaviors and outcomes contributed to the emergence of the field, as did the recognition that the impact of early adversity on lifelong health was not being captured by prevailing biomedical and biopsychosocial models that ignored the timing and influences of social and environmental factors on health development. David Barker et al.'s (1989) pathbreaking research describing the long-term associations between perinatal health conditions, such as birthweight, and adult chronic disease decades later provided an important empirical nudge for considering a new form of life course epidemiological research.

More recently, chronic disease epidemiologists have teamed up with neurobiologists and molecular biologists to elucidate the biological mechanisms for the effects of early childhood exposures and experiences on later and lifelong health. While these largely biomedical research studies were being done, a parallel set of investigations in sociology and psychology examined how mental health develops over the life course in response to interpersonal and environmental interactions. The convergence of life course epidemiology, biology, life course sociology, and life span human development psychology has established the contours of a multidisciplinary field of life course health development (Kuh and Ben-Shlomo 2004; Ben-Shlomo and Kuh 2002; Halfon et al. 2014a) that is in the process of maturing into a unified, transdisciplinary field with a unique set of theoretical constructs, frameworks, models, and methodologies.

By integrating evolutionary and developmental perspectives, the life course health development framework also spans the gap between these two fields of research that emerged with the post-Darwinian synthesis of evolution and heredity, coupled with advances in human genetics and epigenetics. As the LCHD framework began to take shape, it helped support the growing recognition that (1) health development is a complex adaptive process that emerges out of the dynamic coactions between an organism and its environments, (2) this emergent process is mediated by different types and levels of plasticity that evolution has engineered into the human developmental process to optimize a range of adaptive responses to diverse environments, and (3) the synchronization and harmonization of different embedded time frames must be considered, assessed, and understood (Hochberg 2009).

LCHD as a discrete, multidisciplinary field of inquiry is young. Irrespective of how conceptually attractive constructs such as sensitive periods or biological conditioning might be, it is important that the field be appropriately self critical in determining how strong the evidence really is for these notions. The biological plausibility of many of the LCHD hypotheses about the role and impact of different types of plasticity on the development of health and disease needs to be tested and strengthened by carefully designed and implemented research. The tension between advancing the field and ensuring sufficient awareness and reflection about whether and how it challenges the prevailing orthodoxy of biomedical research requires more careful analysis.

Hanson and Gluckman have highlighted the reasons behind the delayed acceptance of the concept of the Developmental Origins of Health and Disease (DOHaD), including a lack of conceptual framework, confusion between factors correlated with disease risk and those involved with causation, assumptions that all of the DOHaD effects were operating only through the pathway of lower birthweight, lack of plausible biological mechanisms, failure to recognize the importance of the DOHaD concept under normal developmental conditions as opposed to extreme conditions, lack of evidence of its relative importance in relation to other risk factors (i.e., population attributable risk analysis), and lack of plausible ways to use the concept clinically and in public health (Hanson and Gluckman 2014). Many of the barriers that Hanson and Gluckman describe are part of the impetus and genesis for further developing the LCHD framework so that DOHaD concepts—including notions of sensitive periods, biological priming and conditioning, life histories, and evolutionary constraints—can be used to further empirical, analytic, translational, health services, policy, and conceptual research.

The LCHD framework that has been articulated in this volume by Halfon and Forrest (2017), while not a fully developed paradigm, provides a new approach for linking health and developmental processes. The framework challenges the explanatory power of older and more linear biomedical models, as well as multidimensional biopsychosocial approaches. The LCHD framework is portrayed as a dynamic network of interactive and interdependent concepts that are coming of age and formulating this new investigative approach. In spite of the challenges for moving life course health research forward, the amount of consistent evidence, the convergence of several fields of inquiry, and the recognition of common principles are providing the opportunity—and need—for not only a more coherent explanatory framework but for the second generation of priority research topics, questions, activities, and strategies that are presented in the next section.

3 Recommendations

The following recommendations are presented in four main sections: (1) priority research types and topics, (2) priority research capacity-building activities, (3) translational priorities pertaining to the application of current knowledge to practice and policy, and (4) strategies for refining the LCHD theoretical framework.

3.1 Section I: Priority Research Types and Topics

3.1.1 Priority Research Types

Epidemiological Research

There is a growing recognition of the value of life course chronic disease epidemiologic research and its application to understanding the origins, distribution, and patterns of various diseases and health conditions. LCHD epidemiology has benefited from a better appreciation for the timing and time-specific interactions of numerous multilevel factors that influence health development. As the importance of what has been called the exposome (i.e., the set of environmental factors that influence health) become more salient and new measures and approaches for assessing environmental influences are created, a demand will be generated for multilevel epidemiologic studies (Robinson et al. 2015). Better epidemiologic measures, modeling, and analysis will all be needed to understand how different kinds of adversity interact with one another and impact health development (see Buka et al. 2017; Little 2017).

A better, more systematic, and useful understanding of how social adversity stimulates different stress responses, how the development of those stress reactivity patterns are biologically conditioned by other stimuli, and how they cascade, or play forward, requires studies using longitudinal cohorts. Such studies will need to further refine the characterization and measurement of different and specific kinds of environments. This includes better measurement of specific components, experiences, and exposures but also how different elements of that environment are contextually linked and expressed both independently and synergistically. Understanding the interplay of genes and environment, and how different contexts influence the emergence of different trajectories, requires that epidemiologic studies focus on proximal neurobiological processes, including the epigenetic influences on the emergence of behaviors that manifest as endophenotypes and how environmental context influences the progression to full-fledged behavioral or psychiatric disorders (see Boyce and Hertzman 2017). This raises a number of measurement challenges, especially concerning how to assess changes in interacting and interdependent influences from the cellular to the social level.

A new fruitful area of LCHD epidemiologic research will focus on better characterizing the role and impact of the places where children and families live, grow, learn, work, and play (Pearce 2014; Dunn et al. 2015). With the expanding number of place-based interventions that attempt to improve the organization and functioning of entire community ecosystems, there is a mounting interest in how place as an organizing force influences health development at both the individual and population levels. The notion that multiple risk and protective factors are uniquely organized and deployed by a particular place provides new ways of understanding how to design and implement place-based interventions that strategically aggregate services, programs, and systems into a more coordinated approach to optimizing health development (Pearce et al. 2016).

Given the role that different mediators and modifiers can play at different ages and with different subgroups, more research is needed to determine how both normal and disordered development unfolds in relationship to nested exposures and experiences. Such research should also include a more strategic focus on how mutable these relationships might be. Specific interventions have been developed to modify family relationships, including interventions focused on parent-child relational content, maternal and infant bonding, or the capacity of mothers and fathers to co-parent (Leslie et al. 2016). How these interventions transform the ecosystem in which the child is developing, and how these alterations track over chronological and developmental time frames, requires further study.

While developmental trajectories are routinely used by developmental psychologists to describe the patterns and contours of developmental pathways and how they change over time, the measurement of health development trajectories in relationship to different proximal (maternal depression) and distal (violent neighborhood) risks, as well as different proximal (supportive grandmother) and distal (strong faith community) protective factors, is sorely lacking. A better understanding of how these different risk and protective factors interact and influence, both individually and in combination, health development requires different measurement and study design strategies than are routinely incorporated into cohort studies where exposures are evaluated as independent influences and causal attribution is often oversimplified (Dunn et al. 2014).

LCHD epidemiologic studies should also focus on better characterization of the role that differential timing of exposures to risk and protective factors has on the emergent quality and function of developmentally contingent hormonal systems and on the development of superordinate behavioral capacities including executive functioning, empathy, and perseverance. In addition, there is also a great need to focus on how multitiered pathways emerge, how they are influenced by different interventions, and how those influences affect outcomes over years and decades.

Mechanism Research

As the life course health sciences mature, they are more fully embracing the complexity of health development. There is a growing realization that health development is a complex adaptive nonlinear, multilevel, and multidirectional process in which the timing, patterning, and interactions of exposures and experience play out against a set of evolutionarily influenced developmental processes, each with its own sequencing and time signature. Throughout this volume, the need for better and more precise mechanism research has been emphasized, such as:

- Elucidating the nature and role of, and the mediators that influence, how sensitive periods emerge, develop, and manifest
- Developing a better understanding of how family- and community-level factors interact and influence each other over time
- Evaluating how the health capital that mothers bring to conception influences prenatal as well as postnatal child health development
- Assessing how biological sensitivity to context emerges and is modified by different signals and cues from both slowly and rapidly changing environmental influences

Biological conditioning—also sometimes referred to as biological priming or, more deterministically, biological embedding—includes the various ways in which environmental influences either exert transitory or more long-lasting impacts on developing biobehavioral regulatory systems. This is a high-value target for future research. Key questions include: What are the specific biological, neurologic, epigenetic, and physiologic mechanisms that are most important for altering biobehavioral regulatory systems? What is the mutability of these mechanisms? Do certain key factors act as "triggers," setting in motion a cascade of future biological response patterns? Biological conditioning processes can range from the exposure to a specific nutrient like folate and its influence on epigenetic methylation based on availability in indigenous diets (see Herman and Taylor Baer 2017) to the role that different patterns of sleep and sleep duration have on cycling of neuroendocrine hormones that serve to prime other factors related to growth, metabolism, and the biological underpinning of behavioral response systems (see Mummert et al. 2017; Hawkins et al. 2017).

Given worldwide rising rates of neurological, mental health, developmental, and substance abuse (NMDS) disorders, the international health community has prioritized developing a better understanding of the epigenetic effects of nutrition, infections, a range of environmental exposures, and psychosocial factors on developing nervous systems, especially the role early exposures and experiences have on later onset neurological conditions (Silberberg et al. 2015). Included in this prioritization is the recognition that adolescents are particularly at risk for developing neurocognitive deficits and mental health problems. Given that 50–75% of lifetime mental health disorders have their onset before age 24, a focus on better understanding the mechanisms that create this long-lasting vulnerability and how it can be addressed is also a high priority (Davidson et al. 2015). The life course health sciences should capitalize on worldwide interest in NMDS by highlighting the importance of life course approaches to understanding how NMDS develops (Birbeck et al. 2015).

Several chapters in this book emphasized the role of biological and behavioral transitions as sensitive periods and how they may afford leverage to alter developmental trajectories (see DelGiudice 2017; Boyce and Hertzman 2017; Wood et al. 2017). Similarly, interactions between the hypothalamic-pituitary-adrenal axis and basic energy metabolism that are also controlled by the hypothalamus may be relevant to the development of both physical and mental health, and understanding these interactions holds promise in better understanding why conditions like attention-deficit hyperactivity disorder (ADHD) and obesity cluster together (Halfon et al. 2013).

The way in which one sensitive period emerges and influences the development of subsequent sensitive periods also bears further investigation. This includes how the preconception period serves as an important platform for the creation and management of health development capital, and how the preconception period organizes and influences the prenatal and subsequent postnatal periods, each with its own defining characteristics, functions, and sensitivities. As more attention focuses on the prevention of adverse birth outcomes and the promotion of equity from the start of life, our understanding of the role and function of the preconception and prenatal periods in lifelong health will become all the more important. As capacity improves to identify, measure, differentiate, and understand the relationships between different sensitive periods of health development, our ability to devise and test more longitudinally integrated health-optimizing interventions will also assume greater importance.

Many of the chapters emphasized the need for research designs that specifically target multi-level influences, multilevel measurement, and analytic techniques that focus on multilevel interactions and modifications. They also suggested extant data limitations and methodological challenges that pose barriers to measuring and modeling the complexity of these influences and interactions. A whole new set of analytic tools and modeling techniques are emerging from the world of complex systems science. Their adaptation and application to the complex multilevel and life course health development processes is likely to be very fruitful and illuminating (Osypuk 2013; El-Sayed et al. 2013).

Evolutionary perspectives on how adversity, stress, and complex evolving cultural structures (e.g., educational and religious institutions) have shaped selection of human development priorities are also ripe for further cross-disciplinary research. The chapters by Boyce and Hertzman (2017) and DelGiudice (2017) in this volume emphasize the importance of how environmental stressors can lead to diverse adaptive responses that can manifest at different levels of impact depending on other contextual factors. They suggest that in advancing life course health development research, we recognize the value of cross-species, comparative studies that can shed light on the relationship between evolutionary biology and social environments and their consequences on human developmental adaptation and environmental mismatches.

Lastly, the evidence reviewed in several of the chapters suggest the potential value of a more integrative developmentally nuanced systems-physiology approach to understanding how co-occurring risks manifest in developmentally comparable changes across multiple physiological systems (Singer and Ryff 2001). For example, while it is well established that exposure to aminoglycoside antibiotics early in life can have detrimental and potentially devastating effects on both auditory and renal function, the chapters in this volume by Russ and colleagues (Russ et al. 2017) on hearing and Brophy and colleagues (Brophy et al. 2017) on chronic kidney disease (CKD) suggest that there are ways that the developing sensory apparatus in the ear and the developing filtration apparatus in the kidney may share other potential vulnerabilities across the life course. Future research on how risks and protective factors influence multiple systems will potentially lead to multi-solving interventions that can optimize health development across several discreet physiological systems. Better modeling of how seemingly distinct biological and behavioral systems develop holds promise to understanding how they develop their inherent robustness, where they share similar vulnerabilities, and how they might be buffered and protected from undesirable insults and risks (Kitano 2004; Cohen 2016).

Intervention Research

Our understanding of the impact of life course risks will be improved by better intervention research that targets key developmental processes and time periods. Throughout this volume, authors have highlighted the important role of intervention research for better understanding not only how to intervene, but also when. For example, the chapter by Hawkins and colleagues (Hawkins et al. 2017) suggests that a key to reducing childhood obesity is finding the right level and time in the life course to intervene for the maximal effectiveness and efficiency of interventions. However, the challenge of mounting programs designed to modify obesogenic health development pathways may be quite complex, involving multiple settings (e.g., medical care, homes, child care, school) (Taveras, Blackburn, et al. 2011a; Taveras, Gortmaker, et al. 2011b; Taveras et al. 2012), or components (e.g., system redesign, individual behavior change strategies including e-technology) (Lubans et al. 2010; Taveras et al. 2012), and targeting single or multiple factors (Taveras, Gortmaker, et al. 2011b; Vesco et al. 2012).

The chapter in this volume by Kim and colleagues (Kim et al. 2017) highlights how new insights into multilevel influences on health development pave the way for a range of different interventions that will further clarify these relationships. New research on pregnancy and the first years of a child's life indicate not only that this is a sensitive period for child neurological development but that it is a period when a parent's brain may demonstrate higher levels of plasticity and undergo changes to support the parental role (Kim et al. 2016). Given that parental brains are being remodeled at the same time that children's brains are developing, there are several potential ways to intervene so that parents modify home environments in developmentally optimizing ways for both their children and for themselves. Many potential interventions that span from cells to society have been studied in isolation, ranging from those that attempt to modify socioeconomic position via cash transfers to those that focus on harmonizing parenting approaches via co-parenting skills training (see Kim et al. 2017; Duncan et al. 2011; Feinberg et al. 2009). Less research has been done to better understand how best to combine interventions into a more integrated, sustained, and sustainable developmentally optimizing strategy.

The chapter in this volume by Boyce and Hertzman (2017) suggests that more effective prevention science demands new and innovative intervention designs that are responsive to the emerging science of health development. Highlighting how the Nurse Family Partnership broke new ground when it was first conceived and launched, the authors point to the need for ambitious and "more radical departures ... from the conventions of traditional early development programs, including careful consideration of how complex dynamic systems thinking might be wed to novel, preventive interventions."

The chapter in this volume by Larson and colleagues (Larson et al. 2017) similarly focuses on the importance of intervention research to better understand the origins, impact, and mutability of health disparities that arise from different health development pathways. They argue that a multilevel intervention research strategy is needed. Intervention research on decreasing disparities in health development could focus on a range of possible sensitive periods, examining the possible and potential benefit of and best timing for interventions in the preconception period for improving birth. They also suggest that new social interventions, designed to alter specific short-term health outcomes (e.g., asthma or early stress reactivity) in at-risk populations, should be designed and tested in relation to how they modify long-term health and well-being outcomes in adulthood. For example, can population-level interventions like teaching young children yoga and other mindfulness techniques serve to "inoculate" them against elevations in allostatic load due to stressful and chaotic family environments?

Questions about the best timing for intervention are important. Cost-effectiveness studies can be used to compare the value of interventions at different life stages. In addition to interventions at the individual level, interventions focused on the multilevel determinants of health (e.g., neighborhood-level interventions) will also be important. Lastly, the chapter by Larson and colleagues (Larson et al. 2017) suggests that research should focus on the impact of new policies and programs at the local, state, and national levels to reduce health disparities across the life course. The authors also make an important distinction between research focused on minimizing risk and preventing poor health and interventions aimed at optimizing health and developmental potential.

3.1.2 Priority Research Topics

The Impact of Adverse Experiences on Health Development and the Origins and Implications of Health Disparities

Because of growing and persistent income inequality, high rates of child poverty, and associated levels of adversity, there is a pressing need to better understand the impact of adversity on health development, as well as ways of mediating and modifying its influence. Recent data from the National Survey of Children's Health reveals that the experience of adversity is not confined solely to children living below the federal poverty level, but extends up the income ladder (Halfon et al. 2014c). With nearly half of all children living in low income families with earnings below 200% of the Federal Poverty Level, these are concerns that now affect a majority of children. Related to the greater prevalence and experience of adversity in children from low income families is the relationship that the experience of adversity has to the development of a range of phenotypic responses.

Research on childhood adversity has been highly influenced by the conceptualization of adversity advanced by Felitti et al. (1998) in the original Adverse Childhood Experiences (ACE) Study. This retrospective cohort study of patients attending a weight reduction clinic at a southern California Kaiser Permanente facility in the 1990s has provided important information on the relationship between adversity early in life and the subsequent occurrence of a range of chronic diseases. However, it has also limited the conceptualization of adversity and how it is measured. Moving forward, it will be important to refine our definition and measurement of adversity, as well as the patterns and variations in its occurrence. The recognition and description of how specific types of adversity can be traumatic, and how that trauma can in turn lead to different kinds of stress response patterns, also call for a better understanding of the relationship between adversity, trauma, and stress. Given that all adversities are not equal, and that not all adversity is experienced as trauma, it is important to develop better measures of the experience of adversity, as well as to examine how that adversity is transduced by the brain and other body systems, including behavioral response patterns, proximal neurobiological processes, and epigenetic and other molecular changes (Hane and Fox 2016).

The chapter by DelGiudice (2017) in this volume warns that researchers should exercise caution in assuming that undesirable developmental outcomes reflect dysregulation of biological systems, and should remain open to the possibility that those outcomes may be part of adaptive (or formerly adaptive) strategies for survival and reproduction. He argues here and elsewhere (Del Giudice 2014b, c) that a life history framework is especially useful in teasing out the logic of potentially adaptive combinations of traits, highlighting critical factors in the environment, and bridging behavioral development with physical growth trajectories. A similar observation is made in the chapter in this volume by Lerner et al. (2017) in their analysis of adolescent health development, highlighting the context dependency of adaptive developmental regulation and how such regulation may vary by specific social situations, times, and places.

Related to the experience of adversity is the capacity for resilience among individuals and populations that experience it. The chapter by Larson and colleagues (Larson et al. 2017) suggests that additional research is needed to not only identify individuals with exceptional health resilience but to better understand the health development pathways that lead to more resilient phenotypes. Studies that examine the cultural, social, and psychological resources that can lead to thriving and better-than-expected health outcomes for individuals from disadvantaged social groups should also receive priority consideration, along with studies that lead to a better understanding of how those resources affect entire populations.

A basic notion of the life course health development framework is that the balance and interplay of risk and protective factors influence health development trajectories. Children living in environments with many more risk factors than protective factors will have a greater propensity for delayed or disordered health development trajectories, while those growing and developing in environments with more protective and health-promoting factors will achieve more optimal developmental pathways and trajectories. However, this simple characterization of the distribution of risk and protective factors in low- versus high-income communities obscures more complex and dynamic processes, a high degree of variability, and other deeper dynamics that might not be readily apparent and need to be considered and measured more directly. As the chapter in this volume by Mummert et al. (2017) points out, the ecosystems in which today's children are developing are novel when conceptualized across evolutionary timescales, with our manmade environments posing additional biological and behavioral challenges to developing humans that can both mediate and exacerbate other forms of more readily observable and measurable adversity.

While the experience of adversity has been directly related to the onset and development of different health outcomes that range from heart disease to depression, the relationships and variability at a population level is less well defined. The chapter in this volume by Larson and colleagues (Larson et al. 2017) suggests that it is important to continue to investigate the underlying biological processes that contribute to health disparities in human populations, and to better understand the role of protective factors and resilience on positive health outcomes for individuals from disadvantaged backgrounds. They also suggest more attention to parental preconception health and other intergenerational mechanisms that may contribute to early health disparities. To inform public policy and further elucidate the link between adversity and health disparities, they suggest additional investigations of the dynamic multilevel contributors to health status disparities across the life course.

The Impact of Family- and Community-Level Factors on Health Development

The LCHD framework highlights how the importance of understanding how health development processes is influenced by multiple factors at multiple levels in dynamic, transactional ways. Of particular salience to practitioners is the role that family- and community-level factors may have on health development. Related to the independent impact of these factors is their combined impact, as well as the impact that comes when these factors are considered in relationship to a particular ecosystem or place. This kind of multilevel and integrative analysis is important in a world where place-based strategies aimed at creating multiple potential opportunities for health improvement are routinely deployed.

Several of the chapters emphasize the importance of multilevel contributors to health status disparities over the life course, with a particular emphasis on upstream structural factors and neighborhood-level determinants. Multilevel studies can help examine the impact of neighborhood-level factors on health disparities by socioeconomic status, race, and ethnicity. Also needed are studies that incorporate longitudinal or life course measures of neighborhood and environmental exposures. At the population level, studies are needed to examine the natural environment, built environment, and social environment exposures that contribute to geographic differentials in rates of health and disease, as well as how variation in health policies contribute to disparities. To the greatest extent possible, research studies that examine lifelong contributors to sociodemographic health disparities should investigate the importance of the timing of key environmental and social exposures.

There is also a need to better understand the role that family and community risk and protective factors play in mediating influences at different levels. For example, how do positive health development enhancing family routines and other family-centric protective factors insulate or buffer a child's response patterns in a community where violence, social chaos, and family isolation are the norm? Evaluating the contribution of family capacities and routines—as well as social isolation, social relationships, and social support—is a fertile and strategically important area for further research. This kind of research is particularly important for a health-care arena in which "care bundles" are being developed to address both the medical and non-medical social, family, and behavioral influences on health.

The Impact of Specific Exposures and Experiences, the Importance of Various Life Stages, and the Development of Health Conditions

There are dynamic developmental relationships between different kinds of experiences and exposures that can be better understood from a life course perspective. For example, the chapter in this volume by Lerner and colleagues (Lerner et al. 2017) suggests profiling how different patterns of nutrition develop and influence a range of related behaviors and outcomes during adolescence. How do adolescents' diets influence their cardio-metabolic risk as adolescents and adults? Do adolescents maintain a healthy diet across different settings involving peers and family members? Is there age-associated variation in answers to this question, for instance, variation associated with pubertal development or pubertal status/stage (e.g., early, on time, or late)? Do answers to these questions vary in relation to gender? As well, do they vary in relation to normative social transitions (e.g., moving from elementary school to middle school)? How do peer social networks influence these behaviors or family mealtime behaviors? Are answers moderated or changed by the socioeconomic, cultural, religious, or national contexts of youth? In turn, do answers here vary in relation to media exposure about eating and about desirable body types that may be prevalent for youth living in particular settings at particular times in history? Given the synchronization issues raised by the seventh life course health development principle (see Halfon and Forrest 2017), how are all these answers moderated or changed by what may be nonnormative life events in the lives of adolescents? Examples here may be the death of a parent or deployment in the military (Cozza and Lerner 2013), family disruption due to divorce or separation, or family challenges in the face of environmental tragedies such as weather.

Important New Epidemics or Emerging Changes in Population Epidemiology

Rapidly changing environmental conditions and exposures have resulted in a variety of epidemiological transitions that yield new patterns of health and disease. Perhaps the most dramatic epidemiologic transition is the one that took place as a result of improvement in sanitation and public health—from mortality due to infectious or communicable disease to mortality due to non-communicable chronic health conditions like diabetes, hypertension, heart disease, and cancer. This transition has been well described and appreciated, although not without controversy as to its origins and drivers. In the past several decades, we have witnessed increased rates of child obesity and child and adolescent mental health disorders. While there have been relatively simple notions about the origins and drivers of the obesity epidemic, the chapter by Hawkins and colleagues in this volume (Hawkins et al. 2017) highlights the developmental complexity underlying this major epidemiologic change.

There has been far less focus and research on the developmental origins and patterns of manifestation of a range of mental health problems that appear to be rapidly increasing in children and adolescents. Recent epidemiologic surveys suggest that over 20% of adolescents now have a mental health disorder with impaired functioning (Merikangas et al. 2010). A better understanding of the mechanisms, causal factors, mutability, and lifelong consequences of these disorders is sorely needed. While there has been some research on whether mental health disorders arising in adolescence persists into adulthood, there is evidence that when they do, the impact on functioning and lifelong success can be more debilitating than the lifelong impact of chronic medical conditions (Moffitt 1993; Currie and Stabile 2006). While there have been studies that have begun to link increasing rates of media and television exposures to the development of attentional problems, the nature and impact of this rapidly changing epidemiology calls out for better life course health development research (Zimmerman and Christakis 2007).

The Health Development of Particularly Vulnerable Populations

The health development of particularly vulnerable populations of children demands more life course focused research. The chapter in this volume by Msall and colleagues (Msall et al. 2017) highlights the impact of socioeconomic-associated risks on the health development of premature infants. While there have been many longitudinal follow-up studies of premature infants, few have adopted a health development perspective or examined the role that other risk and protective factors play in shaping the developmental trajectories of this very vulnerable population. The same can be said for individuals with autism spectrum disorder, CKD, or most other chronic health conditions. In their chapter on autism spectrum disorder (ASD), Drmic, Szatmari, and Volkmer highlight how little that is known about the trajectories of children and adolescents with ASD and how studies focused on optimizing the health development of individuals with ASD could provide critical information. They highlight how adolescents with ASD who are clearly benefiting from participating in school and other educationally related activities experience a functional downturn once the developmental scaffolding that school provides is no longer available. The suggestion that individuals with ASD have delayed maturation of key developmental processes also argues for a more developmentally attuned and integrated understanding of how to optimize outcomes. The chapter on CKD by Brophy and colleagues (Brophy et al. 2017) also connects the dots between prematurity and other insults that may lead to decreased number of functional kidney filtration units (nephrons) and the time-specific and cumulative insults that are increasingly understood as the life course developmental pathway to CKD.

There are several other vulnerable populations of children where a life course health development perspective could be very illuminating and more importantly could shape the services and interventions that are provided. For example, it is well known that children who are abused, neglected, and placed into the foster care system can experience dramatically altered life course trajectories (Zlotnick et al. 2012; Tyler and Schmitz 2013; Patterson et al. 2015). Initial studies examining the impact of adversity, institutional placement, and out-of-home care have suggested how such experiences can alter neurobiological functioning and cellular processes associated with the regulation of cellular aging and longevity (Drury et al. 2012; Karatsoreos and McEwen 2013). Life course health development research could improve these interventions in regard to their capacity to improve long-term trajectories for children in foster care and other vulnerable populations, including young people involved in the juvenile justice system and children with chronic and debilitating medical conditions and impairments (Zlotnick et al. 2012). In each case, better understanding the health, growth, and developmental trajectories—and the factors and experiences associated with optimal health development outcomes—is sorely needed.

3.2 Section II: Priority Research Capacity-Building Activities

3.2.1 Advance LCHD Measurement Capacity and Improve Study Design to Provide Useful Data and Promote Greater Collaboration Across Disciplines

Throughout this volume, the authors have emphasized the importance of new and better measures of health and health development, with specific reference to developing and aging body systems (e.g., kidney health, hearing health). Closely related to measurement research are new and better analytic strategies that utilize data in more creative ways. Several chapters emphasize the need for better measures of "positive health." For example, Russ and colleagues' chapter on hearing (Russ et al. 2017) suggests that researchers need operational measures of positive hearing health to enable better measurement of treatment outcomes and functional hearing ability. Measures of positive health—including oral health, nutritional health, and mental health - as well as measures of positive health trajectories in these and other areas provide an empirical way of measuring both general and targeted health-optimizing strategies. Such measures might be composed of several different related measures and biomarkers that could be used to profile a specific health development capacity.

Measures of positive health development are not only important for assessing the health status and trajectories of individuals but also for use in assessing populations. The Early Development Index is a measurement tool that is used in Canada, Australia, and the USA to assess healthy development and school readiness for 4–6-year-olds (Janus et al. 2016). The EDI is composed of 110 items that span 5 dimensions and 16 subdomains of functioning. It is routinely collected and mapped at the neighborhood level to provide a population measure of health development. It has been used to predict early language and cognitive development and to examine differences in cognitive and emotional development in populations of children (Brownell et al. 2016). It is part of an evolving set of population health development measurement tools that now includes the Middle Development Index that was designed to measure similar dimensions in 9–11-year-olds (Schonert-Reichl et al. 2013; Guhn et al. 2016a). The same Canadian team that created the EDI and MDI is in the process of developing health development indices covering the entire child span, using the EDI to develop a pan-Canadian population health monitoring system (Guhn et al. 2016b). In addition, the EDI has also been used as a measure in "cells to society" research that is examining the impact of social gradients and how that manifests in relationships to social epigenetics (Hertzman and Boyce 2010).

Enhanced data collection of individual behaviors, traits, and biomarkers is now possible using low-cost, readily available technologies like smartphones and self-reported questionnaires. The National Institutes of Health have invested millions of dollars into the creation of state-of-the science self-reported measures of physical, mental, and social health as part of its program called the Patient Reported Outcome Measurement Information System (PROMIS, see www.healthmeasures.net for more information). These assessments of health can be combined with a wide array of environmental sensor assessments that can measure macro and micro fluctuations in the local environments, as well as clinical data stored in electronic health records and other molecular data such as genetics and epigenetics.

Aggregation of large amounts of data of these types can be done to create *big health development data* resources that can be mined and used to elucidate novel, unanticipated associations to inform future causal modeling and interventions.

Advances in life course health sciences have depended on the creation of longitudinal data collection efforts over the past century, most of which have been undertaken in countries located in Europe and Oceania. Recognizing the value of these longitudinal studies, several nations launched millennial cohort studies. This volume profiles several existing longitudinal surveys that can be used for examining life course impacts of different social and environmental factors (see Geller et al. 2017; Sastry et al. 2017; Cooksey 2017).

Longitudinal life course studies are important for capturing the dynamics of intra-individual health development trajectories and their environmental influences and epigenetic profiles. Because longitudinal cohort studies capture temporal relationship between exposures and outcomes, they can assist in defining causality and also in identifying predictive epigenetic biomarkers that may be used clinically and for targeted and more precise public health interventions.

There is also growing recognition that existing longitudinal and disease focused cohorts could be more effectively used to investigate specific questions by increasing sample sizes to enhance statistical power to examine interactions. Work is underway both in the USA and Europe to align and link cohorts, recognizing that the heterogeneity of the different studies will require conceptual and analytic harmonization to allow data to be pooled. Existing cohort studies are being encouraged to not only collect genetic information but to obtain detailed phenotype data—along with broader and more detailed information on environmental, behavioral, and lifestyle measures—in order to improve the capacity to link data sets for new kinds of analysis. Given the growing prevalence of a range of neurodevelopmental disorders in adults, there is an increasing interest collecting early cognitive, behavioral, metabolic, and epigenetic markers that might herald the onset and development of these diseases.

3.2.2 Develop and Apply New and Improved Methodologies to Reflect a Complex Systems Approach and Enable Causal Inference

As an emerging transdisciplinary field, LCHD research is typically done with scientific teams that include several methodologists and analysts to address the complex and multifaceted biological variation that epitomizes human health, but also the many and multilevel relational influences that are interacting and inducing changes in this continuously unfolding biological matrix. The complex and interconnected relationships of factors contributing to the development of obesity, mental health disorders, and other conditions with multiple complex causes typify the challenges that confound many common analytic approaches. Conventional longitudinal analyses, even those that account for multiple levels of influence, are often not powerful enough to account for the complexity and interconnectedness of obesity. Little's chapter in this volume (Little 2017) explains that several new techniques are available to improve estimation and causal inference for study designs with a multitude of time-varying covariates that interact across multiple levels. These include, among others, longitudinal structural equation modeling which can model hierarchically nested contextual influences on health over time. In addition, an emerging set of analytic tools from the systems sciences including agent-based and system dynamics modeling can be utilized to examine longitudinal relationships over multiple levels and, at the same time, account for more complex features of relationships like nonlinearity, path dependence, loops, and tipping (Hammond 2009; Huang, Drewnosksi, Kumanyika, and Glass 2009).

Several authors reference the need for better community-based participatory research involving collaboration and partnership between community leaders, residents, and academic researchers. This kind of research can be used to help design assessments of living conditions (i.e., risk factors and influences) that are richer in content and more appropriately reflect the complex interactions that take place in family and community settings. It can also help to design interventions that are responsive to local needs and promote policy advocacy in disadvantaged neighborhoods. As place-based efforts attempt to transform the basic conditions in a community, they have often taken a life course approach to improve cradle-to-career trajectories with attention paid to what works in different kinds of communities and microenvironments.

3.2.3 Build, Strengthen, and Improve Institutional Capacity to Conduct LCHD Research

Increasing our capacity to conduct life course health science research requires a systematic and purposeful effort that focuses on human skills and talent, infrastructure, and institutional capacity, as well as state-of-the-art life course research tools and methods. Capacity building at the individual level requires mentoring, career guidance, research opportunities, and research pathways that are transdisciplinary and designed to promote optimal development of a life course health development researcher. At an institutional level, advancing life course health science research requires an appreciation for its importance, as well as prioritization of resources allocated for integrative approaches that characterize LCHD research.

Current major research infrastructure building and reform efforts like the Clinical Translational Science Institutes (CTSIs) permit institutions to use life course health development as an integrating strategy for building cross-disciplinary research teams and for focusing research priorities on key health development strategies. The CTSIs have also encouraged approaching diseases and health conditions in a more holistic manner, moving beyond traditional clinic-based models to engage individuals and families in the context of their own lives and life course goals. Similarly, the Patient-Centered Outcome Research Initiative has spearheaded research from a patient's perspective that also lends itself to life course consideration, including challenges presented by specific life course transitions. Life course health science requires team-based, often multi-institutional approaches to research, which is rapidly becoming the norm in the natural, biomedical, and social sciences.

3.3 Section III: Translational Priorities

Efforts are needed to identify existing knowledge that is ready for translation to concrete practice guidelines, programs, and policies aimed at improving health trajectories and alleviating disparities in health. Bringing this life course health development lens to the current healthcare system permits a critical review of how medical care clinics are organized, how healthcare systems organize care pathways, and more. Perhaps the greatest practical clinical and programmatic realization coming from LCHD research is the value of care delivery pathways and systems that are purposeful in their horizontal integration across all of the social ecological domains that influence health development and that are inclusive of all of the sectors and potential influencers on the whole person's health. The other important integration strategy is one that focuses on longitudinal or life course integration, not only anticipating future needs and concerns but designed to optimize life course-organized transitions and challenges. For example, life course-oriented research focused on optimizing health development could be used to redesign the healthcare system with a greater emphasis on promoting optimal health throughout the life course from birth through death, instead of focusing on disease management alone (Halfon et al. 2014b, c). Continued efforts are needed to identify ways in which life course research on health disparities can be integrated into medical, social welfare, education, and public health practice, as well as social and health policies at the local, state, and national levels.

There is also a great need to begin to explore how different periods of the life course have been underappreciated for their potential influence and leverage on downstream outcomes. For example, the chapter in this volume by Del Giudice (2017) calls attention to the juvenile transition and how this underappreciated and virtually unexplored period may be an important developmental window for intervention. The author suggests that interventions focused on optimizing transitions and occurring during these grammar school years can have an important priming and long-term influence on adolescent development. The idea that intervening *during* a biological transition may afford more leverage to alter developmental trajectories resonates with recognizing the nonlinearity of developmental processes and their time sensitivity.

Several of the chapters focused on better screening and assessment tools and approaches that attempt to capture key emergent characteristics and needs so that families can be provided with information about the consequences of decisions being made for a child early in his or her life. Local, state, and national governments also need policies in place that enhance child health development throughout childhood.

Improving public health messaging regarding health development across the life course with specific messaging about healthy hearing trajectories, healthy growth and nutrition trajectories, healthy teeth, and healthy family trajectories can all begin to build awareness and insights into the importance of health development goals, pathways, and trajectories. These include providing growth standards to help individual families implement health-promoting activities, exercise standards, sleep standards, and the like. Such an effort could include both family- and practitioner-based education programs to promote more robust efforts surrounding nutrition and exercise recommendations.

Better ways of sharing life course health development information should also extend to communities so that the optimizing health development of children can be built into the community ethos and appropriate educational materials and policy initiatives developed. Many communities have launched initiatives to promote health development and well-being across the life course. For example, the city of Santa Monica, California, has a lifelong learning system in place and a well-being index that is designed to highlight life course specific health data (Warner and Kern 2013). These kinds of initiatives can promote the importance of life course health science and can mobilize ingenuity and resourcefulness at local and national levels.

3.4 Section IV: Refinement of the LCHD Theoretical Framework

As the chapter by Halfon and Forrest (2017) in this volume indicates, the LCHD framework is an initial version of what may become a new scientific paradigm. As such, LCHD is synthesizing research from a range of different disciplines in ways that will guide the development and testing of new theories of health development and organize future research based on principles established by the field. As the field matures, it will be important to update the framework and its principles, and to consider research approaches, methods, and questions that will further elaborate the framework, moving toward the creation of a model that helps guide future hypothesis-driven research. Important considerations are further developing the explanatory power of the overall framework and interrogating the veracity of the principles that structure the network of ideas, theories, hypotheses, and research questions.

Halfon and Forrest present seven principles that structure the contours of the LCHD framework. They have conceived of these principles not as a linear sequence of defining characteristics but as network of high-level, interconnected generalizations that are empirically supported, logically consistent, and holistically justified. The network presentation suggests that these different principles are distinct but not independent of each other and that judging their explanatory robustness often requires that we consider not the principle in isolation but in relationship to other principles. In keeping with our systems approach to understanding human health development, the system of interconnected and interdependent explanatory principles suggests a dynamic and flexible network of concepts that can be used to build and test theories of causation, interactions, and relational importance. Because some of the principles are not as well supported by a robust empirical literature, some priority should be given to focusing research that addresses areas where additional research is needed.

Further development of the LCHD framework, using it to define the scope and level of life course health development inquiry, and applying it as an organized approach to theory testing will all require continued knowledge synthesis. Because the LCHD framework incorporates a diverse set of factors which interact with each other over significant and variable time horizons, there is a growing need to more systematically analyze and synthesize this information with reference to the overall framework. Greater synthesis of existing cross-disciplinary knowledge of different aspects of LCHD is also necessary for more precise investigation of pathophysiologic mechanisms.

3.4.1 The LCHD Framework, Precision Medicine, and Population Health

As the chapter by Halfon and Forrest suggests, the LCHD framework grew out of recognition that health development is a complex adaptive response of a dynamic, multidimensional, and multilevel system comprising individuals and their contexts codeveloping over time. Adopting the holism of systems biology and other systems sciences, the LCHD framework places more emphasis on the relationship between different components of the system (holism) than on describing the component parts (reductionism). In keeping with emerging notions of precision medicine and precision population health, not only are the insights from systems biology important but also understanding and integrating panomics—the interdependent interactions between the genome, epigenome, microbiome, virome, and exposome. The dynamics, patterns, and predictability of these panomic relationships are not only important for better targeting cancer therapy or customizing the treatment of inflammatory bowel disease but also for creating more effective, efficient, and responsive prevention and health promotion strategies at the population level that are not based on simple notions of risk and dependent on one-size-fits-all interventions (Halfon 2016).

The LCHD framework not only provides a powerful process and tool for knowledge integration but importantly introduces novel and important considerations of emergent developmental processes and developmentally contingent time frames that are important for the synchronization and integration of particular influence, as well as the interactions, flexibility, and dynamics of these relationships across the different combined influences. As the healthcare system focuses more on precision medicine and precision population health, there will be a growing interest in better characterizing health development processes at the individual and population level.

As research using the LCHD framework gallops forward, attention should be paid to how to further develop this framework. Is there an emergent and adaptive strategy to enable the LCHD framework to grow, develop, mature, and evolve as the field of LCHD research moves forward? As LCHD evidence accumulates, is analyzed, and is synthesized, the number of LCHD principles may grow or shrink, and the relationship of the LCHD principles between the principles should become clearer and more useful as a more fully articulated LCHD paradigm emerges. Halfon and Forrest have conceptualized the principles as a network of conceptual nodes whose explanatory utility and robustness is only fully realized in relationship to each other. Modeling and more fully exploring the relationships between the principles can also help test whether this conceptualization of how the principles manifest has explanatory value. As an overarching meta-framework, it will also be useful to examine how the LCHD framework can inform new notions of precision medicine and emerging notions of precision population health.

3.4.2 LCHD and Health System Transformation

Halfon and Forrest also suggest that the LCHD framework is not only strategically responding to a large body of empirical work that challenges long held notions of the causal mechanism responsible for disease causation and the production of different levels of health, but that by focusing on how to optimize health development, it includes considerations of the complex health influencing ecosystem and how that health development ecosystem evolves and changes over time. The framework suggests that health development does not occur solely within an individual or even as a result of an individual's exposure to certain environmental factors, but rather results from continuous coactions between persons and their environments, which we have represented as P⇔E. Thus, individuals are affected by their environments, but they also shape their environments, and the focus on health development is on individual's health assets, their environmental influences, and the ⇔ as well—that is, the relational mechanisms by which persons influence and are influenced by their environments (and vice versa). These insights not only challenge the simpler biomedical and biopsychosocial models of health and disease causation, but challenge the appropriateness, utility, effectiveness, and efficiency of a healthcare system that is largely built on a biomedical chassis and is just now in the process of upgrading its engine to accommodate psychosocial "upstream influences."

The LCHD framework implies that this new and more evolved paradigm of health development and disease causation provides the explanatory rational for how the healthcare delivery system evolves and is organized. The simple linear biomedical framework underwrote the rational for much of the 1.0 acute care focused medical care system with its focus on providing time-limited and rescue care for specific medical conditions over short time horizons. Similarly, the scientific advances and research that led to the development of the more dynamic and multilevel biopsychosocial framework begin to underwrite the upgrade and reengineering of the 2.0 chronic disease system with its greater focus on managing behavioral and lifestyle influences on chronic disease over longer time horizons. The emergence of the LCHD framework is already providing a way of underwriting the need for a more horizontally and longitudinally integrated, anticipatory, and developmentally primed health system (3.0 health system) that is structured to optimize health and health-promoting environments over the life span (Halfon et al. 2014b). Moving forward, it will be important to consider how the LCHD framework can be more fully exploited to inform healthcare innovations and health systems transformation. By fortifying a 3.0 operating system, can LCHD principles be translated into new healthcare system design concepts and innovation strategies? For example, does a better understanding of the potential vulnerability associated with the transition from homecare to preschool suggest a way in which services and supports should be developmentally organized to optimize this transition and support necessary adaptation on the part of the child as well as those in the family?

3.4.3 The LCHD Framework and the Measurement of Health Development

Health in the LCHD framework is defined as an emergent adaptive response to environmental (e.g., biological, behavioral, family, social, physical) challenges. The dynamics of health development and the emergence of diseases, dysfunction, or disintegration depend on dynamic processes and patterns of responses that typically span from the cellular to the whole person level. Because no component of this cluster of interdependent processes and purposeful relationships is ever standing still but is in a constant state of dynamic fluctuations, health is recognizable in the organism's dynamic developmental adaptability and their capacity to strategically respond to different environmental challenges. Because health is conditional on these different environments, measures of health development must be able to capture an individual and populations capacity to dynamically respond when an individual, population, or ecosystem is "out of balance." It also suggests the importance of capturing levels (cellular to ecosystem) of flexibility and resilience that are necessary and manifest to rebalance and achieve not only renewed level of health but an optimal level of health development. Our current measures of health and health development at an individual level are sorely lacking the capacity to sense and integrate signals from the cellular to the whole person level, across physiological systems and response patterns, and across developmentally significant time horizons. At a population level, there are similar conceptual and measurement gaps in how health development is measured and how to capture the developmentally contingent aspects of health development for different populations in facing different ecosystem contexts.

4 Conclusions and Next Steps

This volume has attempted to highlight the importance of the rapidly evolving field of life course health science and its potential impact on improving the lifelong health trajectories. We have used the life course health development framework as a way of organizing inquiry and understanding the relationship between a diverse but converging set of empirical findings. We have proposed a set of LCHD principles that are emerging and, we contend, on their way to describing a new paradigm of scientific investigation and can be used to organize and explain what has been learned and to guide and organize future inquiry (Ostrom 2009; Gatzweiler and Baumuller 2014). This volume has also begun to link and network related areas of inquiry, utilizing these common principles and what they illuminate about deeper and more complex processes of health development. Lastly, we have attempted to relate LCHD research to the field of maternal and child health and to explore how life course enlightened knowledge of health development can be used to improve the health of mothers and children and achieve greater health equity from the start of life.

In this volume, different teams of scholars have analyzed and synthesized the current state of knowledge and research progress in a range of important areas of health development. Spanning topics as diverse as hearing health, kidney health, metabolic health, and oral health across different developmental stages from preconception to emerging adulthood, the chapters examine the health development contribution of different life stages, revealing new considerations for how to prevent losses in health potential, as well as how to optimize lifelong health development. Through the process of writing their chapters, the authors have analyzed and synthesized what is currently known and have begun to shine a light on the way forward by identifying specific research questions and strategies intended to advance research productivity and impact, as well as translation to programs, policy, and practices.

4.1 What's Next?

There are several important national trends that make life course health science and future research on life course health development particularly salient and important at the present time (McGinnis et al. 2016). First are the growing concerns about persistent and structural inequalities in the USA. The life course health sciences have already contributed to the growing recognition of the lifelong health, social, and economic impacts of poverty-associated adversity early in life. Additional research focused on the impact of the early years on future health development will continue to play an important role in refocusing policy, programs, and practices on addressing and leveraging what is at stake in these early years (Halfon et al. 2014c).

Second are the opportunities provided by the implementation of the Affordable Care Act (ACA) and related initiatives designed to move healthcare upstream and to focus more attention and resources on prevention and population health. The life course health sciences are illuminating how such upstream strategies must focus not only on the social and environmental causes of health outcomes but in particular on the upstream influences on costly and preventable adult health outcomes (Wise 2016). As post-ACA policy attempts to steer healthcare financing from a focus on volume (outputs) to value (outcomes), there is a real opportunity to demonstrate how health development value chains begin early in life and how investments in health development capital can be leveraged into significant long-term value results (McGinnis et. al. 2016). ACA-stimulated health system reform is also accelerating the consideration of transformational strategies that are challenging the dominant 2.0 operating logic, structure, and organization that arose to address the diagnosis, treatment, and management of adult chronic health conditions. What is now emerging is a new 3.0 operating logic aimed at optimizing lifelong health by leveraging the new science of life course health development (Halfon et al. 2014b). The findings from the life course health sciences can continue to support this transition from 2.0 to 3.0 by providing the empirical basis for justifying healthcare systems that are more horizontally integrated to address multiple interacting dimensions and influences on health development, as well as longitudinally integrated to anticipate future health development scenarios and build long-term pull strategies into the structure and design of health and health-related social and educational services.

Third are the opportunities and challenges posed by major federal research initiatives, like those focused on precision medicine and clinical translational science and the lag from discovery to wide scale implementation. While both of these National Institutes of Health (NIH)-funded efforts begin with a biomedical orientation—with precision medicine focused on specifying the biological characteristics (phenotype) that will assist in pinpointing pharmacological interventions with greater accuracy and translational science focused on moving from the discovery of a new molecule in a laboratory and more rapidly and efficiently testing it at the hospital bedside and in the clinic making it widely available on a population basis—there is a critical need to inform these and other traditionally biomedically oriented research efforts with life course health science thinking and approaches.

Fourth is the fact that the national health policy focus on improving population health and reducing health disparities can benefit from the LCHD framework and life course health science results. As Larson and colleague (Larson et al. 2017) argue in this volume, "the LCHD framework emphasizes the importance of addressing disparities from preconception onward; understanding that early exposure to multiple stresses may produce biological changes that are difficult, if not impossible, to eradicate later; and acknowledging that adults who experienced the most extreme disparities as young children are likely to develop the worst health in adulthood and require the most expensive interventions. Life course-oriented health disparities research provides an opportunity for large potential savings associated with the development of strategies to intervene early in optimizing human health." Real headway in not only addressing health disparities but reducing these inequalities in health development will arise by taking advantage of the life course health science along with the opportunities afforded by ACA-induced health system transformation to focus greater attention and the role of the early years in reducing disparities, decreasing the prevalence and impact of chronic illness, and saving healthcare costs.

As a product of the Life Course Research Network (LCRN) that is funded by the Department of Health and Human Services (DHHS) Health Resources and Services Administration (HRSA) Maternal and Child Health Bureau (MCHB), this volume is meant—in addition to serving as a catalyst and tool for advancing the LCHD field—to inform MCHB's thinking, planning, and funding of future research. To this end, the content of this chapter will be used to create a more traditionally structured research agenda containing specific research questions that the members of the LCRN (see lcrn.net to learn more and join) and the broader community of LCHD stakeholders will be invited to participate in refining and prioritizing among. Over time, the LCRN—which was recently awarded another 3 years of funding from MCHB—will produce, commission and/or solicit additional research agenda-setting papers on topics missing from the present volume in order to enable the periodic updating of the LCRA and enhance the dissemination and synthesis of emerging findings. Taken together, these efforts will help to advance both the life course health sciences and our understanding of their importance for optimizing life course health development.

References

Barker, D. J., Osmond, C., Winter, P. D., Margetts, B., & Simmonds, S. J. (1989). Weight in infancy and death from ischaemic heart disease. *The Lancet, 334*(8663), 577–580.

Ben-Shlomo, Y., & Kuh, D. (2002). A life course approach to chronic disease epidemiology: Conceptual models, empirical challenges and interdisciplinary perspectives. *International Journal of Epidemiology, 31*(2), 285–293.

Birbeck, G. L., Meyer, A.-C., & Ogunniyi, A. (2015). Nervous system disorders across the life course in resource-limited settings. *Nature, 527*(7578), S167–S171.

Boyce, W. T., & Hertzman, C. (2017). Early childhood and the life course: The state of the science and proposed research priorities. In N. Halfon, C. B. Forrest, R. M. Lerner, & E. Faustman (Eds.), *Handbook of life course health-development science*. Cham: Springer.

Brophy, P. D., Charlton, J. R., Carmody, J. B., Reidy, K. J., Harshman, L., Segar, J., Askenazi, D., & Shoham, D. (2017). Chronic kidney disease: A life course health development perspective. In N. Halfon, C. B. Forrest, R. M. Lerner, & E. Faustman (Eds.), *Handbook of life course health-development science*. Cham: Springer.

Brownell, M. D., Ekuma, O., Nickel, N. C., Chartier, M., Koseva, I., & Santos, R. G. (2016). A population-based analysis of factors that predict early language and cognitive development. *Early Childhood Research Quarterly, 35*, 6–18.

Buka, S. L., Rosenthal, S. R., & Lacy, M. E. (2017). Epidemiological study designs: Traditional and novel approaches to advance life course health development research. In N. Halfon, C. B. Forrest, R. M. Lerner, & E. Faustman (Eds.), *Handbook of life course health-development science*. Cham: Springer.

Cohen, A. A. (2016). Complex systems dynamics in aging: New evidence, continuing questions. *Biogerontology, 17*(1), 205–220.

Cooksey, E. (2017). Using the National Longitudinal Surveys of Youth (NLSY) to conduct life course analyses. In N. Halfon, C. B. Forrest, R. M. Lerner, & E. Faustman (Eds.), *Handbook of life course health-development science*. Cham: Springer.

Currie, J., & Stabile, M. (2006). Child mental health and human capital accumulation: The case of ADHD. *Journal of Health Economics, 25*(6), 1094–1118.

Davidson, L. L., Grigorenko, E. L., Boivin, M. J., Rapa, E., & Stein, A. (2015). A focus on adolescence to reduce neurological, mental health and substance-use disability. *Nature, 527*(7578), S161–S166.

DelGiudice, M. (2017). Middle childhood: An evolutionary-developmental synthesis. In N. Halfon, C. B. Forrest, R. M. Lerner, & E. Faustman (Eds.), *Handbook of life course health-development science*. Cham: Springer.

Drury, S. S., Theall, K., Gleason, M. M., Smyke, A. T., De Vivo, I., Wong, J. Y., Fox, N. A., Zeanah, C. H., & Nelson, C. A. (2012). Telomere length and early severe social deprivation: Linking early adversity and cellular aging. *Molecular Psychiatry, 17*(7), 719–727.

Duncan, G. J., Morris, P. A., & Rodrigues, C. (2011). Does money really matter? Estimating impacts of family income on young children's achievement with data from random-assignment experiments. *Developmental Psychology, 47*(5), 1263.

Dunn, E. C., Masyn, K. E., Yudron, M., Jones, S. M., & Subramanian, S. V. (2014). Translating multilevel theory into multilevel research: Challenges and opportunities for understanding the social determinants of psychiatric disorders. *Social Psychiatry and Psychiatric Epidemiology, 49*(6), 859–872.

Dunn, E. C., Richmond, T. K., Milliren, C. E., & Subramanian, S. V. (2015). Using cross-classified multilevel models to disentangle school and neighborhood effects: An example focusing on smoking behaviors among adolescents in the United States. *Health & Place, 31*, 224–232.

El-Sayed, A. M., Seemann, L., Scarborough, P., & Galea, S. (2013). Are network-based interventions a useful antiobesity strategy? An application of simulation models for causal inference in epidemiology. *American Journal of Epidemiology, 178*(2), 287–295.

Feinberg, M. E., Kan, M. L., & Goslin, M. C. (2009). Enhancing coparenting, parenting, and child self-regulation: Effects of family foundations 1 year after birth. *Prevention Science, 10*(3), 276–285.

Felitti, V. J., Anda, R. F., Nordenberg, D., Williamson, D. F., Spitz, A. M., Edwards, V., Koss, M. P., & Marks, J. S. (1998). Relationship of childhood abuse and household dysfunction to many of the leading causes of death in adults: The adverse childhood experiences (ACE) study. *American Journal of Preventive Medicine, 14*(4), 245–258.

Gatzweiler, F. S., & Baumuller, H. (2014). Marginality-a framework for analyzing causal complexity of poverty. In J. von Braun & F. W. Gatzweiler (Eds.), *Marginality: Addressing the nexus of poverty, exclusion, and ecology*. Dordrecht: Springer.

Geller, A., Jaeger, K., & Pace, G. (2017). Using the Fragile Families and Child Wellbeing Study (FFCWS) in life course health development research. In N. Halfon, C. B. Forrest, R. M. Lerner, & E. Faustman (Eds.), *Handbook of life course health-development science*. Cham: Springer.

Guhn, M., Gadermann, A. M., Almas, A., Schonert-Reichl, K. A., & Hertzman, C. (2016a). Associations of teacher-rated social, emotional, and cognitive development in kindergarten to self-reported wellbeing, peer relations, and academic test scores in middle childhood. *Early Childhood Research Quarterly., 35*, 76–84.

Guhn, M., Janus, M., Enns, J., Brownell, M., Forer, B., Duku, E., Muhajarine, N., & Raos, R. (2016b). Examining the social determinants of children's developmental health: Protocol for building a pan-Canadian population-based monitoring system for early childhood development. *BMJ Open, 6*(4), e012020.

Halfon, N. (2016). More precisely targeting the coal mine of social adversity. *JAMA Pediatrics, 170*(11), e162523.

Halfon, N., & Forrest, C. B. (2017). The emerging theoretical framework of life course health development. In N. Halfon, C. B. Forrest, R. M. Lerner, & E. Faustman (Eds.), *Handbook of life course health-development science*. Cham: Springer.

Halfon, N., Larson, K., & Slusser, W. (2013). Associations between obesity and comorbid mental health, developmental, and physical health conditions in a nationally representative sample of US children aged 10 to 17. *Academic Pediatrics, 13*(1), 6–13.

Halfon, N., Larson, K., Lu, M., Tullis, E., & Russ, S. (2014a). Lifecourse health development: Past, present and future. *Maternal and Child Health Journal, 18*(2), 344–365.

Halfon, N., Long, P., Chang, D. I., Hester, J., Inkelas, M., & Rodgers, A. (2014b). Applying a 3.0 transformation framework to guide large-scale health system reform. *Health Affairs, 33*(11), 2003–2011.

Halfon, N., Wise, P. H., & Forrest, C. B. (2014c). The changing nature of children's health development: New challenges require major policy solutions. *Health Affairs (Millwood)., 33*(12), 2116–2124.

Hammond, R. A. (2009). Peer reviewed: complex systems modeling for obesity research. *Preventing Chronic Disease, 6*(3), A97.

Hane, A. A., & Fox, N. A. (2016). Early caregiving and human biobehavioral development: A comparative physiology approach. *Current Opinion in Behavioral Sciences, 7*, 82–90.

Hanson, M. A., & Gluckman, P. D. (2014). Early developmental conditioning of later health and disease: Physiology or pathophysiology? *Physiological Reviews, 94*(4), 1027–1076.

Hawkins, S. S., Oken, E., & Gillman, M. W. (2017). Early in the life course: Time for obesity prevention. In N. Halfon, C. B. Forrest, R. M. Lerner, & E. Faustman (Eds.), *Handbook of life course health-development science*. Cham: Springer.

Herman, D., & Taylor-Baer, M. (2017). From epidemiology to epigenetics: Evidence for the importance of nutrition to optimal health development across the life course. In N. Halfon, C. B. Forrest, R. M. Lerner, & E. Faustman (Eds.), *Handbook of life course health-development science*. Cham: Springer.

Hertzman, C., & Boyce, T. (2010). How experience gets under the skin to create gradients in developmental health. *Annual Review of Public Health, 31*, 329–347.

Hochberg, Z.'e. (2009). Evo–devo of child growth II: Human life history and transition between its phases. *European Journal of Endocrinology, 160*(2), 135–141.

Huang, T. T., Drewnowski, A., Kumanyika, S. K., & Glass, T. A. (2009). A systems-oriented multilevel framework for addressing obesity in the 21st century. *Preventing Chronic Disease, 6*(3), A82.

Janus, M., Harrison, L. J., Goldfeld, S., Guhn, M., & Brinkman, S. (2016). International research utilizing the early development instrument (EDI) as a measure of early child development: Introduction to the special issue. *Early Childhood Research Quarterly., 35*, 1–5.

Karatsoreos, I. N., & McEwen, B. S. (2013). Annual research review: The neurobiology and physiology of resilience and adaptation across the life course. *Journal of Child Psychology and Psychiatry, 54*(4), 337–347.

Kim, P., Strathearn, L., & Swain, J. E. (2016). The maternal brain and its plasticity in humans. *Hormones and Behavior, 77*, 113–123.

Kim, P., Evans, G. W., Chen, E., Miller, G., & Seeman, T. (2017). How socioeconomic disadvantages get under the skin and into the brain to influence health-development across the lifespan. In N. Halfon, C. B. Forrest, R. M. Lerner, & E. Faustman (Eds.), *Handbook of life course health-development science*. New York: Springer.

Kitano, H. (2004). Biological robustness. *Nature Reviews Genetics, 5*, 826–837.

Kuh, D., & Shlomo, Y. B. (2004). *A life course approach to chronic disease epidemiology*. Oxford: Oxford University Press.

Larson, K., Russ, S. A., Kahn, R. S., Flores, G., Goodman, E., Cheng, T. L., & Halfon, N. (2017). Health disparities: A life course health development perspective and future research directions. In N. Halfon, C. B. Forrest, R. M. Lerner, & E. Faustman (Eds.), *Handbook of life course health-development science*. Cham: Springer.

Lerner, R. M., Brindis, C. C., Batanova, M., & Blum, R. W. (2017). Adolescent health: A relational developmental systems perspective. In N. Halfon, C. B. Forrest, R. M. Lerner, & E. Faustman (Eds.), *Handbook of life course health-development science*. Cham: Springer.

Leslie, L. K., Mehus, C. J., Hawkins, J. D., Boat, T., et al. (2016). Primary care: Potential home for family focused interventions. *American Journal of Preventive Medicine, 51*(4), S106–S118.

Little, T. D. (2017). Core principles of life course health development methodology and analytics. In N. Halfon, C. B. Forrest, R. M. Lerner, & E. Faustman (Eds.), *Handbook of life course health-development science*. Cham: Springer.

McGinnis, J. M., Diaz, A., & Halfon, N. (2016). Systems strategies for health throughout the life course. JAMA, 316(16), 1639–1640.

Merikangas, K. R., He, J. P., Burstein, M., Swanson, S. A., Avenevoli, S., Cui, L., Benjet, C., Georgiades, K., & Swendsen, J. (2010). Lifetime prevalence of mental disorders in US adolescents: Results from the National Comorbidity Survey Replication–Adolescent Supplement (NCS-A). *Journal of the American Academy of Child and Adolescent Psychiatry, 49*(10), 980–989.

Moffitt, T. E. (1993). Adolescence-limited and life-course-persistent antisocial behavior: A developmental taxonomy. *Psychological Review, 100*(4), 674.

Msall, M. E., Sobotka, S. A., Dmowska, A., Hoga, D., & Sullivan, M. (2017). Life course health development outcomes after prematurity: Developing a community, clinical, and translational research agenda to optimize health, behavior and functioning. In N. Halfon, C. B. Forrest, R. M. Lerner, & E. Faustman (Eds.), *Handbook of life course health-development science*. Cham: Springer.

Mummert, A., Schoen, M., & Lampl, M. (2017). Growth and life course health development. In N. Halfon, C. B. Forrest, R. M. Lerner, & E. Faustman (Eds.), *Handbook of life course health-development science*. Cham: Springer.

Ostrom, E. (2009). A general framework for analyzing sustainability of social-ecological systems. *Science, 325*(5939), 419–422.

Osypuk, T. L. (2013). Invited commentary: Integrating a life-course perspective and social theory to advance research on residential segregation and health. *American Journal of Epidemiology, 177*(4), 310–315.

Patterson, M. L., Moniruzzaman, A., & Somers, J. M. (2015). History of foster care among homeless adults with mental illness in Vancouver, British Columbia: A precursor to trajectories of risk. *BMC Psychiatry, 15*(1), 1.

Pearce, J. (2014). Invited commentary: history of place, life course, and health inequalities—historical geographic information systems and epidemiologic research. *American Journal of Epidemiology, 181*(1), 26–29.

Pearce, J., Shortt, N., Rind, E., & Mitchell, R. (2016). Life course, green space and health: Incorporating place into life course epidemiology. *International Journal of Environmental Research and Public Health, 13*(3), 331.

Robinson, O., Basagaña, X., Agier, L., et al. (2015). The pregnancy exposome: Multiple environmental exposures in the INMA-Sabadell birth cohort. *Environmental Science & Technology, 49*(17), 10632–10641.

Russ, S. A., Tremblay, K., Halfon, N., & Davis, A. (2017). A life course approach to hearing health. In N. Halfon, C. B. Forrest, R. M. Lerner, & E. Faustman (Eds.), *Handbook of life course health-development science*. Cham: Springer.

Sastry, N., Fomby, P., & McGonagle, K. (2017). Using the Panel Study of Income Dynamics (PSID) to conduct life course health development analysis. In N. Halfon, C. B. Forrest, R. M. Lerner, & E. Faustman (Eds.), *Handbook of life course health-development science*. Cham: Springer.

Schonert-Reichl, K. A., Guhn, M., Gadermann, A. M., Hymel, S., Sweiss, L., & Hertzman, C. (2013). Development and validation of the middle years development instrument (MDI): Assessing children's well-being and assets across multiple contexts. *Social Indicators Research, 114*(2), 345–369.

Silberberg, D., Anand, N. P., Michels, K., & Kalaria, R. N. (2015). Brain and other nervous system disorders across the lifespan [mdash] global challenges and opportunities. *Nature, 527*(7578), S151–S154.

Singer, B. H., & Ryff, C. D. (Eds.). (2001). *New horizons in health: An integrative approach* (Vol. 277). Washington, D.C.: National Academies Press.

Taveras, E. M., Blackburn, K., Gillman, M. W., Haines, J., McDonald, J., Price, S., & Oken, E. (2011a). First steps for mommy and me: a pilot intervention to improve nutrition and physical activity behaviors of postpartum mothers and their infants. *Maternal and Child Health Journal, 15*(8), 1217–1227.

Taveras, E. M., Gortmaker, S. L., Hohman, K. H., Horan, C. M., Kleinman, K. P., Mitchell, K., & Gillman, M. W. (2011b). Randomized controlled trial to improve primary care to prevent and manage childhood obesity: The high five for kids study. *Archives of Pediatrics & Adolescent Medicine, 165*(8), 714–722.

Taveras, E. M., McDonald, J., O'Brien, A., Haines, J., Sherry, B., Bottino, C. J., & Koziol, R. (2012). Healthy Habits, Happy Homes: Methods and baseline data of a randomized controlled trial to improve household routines. *Preventive Medicine, 55*(5), 418–426.

Tyler, K. A., & Schmitz, R. M. (2013). Family histories and multiple transitions among homeless young adults: Pathways to homelessness. *Children and Youth Services Review, 35*(10), 1719–1726.

Warner, K., & Kern, M. (2013, December). A City of Wellbeing: The what, why & how of measuring community wellbeing. The City of Santa Monica Office of Wellbeing.

Wise, P. H. (2016). Child poverty and the promise of human capacity: Childhood as a foundation for healthy aging. *Academic Pediatrics, 16*(3), S37–S45.

Wood, D., Crapnell, T., Lau, L., Bennett, A., Lotstein, D., Ferris, M., & Kuo, A. (2017). Emerging adulthood as a critical stage in the life course. In N. Halfon, C. B. Forrest, R. M. Lerner, & E. Faustman (Eds.), *Handbook of life course health-development science*. Cham: Springer.

Zlotnick, C., Tam, T. W., & Soman, L. A. (2012). Life course outcomes on mental and physical health: The impact of foster care on adulthood. *American Journal of Public Health, 102*(3), 534–540.

9

Emerging Adulthood as a Critical Stage in the Life Course

David Wood, Tara Crapnell, Lynette Lau, Ashley Bennett, Debra Lotstein, Maria Ferris, and Alice Kuo

1 Introduction to Emerging Adulthood

The path that individuals take from dependency in childhood to independence in adulthood is now a longer and more complicated one than at any other point in history (Arnett 2014). From the mid- to late twentieth century and extending into the twenty-first century, industrial societies have experienced a surge in the concept of individualism and increased salience of self-realization and personal expression (Arnett 1998). Moreover, we have seen a dramatic increase in the number of youth seeking post-high school education, which is required for success as the economy transitions from an industrial to an information-based economy (Rifkin 2011). However, stagnation of wages for low-skilled workers and the lack of work opportunities for youth and young adults, combined with the increased costs of education and independent living, have made the pathway to independence and adulthood prolonged, complex, and varied, creating a new stage in the life course that has been labeled *emerging adulthood* (EA). While not all life course or developmental scientists agree that emerging adulthood constitutes a new developmental stage, there is agreement that social and economic forces have prolonged entry into adulthood and with significant role and developmental challenges beyond the traditional adolescent years (Cote 2014).

At the beginning of this stage, 17–18 years of age, emerging adults are generally dependent, living with their parents or caretakers, beginning to engage in romantic relationships, and attending high school. At the end of this stage, mid- to late 20s, most emerging adults live independently, are in long-term relationships, and have clear career paths ahead of them. How they traverse this life stage is dependent upon the personal, family, and social resources they possess as they enter this stage of life, dynamic and reciprocal interaction between the emerging adult and their environment, and the supports they receive during this stage. The result is that there are many pathways that youth and young adults pursue through this stage to achieve stable adulthood. For example, 40% do not

The original version of this chapter was revised. An erratum to this chapter can be found at https://doi.org/10.1007/978-3-319-47143-3_27

D. Wood, MD, MPH (✉)
Department of Pediatrics, ETSU College of Medicine, PO Box 70578, Johnson City, TN 37614, USA
e-mail: wooddl@etsu.edu

T. Crapnell, OTD, OTR/L • L. Lau, PhD
D. Lotstein, MD, MPH • M. Ferris, MD, PhD, MPH
A. Kuo, MD, PhD
UCLA, Department of Pediatrics, Los Angeles, CA, USA

A. Bennett, MD
Department of Pediatrics, USC, Los Angeles, CA, USA

pursue post-high school education. While 60% entered college immediately after graduating high school, many drop out or interrupt their college education with periods of work. Some 33% in this stage remain unmarried; however, 67% of them achieve stable domestic partners. Importantly, only a minority of emerging adults are employed in full-time jobs, limiting the economic opportunities they experience (U.S. Census Bureau. American Community Survey 2006).

Emerging adulthood is considered to be the *volitional years*, as it offers the most opportunity for identity exploration in the areas of love, work, and worldviews (Arnett 2000). During this time, individuals begin to develop the characteristic qualities necessary for becoming self-sufficient, engage in mature, committed relationships, assume more adult roles and responsibilities, and obtain a level of education and training that sets the foundation for work during the adult years. Characterizing emerging adulthood as a stage in the life course has proven to be beneficial to explain the social, cognitive, and psychological development that occurs during this stage. Research demonstrating continued brain development into the late 20s provides further justification for viewing emerging adulthood as a stage in the life course (Spear 2000).

2 Conceptual Framework

The Life Course Health Development (LCHD) model posits that myriad factors (e.g., biological, psychological, cultural) on multiple levels (e.g., micro, meso, macro) interact simultaneously in a transactional fashion to influence an individual's LCHD during each stage to determine a "health developmental" trajectory (see also Halfon and Forrest 2017). The Life Course Health Development (LCHD) model further posits that transitions and pivotal points in an individual's life have the potential to influence and alter an individual's developmental pathways. EA is a life stage characterized by changes in person-context cognitive, emotional, physical, and social domains, and the ultimate pathway achieved by the emerging adults during this stage is determined by the ongoing, dynamic, and reciprocal interactions between the individual and their environment. The degree of agency and role exploration that characterizes EA results in the potential for growth in intellectual and emotional functioning (Arnett 2000). EA represents a broad and diverse but fundamentally important area of consideration by virtue of the multiple avenues through which an individual's developmental trajectories and outcomes may be influenced. Important developmental challenges during EA include the continued formation of identity and values, which occur in the midst of frequent changes in personal relationships, living arrangements, vocational and educational pursuits, and social roles (Shanahan 2000).

No stage in life, other than perhaps infancy, experiences such dynamic and complex changes on the personal, social, emotional, neuroanatomical, and developmental levels. For the 10 years between 18 and 28, the vast majority of emerging adults change living situation, change their primary relationships, complete education or vocational preparation, get married, have children, and transition from adolescent/dependent roles to adult/independent roles. This occurs during often volatile emotional, neurodevelopmental, and social development. Increasing agency occurs at the same time as decreasing institutional and family supports. The theoretical framework developed by Learner and others to create the positive youth development theory nicely explains how the developmental trajectories that emerge during the period of EA are dependent upon multiple influential, bidirectional, person-context coactions. Individuals during emerging adulthood act as co-developers of their own developmental pathways, adaptively responding to different biological, social, cultural, and physical environmental contexts that they influence and are also influenced by (Learner and Overton 2008). Successfully navigating the developmental challenges inherent in EA will likely, in large part, influence the developmental trajectory of adulthood because these challenges ultimately influence the important adult outcomes of independent living, committed intimate relationships, and vocational and educational achievement. Youth and young adults with chronic disease or disabilities face additional challenges (disease management, disease complications, limitations in opportunities, etc.) in the context of these multiple domains of growth and development, which impact their pathway through this stage.

The continued positive trajectory of the emerging adult's mental health, identity formation, education achievement, social relationships, and other developmental areas is somewhat dependent on the degree to which there are matches or mismatches between the individual and his/her resources and the environmental challenges and supports. If the transition, such as school to work, provides a reasonable and developmentally appropriate challenge and the emerging adult successfully navigates that challenge, then the developmental trajectory of the emerging adult will be enhanced. In contrast, if the same transition lacks supports or is an inappropriate match for the emerging adult's abilities (e.g., an inadequate vocational program for an emerging adult with a learning disorder or lack of support for chronic disease management) and the emerging adult experiences failure, then the developmental trajectory may be impaired, resulting in significantly less achievement or developmental progression across the lifespan. A major defining characteristic of the stage of EA is that contexts are changing significantly (family to independence or romantic relationships, school to work or disconnected state, dependent living to independent living arrangements). The changes are so significant that emerging adults need substantial supports to navigate the transition successfully. Emerging adults with disabilities or chronic health conditions require more support to maximize their potential development during EA (Table 1).

Table 1 Principles of the Life Course Health Development framework

Principle	Brief description
1. Health development	Health development integrates the concepts of health and developmental processes into a unified whole
2. Unfolding	Health development unfolds continuously over the lifespan, from conception to death, and is shaped by prior experiences and environmental interactions
3. Complexity	Health development results from adaptive, multilevel, and reciprocal interactions between individuals and their physical, natural, and social environments
4. Timing	Health development is sensitive to the timing and social structuring of environmental exposures and experiences
5. Plasticity	Health development phenotypes are malleable and enabled and constrained by evolution to enhance adaptability to diverse environments
6. Thriving	Optimal health development promotes survival, enhances well-being, and protects against disease
7. Harmony	Health development results from the balanced interactions of molecular, physiological, behavioral, cultural, and evolutionary processes

The above table outlines the seven principles of the Life Course Health Development framework. These principles can be applied to the stage of emerging adulthood in a limited fashion due to the limited research literature focused on this life stage. However, conceptually, using the seven principles to view the stage of emerging adulthood can be instructive and can lead to additional research questions (see end of this article). For example, Principle 5 states that health development expressions are malleable and enable and constrain health development pathways and plasticity. According to Bogin's reserve capacity hypothesis, prolonged childhood into adolescence and perhaps emerging adulthood leads to greater biologic and social resilience in adulthood, which leads to enhanced fertility and greater longevity (Bogin 2013). Principle 4 states that health development is sensitive to life course timing and social structuring of the environment. As we described above, this is particularly true of emerging adulthood, where the interaction between age, personal development, and environment (peers, schools, social institutions, etc.) leads to multiple pathways to identify formation and academic and social achievement during this stage (Benson and Elder 2011; Benson et al. 2012).

Multiple factors can influence the life course during EA, including factors at the macro-level (historical and societal influences), meso-level (parent-child relationship, family environment, and socioeconomic status), and microlevel (individual cognitive, personality, and emotional development). The timing of these exposures during EA, which we consider a critical or sensitive period in the life course development, can significantly impact adult outcomes. For example, an emerging adult that engages in criminal activity and is convicted of a felony will suffer repercussions that will greatly diminish their chances of achieving success in relationships and work. In the sections that follow, we review the macro-, meso-, and microlevel influences occurring during EA for emerging adults generally. Next we explore the additional challenges faced by those with selected chronic health or developmental conditions including mental illness or substance abuse, diabetes, chronic renal failure, and autism, to serve as case studies of the increased complexity faced by emerging adults with chronic disease. Finally, we finish up with a set of questions and issues that are research priorities for developing an LCHD research agenda on the stage of emerging adulthood.

3 Macro-level Influences on the Trajectory of Emerging Adulthood

Emerging adulthood, like many other developmental stages, is a period in the life course that is culturally constructed and not universal (Arnett 1998, 2000). Thus, the very existence and trajectory of EA are dependent on macro-level societal expectations and influences. For many years, it was theorized that an individual transitioned from adolescence (which begins in puberty and ends in the late teens) into young adulthood. Over history and cross-culturally, the length of time during which an individual spends in adolescence has been determined by the age at which the person enters marriage or a committed relationship (Schlegel and Barry III 1991, Gilmore 1990). In fact, human life history posits that the life stage of adolescence came into existence about 75,000 years ago due to changes in human societies and cultures associated with pair bonding and living in large groups (Bogin 2013). So massive culture and reproductive change led to a change in life history with the addition of a new period of development. It is theorized by those promoting emerging adulthood as a new life stage that the same kind of massive cultural and reproductive change is happening once again and new social and cultural demands of adult life necessitate a longer and more complex prologue to adult life.

Although the functional outcome of EA, causing a delayed transition to adulthood, appears relatively novel, this practice of prolonging the transition to adulthood may be dated back to early modern English society from the 1500s to 1700s (Ben-Amos 1994). Similar to what generally occurs during EA today, individuals during that era took part in a "life cycle service" between their late teens and 20s, wherein they would engage in developing important vocational skills (e.g., a trade or craft) and marriage was often postponed until the late 20s for both men and women; adult roles and responsibilities for individuals during that era were provided only gradually, as each individual acquired the desired character qualities deemed appropriate by society (Ben-Amos 1994). It was not until industrialization in America began to emerge in the nineteenth century that the concept of individualism developed and strengthened (Rotundo 1994). The twentieth century marked the first time that an individual could obtain and gain control over the resources that would allow them to choose the timing of major life events and personal expression was valued in society (Modell 1991).

As we move forward into the twenty-first century, individualism in contemporary postindustrial society continues to strengthen, while the age at which individuals marry continues to increase, and individuals increasingly seek to pursue other life course events (Modell 1991; Alwin 1988; Bellah et al. 2007). As a reflection of these trends, recent evidence indicates that contemporary postindustrial society considers marriage status of low importance in the determination of whether or not an individual has reached adulthood; rather, societies in developed countries appear to now consider the acquisition of certain character qualities as the most important indicator of having attained adulthood, the top three character qualities of which include (1) accepting responsibility for oneself, (2) making independent decisions, and (3) assuming financial independence – all of which emphasize an individual's ability to be self-sufficient (Scheer et al. 1996; Greene et al. 1992; Arnett 1997, 1998).

4 Meso-level Influences of Life Trajectories During Emerging Adulthood

Earlier life experiences and family environment can impact one's life trajectory from childhood through EA and into adulthood. Longitudinal studies that span early childhood through EA indicate that there is both continuity and discontinuity of healthy and unhealthy paths and outcomes. (Masten et al. 2006, 2005). In this section, we will be discussing the impact of the parent-child relationship, family environment, and other sociodemographic factors, such as socioeconomic status (SES) and its influence in EA.

4.1 Earlier Parent-Child Relationships

The quality of parent-child relationships during EA is, in large part, a function of the history of early parent-child attachment experiences. Attachment theory suggests that positive bonding with an emotionally available adult during early childhood facilitates the development of the child's capacity to bond with others and respond to stressful events. A history of positive attachment experiences will ultimately provide a foundation for positive interactions with others and foster secure, lasting relationships in EA which subsequently influence the LCHD (Mikulincer M and Shaver PR 2009), whereas insecure attachments can result in mistrust or lack of security and reduced sense of self-efficacy and self-esteem. Simultaneously, social learning theory suggests that styles of family interactions learned in early and middle childhood are carried by emerging adults into adulthood (Whitbeck et al. 1994). Familiar patterns of interaction help individuals deal with new situations and have a significant influence on the emerging adult's capacity to deal with the multiple changes that occur during EA. Alternatively, inadequate parenting, disrupted family bonds, and poverty are environmental risks for childhood-onset conduct, behavioral and emotional problems, and educational underachievement that can persist into adolescence and emerging adulthood (Moffit and Caspi 2001).

Adverse events experienced in childhood such as parental divorce or alcoholism or the experience of abuse are major risk factors for the leading causes of illness and death as well as poor quality of life in adults in the USA. Disruptions in the parent relationship (e.g., divorce) can have strong, negative effects on the parent-child relationship (Aquilino 1994) causing significant emotional impact throughout the life course. Parental divorce may influence the emerging adults' ability to form stable romantic relationships and their decision to marry early or may undermine the emerging adult's financial ability to attend college (Jacquet and Surra 2001, Cherlin et al. 1998).

Importantly, parental acceptance and support for independence have been linked to higher self-esteem, individualism, and feelings of worthiness among emerging adults (Ryan and Lynch 1989). Critical to the emerging adult's achievement of independence are feeling connected, secure, understood, and loved in their families and having the willingness to call on parental resources for help in making choices in educational, relationship, living, and other changes that confront the emerging adult. Persistent connectedness to parents facilitates rather than undermines ongoing identity development in emerging adulthood (Grotevant and Cooper 1986; Ryan and Lynch 1989).

4.2 Childhood Socioeconomic Status

Socioeconomic status (SES), family supports, and the neighborhood environment all can contribute to the positive or negative life trajectory prior to and during EA (Galobardes et al. 2008; Gilman 2012; Gilman and Loucks 2012). Socioeconomic status has been identified as one of the most important health determinants throughout the life course (Miller et al. 2015). Low financial resources and all the other exposures that go along with poverty – poor schools, chaotic families, exposure to violence, and victimization – limit opportunities for growth or acquisition of other resources that enhance quality of life (Wadsworth et al. 2016; Kim et al. 2015).

In addition to being an important predictor of disease-specific morbidity and mortality in adulthood, early childhood poverty has been associated with lower adult educational attainment (Duncan and Brooks-Gunn 2000). Educational achievement has a major influence on the life trajectory, including financial stability and health in EA and onward throughout adulthood. Seventy percent of emerging adults who grow up in poverty delay enrollment in postsecondary education, in comparison to 40% who grow up in household of higher SES. Furthermore, research has indicated that individuals who delay enrollment past the age of 22 are less likely to ever enroll in postsecondary education and less likely to complete a degree (Feliciano and Ashtiani 2012). The result is that only 22% of young adults from low-income families earn college degrees, while 48% of young adults from higher-income families earn at least an associate's degree. Earning a college education results in not only higher lifetime earnings but enhancement of multiple aspects of psychosocial development (Evans and Cassells 2014).

However, while SES has been found to be predictive of educational attainment, the impact of poverty can be mitigated by a number of factors such as individual characteristics of self-efficacy and hope. Students from poor families that have high self-efficacy and a similar concept of hope for educational attainment do equally as well in school as their higher SES peers (Osgood et al. 2005). Recent research by Dweck and colleagues indicates that students' mindsets are critically linked to resilience and achievement and that they can be changed through brief interventions, leading to substantial increases in measures of resilience and achievement (Yeager and Dweck 2012). These studies suggest that in addition to SES, individual characteristics also have a large influence on outcomes of EA and that these characteristics can be influenced through individual interventions. Individual characteristics and development are discussed in the next section.

5 Microlevel Influences on the Trajectories During Emerging Adulthood

As discussed in previous sections, individualism and the qualities of character have become increasingly important in the transition to EA and ultimately reaching full adulthood in postindustrial, developed societies. Studies have shown that the ability to accept responsibility for one's self, make independent decisions, and assume financial independence are the top three most important factors in becoming an adult (Arnett 2014). In order to achieve individualism and obtain these important qualities of character, one needs to reach some degree of cognitive and psychological maturity, as well as possess some level of resilience. These individual factors are discussed in this section.

5.1 Cognitive Development

One of the identified qualities of character that is important in EA and reaching full adulthood is independent decision-making. While the ability to make independent decisions is a reflection of one's psychological and moral identity, it also has to do with cognitive maturity and the ability to weigh a variety of considerations before deciding on a choice. Recent neuroscience research indicates that brain development (particularly in the prefrontal cortex) continues well into the third decade of life, ultimately resulting in the integration and coordination of cognitions, emotion and action, and strategic executive control (Luciana et al. 2005). The continuous unfolding and acquisition of specific neurodevelopmental capacities during adolescences and EA influence the acquisition of goal directedness and future orientation that have been observed behaviorally during EA (Dahl 2004; Nelson et al. 2012; Nurmi 1999; Steinberg et al. 2006). As new capacities emerge, they are available to solve problems, delay gratification, and filter unnecessary input. With maturation of these skills, emerging adults are also more capable of reflecting on the influence of their environment and on their internal state, regulate their emotions, and use problem-solving skills to effectively compromise, which is important for the development of meaningful social interactions and personal relationships as well as in the work environment. These skills also support an emerging adult's capacity for optimally interacting with the health-care system, managing their health-care needs, and making decisions that will influence their long-term health outcomes.

However, the preceding paragraph assumes that the individual has experienced optimal neurodevelopment up to the point that they enter the stage of EA. Studies have demonstrated that exposure to chronic stress during childhood (e.g., poverty) or experiencing adverse childhood events (e.g., child maltreatment, neglect, parental divorce, parental substance abuse) may cause detrimental impact to the developing brain. For example, repeated exposure to stressful events has been associated with structural differences in specific brain regions (i.e., amygdala, hippocampus, and prefrontal cortex), which are in turn associated with functional differences in learning, memory, and aspects of executive functioning. Furthermore, preliminary studies go on to suggest that there may be sensitive periods of brain development with increased susceptibility to the effects of stress and adverse events. These environmentally induced modulations in neurodevelopment can impact an individual's cognitive development and their capacity to develop the necessary skills and relationships that will enable them to thrive.

An emerging adult, who has experienced chronic stress or adverse events earlier in childhood and adolescence and is cognitively immature, is more likely, through adverse interaction with their environment, to suffer secondary effects such as school failure, risky/impulsive behaviors, accidental injury, criminal activity, or substance misuse or overuse. These behaviors may in turn interfere with the ongoing development of an optimal pathway to adulthood. Feelings of isolation and rates of substance abuse in individuals often peak during this period as emerging adults are faced with the stresses of having to navigate societal structures that are not adequately informed or equipped to address the needs of an emerging adult population – all while their brains have yet to reach full maturation (Spear 2000). An impulsive emerging adult fueled by alcohol and despair is at high risk for suicide. It is thus apparent that multiple factors related to an individual's cognitive and emotional development may intersect and interact to multiply the likelihood of adverse or positive health outcomes in EA. It is crucial for service providers to recognize the level of cognitive maturation an emerging adult possesses and tailor their interventions and supports based on this.

5.2 Identity Formation

Identity formation is a major developmental activity during EA. Identity development, occurs in a number of dimensions: (1) psychological dimension, or ego identity via a sense of temporal-spatial continuity and its concomitants; (2) the personal dimension, or a behavioral and character repertoire that differentiates the individuals; and (3) the social dimension, or recognized roles within a community. These components come together during the stage of identity formation (adolescence and EA) and stabilization (EA and young adulthood), and once the identity is considered stable, this is when a relatively firm sense of ego identity is developed, behavior and character become stabilized, and community-sanctioned roles are acquired (2002).

Identity formation during adolescence was thought to be a critical milestone in adolescence; however, it has been recognized that in certain societal contexts, identity formation continues beyond adolescence. In the postindustrial society, with the prolongation of educational and vocational attainment, prolongation of identity exploration in the three main areas of love, work, and worldviews into the 20s has become the norm. Identity formation is critical in EA, as it has direct implications on psychological and moral identity and in achieving the three qualities of character deemed as important in the transition to adulthood.

5.3 Resilience in Emerging Adulthood

Resilience is an individual's capacity to adapt to change in healthy and flexible ways during stressful events (Catalano et al. 2004). Resilience can be measured in various ways, including internal adaption (e.g., well-being, happiness, or self-concept) or external adaption (academic achievement, relationship development) to adverse circumstances, such as how well a person navigates and achieves the developmental tasks presented by the external world (e.g., educational achievement, stable work/career, marriage, etc.). Resiliency in adolescence and young adulthood is higher among youth with higher intellectual resources, optimistic future orientation, the presence of caring relationships with positive adult role models, and opportunities to succeed and serve the community. Emerging adulthood is a particularly important stage in the life course to understand resilience because the important changes in functional capacity, educational achievement, and social roles are large and varied and have a significant influence on life course outcomes.

Key individual characteristics that predict resilience during EA are goal-directed motivation and planfulness about the future. In addition, adult support and mentorship are important factors that help promote resilience (Miller GE 2015; Masten et al. 2005; Arnett 2005). Furstenberg, Brooks-Gunn, and others studied young women who became pregnant during adolescence and found that a small proportion with positive adult relationships had dramatic change in trajectory for the better (Furstenberg 2002). Masten, studying a cohort of low-income youth (beginning at ages 8–12) over a 20-year period, found that a number of factors predict competence in EA including higher intellectual capacity, higher parenting quality, and higher SES (Masten and Coatsworth 1998). When they examined resilience between the 10- and 20-year follow-up, they found that youth doing well in EA was predicted from doing well 10 years earlier. In the context of high adversity, childhood IQ was particularly an important moderator and predictor of resilience. During EA, individuals who were doing well from high-adversity backgrounds had significant personal resources in intelligence and personal competence and a history of receiving high-quality parenting (Masten et al. 2004).

6 Trajectories During Emerging Adulthood for Emerging Adults with Chronic Health Condition

Chronic health conditions can significantly impact the developmental trajectory of emerging adults during this life stage. Many types of chronic conditions, including those that impact physical, intellectual, or emotional functioning, may undermine the assumption of adult roles by the emerging adult, undermine success in school, impair the transition to work, and make living independently more of a challenge. Eighteen percent of youth aged 12–17 in the USA are defined as having a special health-care need, meaning they have a chronic physical, medical, emotional, or developmental condition that requires a more intensive use of health-care and related services. Emerging adults with chronic conditions are at risk for a number of problems during transition to adulthood, including experiencing gaps in needed medical and related services and gaps in health insurance (Lotstein et al. 2008, Reiss et al. 2005). Below we review the impact of several specific chronic conditions on the growth trajectory during emerging adulthood.

6.1 Autism Spectrum Disorders (ASDs)

For youth with autism spectrum disorders (ASDs) and their families, the transition from adolescence to emerging adulthood is a time of uncertainty and loss of entitlement to many services that were available while in the public school system under the Individuals with Disabilities Education Act (IDEA). In comparison to childhood, young adults with autism often experience a dearth of appropriate supports and opportunities. Leaving high school is associated with deterioration in ASD symptom presentation, increase in maladaptive behaviors, and worsening family functioning (Taylor and Seltzer 2010, 2011a, b). Many persons with ASD are able to work successfully within the community (Garcia-Villamisar et al. 2000; Mawhood and Howlin 1999); however, the majority experience difficulty securing meaningful employment (Eaves and Ho 2008; Howlin et al. 2004; Newman et al. 2011). A recent study indicated that only 58% have ever worked for pay. In addition, it was found that only one in five individuals ever lived independently (Roux et al. 2015). Even among those employed, their jobs tended to be low level and low income (Cimera and Cowan 2009; Eaves and Ho 2008; Howlin et al. 2004). Jobs often ended prematurely because of social or behavioral difficulties or other work-related difficulties (Mawhood and Howlin 1999).

Young adults on the autism spectrum are reported to experience difficulties in assuming other important adult roles and responsibilities, including attaining postsecondary education and living independently (Roux et al. 2015). A number of studies (Billstedt et al. 2005; Gillespie-Lynch et al. 2012; Howlin et al. 2004) have found that having an IQ of around 70 seemed to be a critical cutoff point for better outcome (e.g., level of independence). A number of comorbid conditions can complicate the trajectory for youth with intellectual disability through adolescence and EA, such as seizure disorder, which substantially increase in prevalence from childhood through adolescence into adulthood. Adults with ASD and related conditions are more vulnerable to anxiety and depression which can require specific treatments (Skokauskas and Gallagher 2010; White et al. 2009). The majority of young adults with ASD remain dependent on parents for support in living, recreation, and occupational situations. The availability of appropriate resources, services, and supports for the individuals with ASD and their families is key for successful transition into adulthood and better outcomes throughout adult life. The following elements are important for high-quality transition services and associated with improved young adult outcomes: (1) individualized services that reflect the strengths of the individual, (2) positive career development and early work experiences, (3) collaboration and interagency involvement, (4) family supports and expectations, (5) fostering self-determination and independence, (6) social and employment-related skill instruction, and (7) establishment of job-related supports. Therefore, outcomes for emerging adults with ASD could be improved if social and institutional supports available through adolescence continued into adulthood.

6.2 Type 1 Diabetes Mellitus (DM)

The study of emerging adults with type 1 DM has elucidated the potential challenges facing emerging adults with diabetes and other chronic health conditions that have significant self-management burden. Emerging adults with type 1 diabetes face extensive behavioral demands in order to maintain their health, including the necessity for precisely scheduled daily insulin injections, blood glucose monitoring, dietary monitoring, regular physical exercise, and the management of DM-related complications. In early adulthood, frequent changes in roles, living situations, educational routines, jobs, friendships, and romantic relationships are common and can undermine the routines and the resolve needed to maintain metabolic control (Anderson and Wolpert 2004).

The developmental tasks of emerging adulthood may be at odds with maintaining the intensive self-care that is required of those with type 1 diabetes and vice versa. For example, the tasks of establishing autonomy and prevailing egocentrism may be associated with the emerging adult not wanting to follow medical advice or advice of his or her family (Masten et al. 1995). Heightened concern for peer acceptance or the establishment of intimate relationships is characteristic of this period of development. Emerging adults may be reluctant to admit to their significant others that they have type 1 diabetes or any other chronic condition that puts them at risk for being rejected (Madsen et al. 2002). Moreover, the major cognitive developmental milestone during the stage of emerging adulthood is the ability to think abstractly (Erikson 1994). Those who have not yet reached this developmental milestone may struggle with taking responsibility to maintain good disease management and understanding the consequences of poor disease management. Lastly, increased rates of drinking, illicit drug use, or other high-risk behaviors may disrupt the emerging adults' lifestyle and negatively impact self-care management of diabetes, resulting in (Madsen et al. 2002) lack of control of diabetes and the resulting physical and mental consequences of hypo- or hyperglycemia, which undermine emerging adults' abilities to perform in school, maintain relationships, or keep employment.

As has been demonstrated in other chronic childhood conditions, the transition from pediatric- to adult-centered medical care for youth with DM is associated with a decline in DM control (Busse et al. 2007; Oeffinger et al. 2006). Adverse health-related outcomes documented in the young adult population with diabetes include a decline in disease self-care behaviors and an increased risk for diabetes-related complications (Bryden et al. 2001; Fredericks et al. 2010; Yeung et al. 2008). In addition, emerging adults with diabetes are at higher than average risk for psychosocial morbidity including social delays and isolation, impaired social competence, and emotional problems such as depression (Helgeson et al. 2007). As in the case in ASD, additional support for an emerging adult with DM during the transition to adult medical care has been shown to help decrease the adverse outcomes seen with usual practice. For example, DM transition programs that include introductions to new adult care providers or intensive care coordination have been found to be protective (Holmes-Walker et al. 2007).

6.3 Chronic Kidney Disease

Chronic kidney disease (CKD) is a condition characterized by disease progression, significant cardiovascular morbidity, growth failure, neurocognitive impairment, and impaired quality of life changes (Sarnak 2003; Copelovitch et al. 2011; Gerson et al. 2006; McKenna et al. 2006). CKD is divided into five stages based on glomerular filtration rate, with stage 1 being the mildest form and stage 5 the worst form, also called end-stage kidney disease (ESKD), requiring renal replacement therapy (dialysis or transplant) (Hogg et al. 2003). The prevalence of pediatric CKD is unknown as it may be silent in early stages. The prevalence of pediatric ESKD is 15 cases per million population (Saran et al. 2015). African-Americans and Latinos are disproportionately affected by CKD in part due to a higher incidence of glomerular conditions (Ferris et al. 2006). While the 10-year survival for adolescent-onset ESKD is 80–85% (much higher than adult-onset ESKD patients), this still represents a 30-fold increase in mortality compared to the general US adolescent population. Survival is better for younger adolescents, males, Caucasians, Asians, and transplant recipients (2006). However, emerging adults with CKD achieve adult milestones (e.g., employment, marriage) less frequently than their healthy peers (Bartosh et al. 2003).

The burden of care directly correlates with the stage of CKD. Based on the mean number of unique medications, those with CKD stages 1–4 take 6.2 ± 4 of medications, those with peritoneal dialysis (CKD 5) take 8.5 ± 2 medications, those with kidney transplant (CKD 5) take 9.7 ± 4.2 medications, and those on hemodialysis (CKD 5) take 11.3 ± 2.1 (So et al. 2011). The complexity of care also include procedures such as self-catheterization several times per day, fluid and dietary restrictions, blood pressure measurements daily, and injections (erythropoiesis-stimulating agents once to thrice weekly, growth hormone daily, or insulin several times per day). The life course of pediatric-onset CKD-ESKD varies by etiology and age at onset of this condition, but once they reach ESKD, most patients share the same comorbidities (hypertension, anemia, acidosis, metabolic bone disease, and growth delay). Patients with greater level of CKD have a decreased sense of self-worth, perceive a poor future, and feel limited in their physical and psychosocial capacities to have the same potential and opportunity as their healthy peers.

While most children and adolescent patients with ESKD will receive a kidney transplant, they likely will experience dialysis prior to receiving an organ. The most common cause of kidney transplant rejection in adolescents and emerging adults is treatment nonadherence (Andreoni et al. 2013). Adherence among adolescents is compromised by poor understanding and poor consequence recognition leading to an inconsistent commitment to the treatment regimens. Once the kidney transplant is lost, patients return to dialysis and likely will not receive another kidney transplant for many years. As in adult patients, cardiovascular disease (CVD) accounts for a majority of deaths in patients with pediatric-onset CKD, but unlike adults, pediatric-onset CKD patients rarely demonstrate symptomatic atherosclerosis (Shroff et al. 2011). Lastly, survivors of pediatric-onset CKD are at greater risk for malignancies and post-transplant diabetes mellitus (Koukourgianni et al. 2010).

Patients who transfer to adult-focused services without transition preparation and support appear to be at greater risk to lose their kidney transplant (Watson 2000, 2005). The international societies of internal medicine and pediatric nephrology have published position statements and policies to promote health-care transition preparation (Watson 2005; Watson et al. 2011). Strategies to increase patient autonomy, health-care transition, and self-management are needed to achieve successful outcomes at the time of transfer to adult-focused providers.

6.4 Mental Health and Substance Use

Emerging adulthood is a time of increased experimentation with tobacco, drugs, and alcohol (Schulenberg et al. 2004; Schulenberg and Maggs 2002), increasing from rates of 12.2% in adolescence to 40.2% in young adulthood for cigarette smoking, from 10.7% to 41.9% for binge drinking, from 11.2% to 20.3% for illicit drug use, and from 2.6% to 14.9% for heavy alcohol use. While cigarette, alcohol, and drug use are normative during adolescence and emerging adulthood, a number of factors predict excessive use rather than experimentation including genetic (e.g., family history of alcohol abuse), biological (e.g., early puberty timing), family (e.g., low parental monitoring), school (e.g., low grade average, school failure), peer (e.g., peer substance use), and youth personality and psychopathology (e.g., depression) factors (Cicchetti 1999). However, the pattern of use/abuse of these substances is influenced by the experience during the stage of EA. For example, increasing responsibility, work, and marriage all are associated with decreased use of these substances (Masten et al. 1999; Bachman et al. 2014). Again, there is great heterogeneity in the trajectories followed by individuals with regard to substance use during this period, all influenced by the multiplicity of factors listed above.

Among young adults, 13.7% experience serious mental illness such as major depressive disorders, schizophrenia, and bipolar disorder (AmericanPsychiatricAssociation 2013). The neuropsychological pathology that has onset during EA has many of the predisposing factors related to family adversities, such as social disadvantage, divorce, dysfunctional parenting, multiple family changes/moves, and peer group choices. The expanded independence and self-reliance during EA may be difficult to handle for youth with preexisting emotional or social challenges or poor attachment. The decrease in supports from school or family during EA may be even further destabilizing, leading to increased emotional and interpersonal difficulties. Young people with serious mental health conditions have difficulty with impulse control and self-regulation (Walker and Gowen 2011). Their apparent immaturity reflects a delay in social and emotional development and undermines progress toward goals in education, relationships, independence in health, and health-care management.

Three-quarters of lifetime cases of mental, emotional, and behavioral disorders begin by age 24 (Kessler et al. 2005). In emerging adults with social, emotional, and behavioral disorders, much higher risk is associated with onset in early adolescence versus onset in late adolescence (Mofitt and Caspi 2001). Dysfunctional family environments and participation in deviant peer group increase the likelihood of early-onset delinquency followed by a long trajectory of social, emotional, and behavioral problems. Youth with later onset of social, emotional, and behavioral problems are more commonly from relatively healthy family backgrounds and more likely to desist from delinquency by age 23 (Roisman et al. 2004). Similar patterns can be seen for major psychiatric disorders such as depression, with early-onset mood disorders being representative of more severe recurrent forms of mood disorders arising from increased severity and complexity of family and biologic risk factors (Fergusson and Woodward 2002) and later-onset disorders reflecting lower levels of risk factors in childhood.

7 Protective and Risk Factors That Impact Emerging Adulthood

The supports, opportunities, and experiences that occur during the stage of EA greatly influence the ultimate outcome of this stage and the ensuing life trajectory into young adulthood. As discussed in this chapter, critical influences during EA include mentoring relationships, socioeconomic supports, and educational and vocational opportunities. Emerging adulthood typically is accompanied by an increase in agency/independence and decrease in social and institutional support (e.g., schools and family), such that most individuals have more choice in day-to-day activities and life decisions. This increase in choice may result in greater success which will likely contribute to well-being. However, increased freedom can result in poor choices (e.g., drug use, criminal activity) that have a negative impact on the developmental trajectory as well (Schulenberg and Maggs 2002; Schulenberg et al. 2004). For example, many relationships and other aspects of life are so unstable during EA that important and powerful negative experiences can occur such as date rape, school failure, and substance addiction. These experiences can have a lasting, if not lifetime, detrimental impact on the developmental and mental health trajectory of the emerging adult. Similarly, many potential powerful positive influences can occur during this period in life (e.g., marriage, educational achievement, mentoring) that can enhance the developmental and mental health trajectory. Therefore, experiences both distal (early childhood) and proximal (during emerging adulthood) can influence, either positively or negatively, the developmental and mental health trajectory of the emerging adult (Miller et al. 2015).

Practical supports during EA provided by families include financial support for education, transportation, independent living, health insurance, and other necessities. The primary determinant of parental support are the level of parental resources. Emerging adults with wealthier parents and those with fewer siblings receive more financial support for education (Steelman and Powell 1991). Divorced parents provide less financial support than parents with intact marriages (Cooney and Uhlenberg 1992). Support from families by parents and grandparents during EA is also provided in the form of guidance or advice, information, and emotional support. Parents of emerging adults may also help the emerging adult negotiate the health-care system, formulate and carry out educational and vocational goals, and acquire leases for apartments and even provide advice for intimate relationships. In short, continued social and financial connection to parents with adequate emotional and financial resources can be a very significant factor in the positive life trajectory during emerging adulthood (Aquilino 2005). Previous studies have found a high correlation between improved EA outcomes and adolescent hope in the future (Bennett 2014). Hope is a form of personal capital that protects youth from social, emotional, and behavioral disorders and correlates with and predicts the rates of many outcomes, including academic achievement, delay of initiation of early sexual activity, and lower likelihood of violent behavior. Hope requires a sense of self-efficacy and knowledge of alternate outcomes. Hope is reflected in adolescent and young adult goals as they reflect and make ongoing assessments of their current and future selves. Individual goals and aspirations relate to the sense of control an individual feels in relation to a particular domain.

Positive youth development (PYD) programs are approaches that provide supports to adolescents and emerging adults to achieve social, emotional, behavioral, and moral competence, foster self-efficacy, a clear and positive identity, and belief in the future; and reinforce pro-social norms (Catalano et al. 2004). Positive development approaches involve a paradigm shift from targeting the risk factors to enhancing the assets and protective factors. The emphasis on hope, empowerment, and well-being resonates with youth and mental health professionals. The PYD approach outlined above suggests that effective programs to support EA would include an individualized approach supporting young people to identify and move toward personally meaningful goals. This begins with envisioning a positive future identity ("Who do I want to become?"). Pursuing goals promotes a sense of purpose, and making progress toward those goals contributes to building feelings of efficacy, empowerment, and self-determination, enhancing the individual's ability to act as the primary causal agent in pursuing personally meaningful goals (Silbereisen and Lerner 2007).

A PYD perspective further suggests that youth and emerging adults will benefit from learning specific strategies for increasing and maintaining interpersonal support from positive peers, family, providers, and people in the community (Guerra and Bradshaw 2008). Young people can learn specific steps and skills that can help them increase the quality and the extent of their interpersonal networks, as well as the amount of emotional, instrumental, and informational support available to them. Using a PYD perspective suggests that the development of assets is an important recovery-oriented outcome in and of themselves, as well as a mediator of longer-term outcomes related to education, employment, mental health, and general quality of life. Indeed, a review of the available research on community-based programs and interventions for EA reveals a common focus on personal asset building (Lerner 2014). Also consistent with the PYD perspective is that many of the programs and interventions include a focus on changing the meso-environment of youth so that it encourages young people to develop or express strengths and assets.

8 Services and Supports

As we better understand the limits of and issues related to EA, it is imperative that we review and revise policy and current social and medical services and supports so they optimally address the current and future needs of individuals during this life stage. Current medical, mental health, and social service delivery models are geared toward either child or adult populations. In other words, individuals generally seek child-serving services between the ages of 0 and 18, and they are subsequently transferred directly to adult-serving services. However, the various biobehavioral and sociocultural factors discussed above make this direct transition from child to adult-centered care ill-suited for optimally addressing the nuances and challenges that individuals may face during EA. For example, an adult-centered medical doctor may regularly treat patients with fixed habits and lifestyles, who may already suffer from a variety of chronic health conditions. However, many such chronic health conditions in adults represent a culmination of experiences from an individual's earlier years, which may not yet be apparent during EA. It is thus strongly recommended that EA service providers reorient themselves using a prevention-based paradigm and familiarize themselves with the possible antecedents to social, emotional, and medical conditions so that they may make health-care or social service recommendations to minimize risk factors and to maximize strengths and assets to facilitate development along optimal health trajectories. EA presents a unique opportunity for service providers to intervene and influence an individual's LCHD before significant social, emotional, and medical pathology fully develops, utilizing existing knowledge of the skills and capacities associated with EA to inform services and interventions.

In addition to training service providers to reorient their approach to care and become more sensitive to antecedents of chronic health conditions in adulthood, the multifactorial nature of the LCHD model suggests that it would be important for service providers to consider horizontal (i.e., cross sector) and longitudinal (i.e., across the lifespan) service integration. Specifically, the current model posits that myriad factors (e.g., biological, psychological, cultural) on multiple levels (e.g., micro, meso, macro) interact simultaneously in a transactional fashion to influence an individual's LCHD and overall health trajectory. However, most current training models which emphasize specialization in their independent fields and opportunities for cross-disciplinary case conceptualization and collaboration with regard to service delivery – particularly with respect to preventive care, which may be of special importance when considering EA as a sensitive period of development – tend to be rare. Such specialization in service delivery may result in service fragmentation. Additionally, adult service providers generally do not work in tandem with child service providers as individuals transition from one care setting to the next, consequently resulting in potential gaps in service delivery and care, which may be exacerbated as individuals work to rebuild rapport with their new service providers. Moreover, health, mental health, social service, and education professionals rarely collaborate to create comprehensive models across the EA stage. Clearly, the current service delivery infrastructure does not adequately support the needs and challenges unique to emerging adult populations. It is thus important to recognize emerging adults as a unique population requiring additional and specialized skills of service providers and the creation of specific pathways for transition which support continuity of care.

The larger sociopolitical and cultural contexts may also facilitate or create challenges which impact service and intervention efforts directed at emerging adults. The majority of individuals in developed nations transitioning through EA, for instance, may be classified as "digital natives," individuals who have been brought up in environments where exposure to digital technology may be normative and who are therefore familiar with computers and the Internet. As emerging adults increasingly turn to digital and mobile solutions to support and enhance their daily routines, it behooves service providers to creatively explore ways of engaging emerging adult populations using technology. Use of social networks, such as Instagram, Twitter, and Facebook, to advance primary prevention efforts, increase awareness of public health issues, and provide basic health and psychological education affords service providers the opportunity to outreach to unprecedented numbers and populations. Use of text messaging may also be effective as a way of engaging with digital native emerging adult populations and promoting engagement and adherence by emerging adults or to promote youth development programs. Also, as service providers keep pace with technological advancements, they may even begin to explore novel methods of service delivery and intervention using digital or Internet-based platforms, which may increase "buy-in" and potentially preventive service utilization, among digitally native emerging adult populations. For example, service providers might potentially leverage the data that digitally native emerging adults might collect as part of the "quantified self" movement (e.g., pedometer information, weight, blood pressure, etc.) in an effort to inform their ongoing care efforts.

On the other hand, due to clinical billing practices and regulations, as well as patient privacy concerns and regulations (e.g., Health Insurance

Portability and Accountability Act, HIPAA), current service delivery models often tend to operate in a fragmented and siloed fashion, which in turn may limit the ability of service providers to develop a holistic treatment plan to address each individual's needs. Further complicating this fragmentation is the restricted access to health records once an individual turns 18 years of age, when parents who may have been primarily responsible for managing their child's health-care needs no longer are able to access their child's medical records (unless explicit permission is granted by the child, who is now an emerging adult). Depending on each family's cultural context and the relationship between the emerging adult and his or her parents, this transition may be a cause for significant stress and/or strife between family members as they work to renegotiate previously familiar boundaries. Mothers of children with diabetes, for example, have indicated feeling increased stress as their children transitioned from pediatric to adult care, particularly if they perceived that their children were not managing their health-care condition as well as they had been when it was previously under greater parent control (Allen et al. 2011). Such stress might result in familial conflict and dysfunction which could subsequently interfere with the emerging adult's willingness or ability to adequately access services. One potential solution to overcoming the issue of patient privacy may be to implement public health programs and tools to educate and empower individuals with respect to managing and taking an active role in their own care. However, it is important to underscore the need for larger, overall systems to change in order to support service providers in working together with individuals and their families to ensure continuity and comprehensiveness of services and health-related information during the transition.

Finally, the implementation of health-care policies may have important implications for service and intervention delivery with an emerging adult population. With the introduction of the Patient Protection and Affordable Care Act of 2010 (ACA), for example, individuals may now remain on their parents' health insurance plans until they turn 26 years of age. While this theoretically affords emerging adults the opportunity to develop the necessary skills for interacting with the health-care system and managing their own care, research indicates that emerging adults frequently perceived themselves as being at lower risk for health problems and the financial burden of health insurance as lacking in value. Consequently, emerging adults may opt for high-deductible catastrophic insurance which generally costs less compared to other health insurance plans, but translates to fewer opportunities for interaction with the health service sector and fewer opportunities for service providers to intervene early during an individual's LCHD trajectory prior to the onset of chronic adult disease. Importantly, research indicates that despite preventive maintenance health visits being mandatory under the ACA, emerging adults were less likely to request health maintenance visits. Thus, it may be important for public health efforts to determine the underlying factors associated with this diminished utilization of health services by emerging adults and subsequently develop health literacy programs to promote prevention mindedness and service utilization in emerging adults.

9 Recommendations for Research Priorities

The following is a list of issues in life course research that are critical for better understanding the positive supports and challenges that influence the trajectory of development of emerging adults organized along the macro-, meso-, micro-framework.

Macro Issues

- What community supports in emerging adulthood enhance health development into adulthood and improve outcomes for an emerging adult with specific health, mental health, and developmental conditions? Is there an "early intervention model" to optimize outcomes for EA? What model should be used for an emerging adult with chronic health, mental health, and developmental conditions?

- What are the historical, economic, and cultural influences on the meaning of EA, adaptation, and maladaptation to the stage and expectations for normative transitions? How have these changed over time? How are they different for an emerging adult with social, health, mental health, and developmental problems?
- How have the delays in marriage/relationship commitment impacted adult life trajectories?
- What are the racial and ethnic differences for how these factors interact to support development during EA?
- How has the information economy and the increased demands for education impacted the life course for youth in upper, middle, and lower socioeconomic strata? Are there regional variations in these outcomes and how can they be improved?

Meso Issues

- Earlier childhood development and family environment are predictors of adult outcomes, but it is unclear how optimizing health development can be achieved with supports during EA.
- What is the interaction between health and social system supports, family supports, youth abilities, cognitive and psychological maturity, and EA outcomes for an emerging adult with and without mental or physical disabilities?
- How can the different support systems be integrated to provide seamless services to youth and emerging adults with significant physical, mental health, or intellectual disabilities?
- Using the model below from the work of Masten et al. (2005), how do these different resources, supports, and personal characteristics interact to promote optimal development during EA? (Fig. 1)
- What factors promote resilience for youth during EA who lack family supports?
- What is the role of extended families in support for EA?
- How can studies of conditions and processes that influence development during EA inform educational/vocational/EA support policies?
- How can data be gathered across this stage in the lifespan given that emerging adults leave school and have many changes in living arrangements, education, relationships, and work?

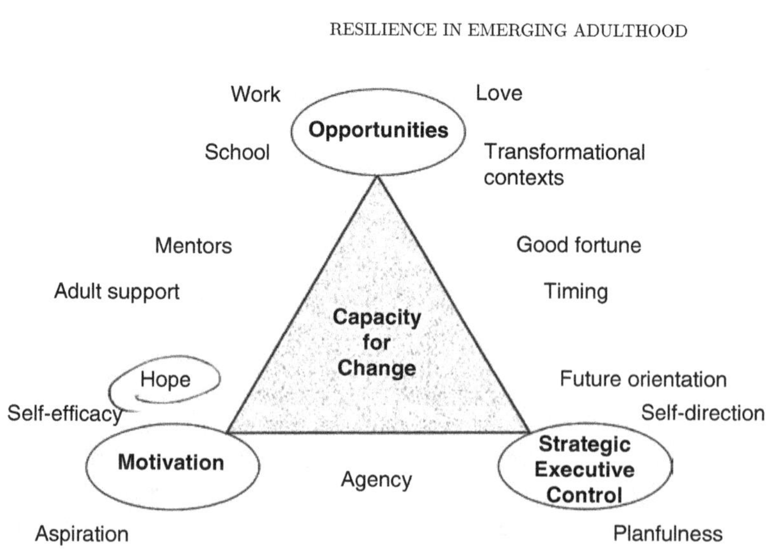

Fig. 1 Moving toward resilience: a model of positive change in emerging adulthood

Micro Issues

- To what degree is cognitive, social, physical, moral, and spiritual development mediated during emerging adulthood? How are these developmental pathways impacted by chronic health, mental health, and developmental conditions?
- How can we optimize the person-context match to promote development during EA with and without chronic health, mental health, and developmental conditions?
- What is the impact of positive turning points in EA compared to early life stages on life trajectories into adulthood?
- During EA, exploration of new experiences is normative. Is more exploration better or worse and for which activities is it better or worse? How is this equation different for an emerging adult with chronic health, mental health, and developmental conditions?
- Do emerging adults with particular health conditions, such as diabetes, spina bifida, solid organ transplant, or cancer survivorship, experience sharply downward trajectories during EA, and what supports are effective to prevent these sharply downward trajectories?
- How does brain development progress during EA? What is the impact of brain development on the factors that influence the developmental trajectory during EA such as executive control (planfulness, future orientation), motivation, self-efficacy, and hope?

References

Allen, D., Channon, S., Lowes, L., Atwell, C., & Lane, C. (2011). Behind the scenes: The changing roles of parents in the transition from child to adult diabetes service. *Diabetic Medicine, 28*(8), 994–1000.

Alwin, D. F. (1988). From obedience to autonomy changes in traits desired in children, 1924–1978. *Public Opinion Quarterly, 52*, 33–52.

American Psychiatric Association. (2013). *Diagnostic and statistical manual of mental disorders*. Arlington: American Psychiatric Publishing.

Anderson, B. J., & Wolpert, H. A. (2004). A developmental perspective on the challenges of diabetes education and care during the young adult period. *Patient Education and Counseling, 53*, 347–352.

Andreoni, K. A., Forbes, R., Andreoni, R. M., Phillips, G., Stewart, H., & Ferris, M. (2013). Age-related kidney transplant outcomes: Health disparities amplified in adolescence. *JAMA Internal Medicine, 173*, 1524–1532.

Aquilino, W. S. (1994). Impact of childhood family disruption on young Adults' relationships with parents. *Journal of Marriage and the Family, 56*, 295–313.

Aquilino, W. S. (2005). Impact of family structure on parental attitudes toward the economic support of adult children over the transition to adulthood. *Journal of Family Issues, 26*, 143–167.

Arnett, J. J. (1997). Young People's conceptions of the transition to adulthood. *Youth & Society, 29*, 3–23.

Arnett, J. J. (1998). Learning to stand alone: The contemporary American transition to adulthood in cultural and historical context. *Human Development, 41*, 295–315.

Arnett, J. J. (2000). Emerging adulthood: A theory of development from the late teens through the twenties. *American Psychologist, 55*, 469.

Arnett, J. J. (2005). The developmental context of substance use in emerging adulthood. *Journal of Drug Issues, 35*, 235–254.

Arnett, J. J. (2014). *Emerging adulthood: The winding road from the late teens through the twenties*. New York: Oxford University Press.

Bachman, J. G., O'malley, P. M., Schulenberg, J. E., Johnston, L. D., Bryant, A. L., & Merline, A. C. (2014). *The decline of substance use in young adulthood: Changes in social activities, roles, and beliefs*. New York: Psychology Press.

Bartosh, S. M., Leverson, G., Robillard, D., & Sollinger, H. W. (2003). Long-term outcomes in pediatric renal transplant recipients who survive into adulthood. *Transplantation, 76*, 1195–1200.

Bellah, E. R. N., Bellah, R. N., Tipton, S. M., Sullivan, W. M., Madsen, R., Swidler, A., Sullivan, W. M., & Tipton, S. M. (2007). *Habits of the heart: Individualism and commitment in American life*. Berkeley: University of California Press.

Ben-Amos, I. K. (1994). *Adolescence and youth in early modern England*. New Haven: Yale University Press.

Bennett, A. (2014). Finding hope in hopeless environments. *International Journal of Child Health And Human Development, 7*, 313.

Benson, J. E., & Elder, G. H. (2011). Young adult identities and their pathways: A developmental and life course model. *Developmental Psychology, 47*, 1646–1657.

Benson, J. E., Johnson, M. K., & Elder, G. H. (2012). The implications of adult identity for educational and work attainment in young adulthood. *Developmental Psychology, 48*(6), 1752.

Billstedt, E., Gillberg, C., & Gillberg, C. (2005). Autism after adolescence: Population-based 13-to 22-year follow-up study of 120 individuals with autism diagnosed in childhood. *Journal of Autism and Developmental Disorders, 35*, 351–360.

Bogin, B. (2013). Chapter 2, Childhood, adolescence and longevity: A chapter on human Evolutionary life history. In B. Hewlett (Ed.), *Adolescent identify: Evolutionary, cultural and developmental perspectives*. New York: Routledge.

Brody, G. H., et al. (2013). Is resilience only skin deep? Rural African Americans' socioeconomic status–related risk and competence in preadolescence and psychological adjustment and Allostatic load at age 19. *Psychological Science*. doi:10.1177/0956797612471954.

Bryden, K. S., Peveler, R. C., Stein, A., Neil, A., Mayou, R. A., & Dunger, D. B. (2001). Clinical and psychological course of diabetes from adolescence to young adulthood a longitudinal cohort study. *Diabetes Care, 24*, 1536–1540.

Busse, F., Hiermann, P., Galler, A., Stumvoll, M., Wiessner, T., Kiess, W., & Kapellen, T. (2007). Evaluation of patients' opinion and metabolic control after transfer of young adults with type 1 diabetes from a pediatric diabetes clinic to adult care. *Hormone Research in Pædiatrics, 67*, 132–138.

Catalano, R. F., Berglund, M. L., Ryan, J. A., Lonczak, H. S., & Hawkins, J. D. (2004). Positive youth development in the United States: Research findings on evaluations of positive youth development programs. *The Annals of the American Academy of Political and Social Science, 591*, 98–124.

Cherlin, A. J., Chase-Lansdale, P. L., & Mcrae, C. (1998). Effects of parental divorce on mental health throughout the life course. *American Sociological Review, 63*(2), 239–249.

Cicchetti, D., et al. (1999). *A developmental psychopathology perspective on drug abuse. Drug abuse: Origins & interventions* (pp. 97–117). Washington, DC: American Psychological Association, xxiii, 492 pp.

Cimera, R. E., & Cowan, R. J. (2009). The costs of services and employment outcomes achieved by adults with autism in the us. *Autism, 13*, 285–302.

Cooney, T. M., & Uhlenberg, P. (1992). Support from parents over the life course: The adult Child's perspective. *Social Forces, 71*, 63–84.

Copelovitch, L., Warady, B. A., & Furth, S. L. (2011). Insights from the chronic kidney disease in children (Ckid) study. *Clinical Journal of the American Society of Nephrology, 6*, 2047–2053.

Cote, J. E. (2014). The dangerous myth of emerging adulthood: An evidence-based critique of a flawed developmental theory. *Applied Developmental Science, 18*(4), 177–188.

Dahl, R. E. (2004). Adolescent brain development: A period of vulnerabilities and opportunities. Keynote address. *Annals of the New York Academy of Sciences, 1021*, 1–22.

Duncan, G. J., & Brooks-Gunn, J. (2000). Family poverty, welfare reform, and child development. *Child Development, 71*, 188–196.

Eaves, L. C., & Ho, H. H. (2008). Young adult outcome of autism Spectrum disorders. *Journal of Autism and Developmental Disorders, 38*, 739–747.

Erikson, E. H. (1994). *Identity: Youth and crisis*. New York: Ww Norton & Company.

Evans, G. W., & Cassells, R. C. (2014). Childhood poverty, cumulative risk exposure, and mental health in emerging adults. *Clinical Psychological Science, 2*(3), 287–296.

Feliciano, C., & Ashtiani, M. (2012). *Postsecondary educational pathways of low-income youth: An analysis of add health data*. Irvine: Uc/Accord.

Fergusson, D. M., & Woodward, L. J. (2002). Mental health, educational, and social role outcomes of adolescents with depression. *Archives of General Psychiatry, 59*, 225–231.

Ferris, M. E., Gipson, D. S., Kimmel, P. L., & Eggers, P. W. (2006). Trends in treatment and outcomes of survival of adolescents initiating end-stage renal disease care in the United States of America. *Pediatric Nephrology, 21*, 1020–1026.

Fredericks, E. M., Dore-Stites, D., Well, A., Magee, J. C., Freed, G. L., Shieck, V., & James Lopez, M. (2010). Assessment of transition readiness skills and adherence in pediatric liver transplant recipients. *Pediatric Transplantation, 14*, 944–953.

Furstenberg, F. F. (2002). How it takes thirty years to do a study. In *Looking at lives: American longitudinal studies of the twentieth century* (pp. 37–57).

Galobardes, B., Lynch, J. W., & Smith, G. D. (2008). Is the Association between childhood socioeconomic circumstances and cause-specific mortality established? Update of a systematic review. *Journal of Epidemiology and Community Health, 62*, 387–390.

Garcia-Villamisar, D., Ross, D., & Wehman, P. (2000). Clinical differential analysis of persons with autism in a work setting: A follow-up study. *Journal Of Vocational Rehabilitation, 14*, 183–185.

Gerson, A. C., Butler, R., Moxey-Mims, M., Wentz, A., Shinnar, S., Lande, M. B., Mendley, S. R., Warady, B. A., Furth, S. L., & Hooper, S. R. (2006). Neurocognitive outcomes in children with chronic kidney disease: Current findings and contemporary endeavors. *Mental Retardation and Developmental Disabilities Research Reviews, 12*(3), 208–215.

Gillespie-Lynch, K., Sepeta, L., Wang, Y., Marshall, S., Gomez, L., Sigman, M., & Hutman, T. (2012). Early childhood predictors of the social competence of adults with autism. *Journal of Autism and Developmental Disorders, 42*, 161–174.

Gilman, S. E. (2012). The successes and challenges of life course Epidemiology: A commentary on Gibb, Fergusson and Horwood (2012). *Social Science & Medicine, 75*, 2124–2128.

Gilman, S. E., & Loucks, E. B. (2012). Invited commentary: Does the childhood environment influence the Association between every X and every Y in adulthood? *American Journal of Epidemiology, 176*, 684–688.

Gilmore, D. D. (1990). *Manhood in the making: Cultural concepts of masculinity*. New Haven: Yale University Press.

Greene, A., Wheatley, S. M., & Aldava, J. F. (1992). Stages on Life's way Adolescents' implicit theories of the life course. *Journal of Adolescent Research, 7*, 364–381.

Grotevant, H. D., & Cooper, C. R. (1986). Individuation in family relationships. *Human Development, 29*, 82–100.

Guerra, N. G., & Bradshaw, C. P. (2008). Linking the prevention of problem behaviors and positive youth development: Core competencies for positive youth development and risk prevention. *New Directions for Child and Adolescent Development, 2008*, 1–17.

Halfon, N., & Forrest, C. B. (2017). The emerging theoretical framework of life course health development. In N. Halfon, C. B. Forrest, R. M. Lerner, & E. Faustman (Eds.), *Handbook of life course health-development science*. Cham: Springer.

Helgeson, V. S., Snyder, P. R., Escobar, O., Siminerio, L., & Becker, D. (2007). Comparison of adolescents with and without diabetes on indices of psychosocial functioning for three years. *Journal of Pediatric Psychology, 32*, 794–806.

Hogg, R. J., Furth, S., Lemley, K. V., Portman, R., Schwartz, G. J., Coresh, J., Balk, E., Lau, J., Levin, A., & Kausz, A. T. (2003). National Kidney Foundation's kidney disease outcomes quality initiative clinical practice guidelines for chronic kidney disease in children and adolescents: Evaluation, classification, and stratification. *Pediatrics, 111*, 1416–1421.

Holmes-Walker, D., Llewellyn, A., & Farrell, K. (2007). A transition care Programme which improves diabetes control and reduces hospital admission rates in young adults with type 1 diabetes aged 15–25 years. *Diabetic Medicine, 24*, 764–769.

Howlin, P., Goode, S., Hutton, J., & Rutter, M. (2004). Adult outcome for children with autism. *Journal of Child Psychology and Psychiatry, 45*, 212–229.

Jacquet, S. E., & Surra, C. A. (2001). Parental divorce and premarital couples: Commitment and other relationship characteristics. *Journal of Marriage and Family, 63*, 627–638.

Kessler, R. C., Berglund, P., Demler, O., Jin, R., Merikangas, K. R., & Walters, E. E. (2005). Lifetime prevalence and age-of-onset distributions of Dsm-iv disorders in the National Comorbidity Survey Replication. *Archives of General Psychiatry, 62*, 593–602.

Kim, P., Neuendorf, C., Bianco, H., & Evans, G. W. (2015). Exposure to childhood poverty and mental health symptomatology in adolescence: A role of coping strategies. *Stress and Health, 32*, 494–502.

Koukourgianni, F., Harambat, J., Ranchin, B., Euvrard, S., Bouvier, R., Liutkus, A., & Cochat, P. (2010). Malignancy incidence after renal transplantation in children: A 20-year single-Centre experience. *Nephrology Dialysis Transplantation, 25*, 611–616.

Lerner, R. M. (2014). Developmental science, developmental systems, and contemporary theories of human development. In *Handbook of child psychology*. New York: Wiley and Sons.

Lotstein, D. S., Inkelas, M., Hays, R. D., Halfon, N., & Brook, R. (2008). Access to care for youth with special health care needs in the transition to adulthood. *Journal of Adolescent Health, 43*, 23–29.

Luciana, M., Conklin, H. M., Hooper, C. J., & Yarger, R. S. (2005). The development of nonverbal working memory and executive control processes in adolescents. *Child Development, 76*, 697–712.

Madsen, S. D., Roisman, G. I., & Collins, W. A. (2002). The intersection of adolescent development and intensive intervention: Age-related psychosocial correlates of treatment regimens in the diabetes control and complication trial. *Journal of Pediatric Psychology, 27*, 451–459.

Masten, A. S., & Coatsworth, J. D. (1998). The development of competence in favorable and unfavorable environments: Lessons from research on successful children. *American Psychologist, 53*, 205.

Masten, A. S., Coatsworth, J. D., Neemann, J., Gest, S. D., Tellegen, A., & Garmezy, N. (1995). The structure and coherence of competence from childhood through adolescence. *Child Development, 66*, 1635–1659.

Masten, A. S., Hubbard, J. J., Gest, S. D., Tellegen, A., Garmezy, N., & Ramirez, M. (1999). Competence in the context of adversity: Pathways to resilience and maladaptation from childhood to late adolescence. *Development and Psychopathology, 11*, 143–169.

Masten, A. S., Burt, K. B., Roisman, G. I., Obradovic, J., Long, J. D., & Tellegen, A. (2004). Resources and resilience in the transition to adulthood: Continuity and change. *Development and Psychopathology, 16*, 1071–1094.

Masten, A. S., Roisman, G. I., Long, J. D., Burt, K. B., Obradović, J., Riley, J. R., Boelcke-Stennes, K., & Tellegen, A. (2005). Developmental cascades: Linking academic achievement and externalizing and internalizing symptoms over 20 years. *Developmental Psychology, 41*, 733.

Masten, A. S., Burt, K. B., & Coatsworth, J. D. (2006). Competence and psychopathology in development. D. Cicchetti, C. Dante, & J. Donald (Eds). *Developmental psychopathology: Risk, disorder, and adaptation* (Vol. 3, 2nd ed., pp. 696–738). Hoboken: John Wiley & Sons Inc, xvi 944 pp.

Mawhood, L., & Howlin, P. (1999). The outcome of a supported employment scheme for high-functioning adults with autism or Asperger syndrome. *Autism, 3*, 229–254.

Mckenna, A. M., Keating, L. E., Vigneux, A., Stevens, S., Williams, A., & Geary, D. F. (2006). Quality of life in children with chronic kidney disease—Patient and caregiver assessments. *Nephrology Dialysis Transplantation, 21*, 1899–1905.

Mikulincer, M., & Shaver, P. R. (2009). The attachment and behavioral systems perspective on social support. *Journal of Social and Personal Relationships, 26*(1), 7–19.

Miller, G. E., Yu, T., Chen, E., & Brody, G. H. (2015 Aug 18). Self-control forecasts better psychosocial outcomes but faster epigenetic aging in low-Ses youth. *Proceedings Of The National Academy Of Sciences., 112*(33), 10325–10330.

Modell, J. (1991). *Into One's own: From youth to adulthood in the United States, 1920–1975*. Berkeley: University of California Press.

Moffitt, T. E., & Caspi, A. (2001). Childhood predictors differentiate life-course persistent and adolescence-limited antisocial pathways among males and females. *Devcelopment and Psychopathology, 13*, 355–375.

Nelson, C. A., Thomas, K. M., & De Haan, M. (2012). *Neuroscience of cognitive development: The role of experience and the developing brain*. Hoboken: John Wiley & Sons.

Newman, L., Wagner, M., Knokey, A.-M., Marder, C., Nagle, K., Shaver, D., & Wei, X. (2011). *The post-high school outcomes of young adults with disabilities up to 8 years after high school: A Report from the National Longitudinal Transition Study-2 (Nlts2). Ncser 2011–3005*. Washington, DC: National Center For Special Education Research.

Nurmi, J.-E. (1999). 15 self-definition and mental health during adolescence and young adulthood. In J. Schulenberg, J. L. Maggs, & K. Hurrelmann (Eds.), *Health risks and developmental transitions during adolescence* (p. 395). New York: Cambridge University Press.

Oeffinger, K. C., Mertens, A. C., Sklar, C. A., Kawashima, T., Hudson, M. M., Meadows, A. T., Friedman, D. L., Marina, N., Hobbie, W., & Kadan-Lottick, N. S. (2006). Chronic health conditions in adult survivors of childhood cancer. *New England Journal of Medicine, 355*, 1572–1582.

Osgood, D. W., Ruth, G., Eccles, J. S., Jacobs, J. E. & Barber, B. L. (2005). *Six paths to adulthood: Fast starters, parents without careers, educated partners, educated singles, working singles, and slow starters.* na.

Reiss, J. G., Gibson, R. W., & Walker, L. R. (2005). Health care transition: Youth, family, and provider perspectives. *Pediatrics, 115*, 112–120.

Rifkin, J. (2011). *The Thired industrial revolution*. New York: St. Martin's Press.

Roisman, G. I., Aguilar, B., & Egeland, B. (2004). Antisocial behavior in the transition to adulthood: The independent and interactive roles of developmental history and emerging developmental tasks. *Development and Psychopathology, 16*, 857–871.

Rotundo, E. A. (1994). *American manhood: Transformations in masculinity from the revolution to the modern era*. New York: Basic Books.

Roux, A. M., Shattuck, P. T., Rast, J. E., Rava, J. A., & Anderson, K.,. A. (2015). *National autism indicators report: Transition into young adulthood*. Philadelphia: Life Course Outcomes Research Program/A.J. Drexel Autism Institute/Drexel University.

Ryan, R. M., & Lynch, J. H. (1989). Emotional autonomy versus detachment: Revisiting the vicissitudes of adolescence and young adulthood. *Child Development, 60*(2), 340–356.

Saran, R., Li, Y., Robinson, B., Ayanian, J., Balkrishnan, R., Bragg-Gresham, J., Chen, J., Cope, E., Gipson, D., & He, K. (2015). US renal data system 2014 annual data Report: Epidemiology of kidney disease in the United States. *American Journal of Kidney Diseases: The Official Journal of the National Kidney Foundation, 65*, A7.

Sarnak, M. J. (2003). Cardiovascular complications in chronic kidney disease. *American Journal of Kidney Diseases, 41*, 11–17.

Scheer, S. D., Unger, D. G., & Brown, M. B. (1996). Adolescents becoming adults: Attributes for adulthood. *Adolescence, 31*, 127.

Schlegel, A., & Barry Iii, H. (1991). *Adolescence: An anthropological inquiry*. New York: Free Press.

Schulenberg, J. E., & Maggs, J. L. (2002). A developmental perspective on alcohol use and heavy drinking during adolescence and the transition to young adulthood. *Journal of Studies on Alcohol, Supplement No. 14*, 54–70.

Schulenberg, J. E., Sameroff, A. J., & Cicchetti, D. (2004). The transition to adulthood as a critical juncture in the course of psychopathology and mental health. *Development and Psychopathology, 16*, 799–806.

Shanahan, M. J. (2000). Pathways to adulthood in changing societies: Variability and mechanisms in life course perspective. *Annual Review of Sociology, 26*, 667–692.

Shroff, R., Weaver, D. J., & Mitsnefes, M. M. (2011). Cardiovascular complications in children with chronic kidney disease. *Nature Reviews Nephrology, 7*, 642–649.

Silbereisen, R. K., & Lerner, R. M. (2007). *Approaches to positive youth development*. Los Angeles/London: Sage.

Skokauskas, N., & Gallagher, L. (2010). Psychosis, affective disorders and anxiety in autistic Spectrum disorder: Prevalence and Nosological considerations. *Psychopathology, 43*, 8–16.

So, T.-Y., Bradley Layton, J., Bozik, K., Farrington, E., Gipson, P. E., Gibson, K., Primack, W., Conley Iii, W., Gipson, D. S., & Ferris, M. (2011). Cognitive pharmacy services at a pediatric nephrology and hypertension clinic. *Renal Failure, 33*, 19–25.

Spear, L. P. (2000). The adolescent brain and age-related behavioral manifestations. *Neuroscience & Biobehavioral Reviews, 24*(4), 417–463.

Steelman, L. C., & Powell, B. (1991). Sponsoring the next generation: Parental willingness to pay for higher education. *American Journal of Sociology, 96*(6), 1505–1529.

Steinberg, L., Dahl, R., Keating, D., Kupfer, D. J., Masten, A. S., & Pine, D. S. (2006). The study of developmental psychopathology in adolescence: Integrating affective neuroscience with the study of context. In D. Cicchetti & D. Cohen (Eds.), *Handbook of developmental psychopathology* (Vol. 2, pp. 710–741). New York: Wiley.

Taylor, J. L., & Seltzer, M. M. (2010). Changes in the autism behavioral phenotype during the transition to adulthood. *Journal of Autism and Developmental Disorders, 40*, 1431–1446.

Taylor, J. L., & Seltzer, M. M. (2011a). Changes in the mother–child relationship during the transition to adulthood for youth with autism Spectrum disorders. *Journal of Autism and Developmental Disorders, 41*, 1397–1410.

Taylor, J. L., & Seltzer, M. M. (2011b). Employment and post-secondary educational activities for young adults with autism Spectrum disorders during the transition to adulthood. *Journal of Autism and Developmental Disorders, 41*, 566–574.

Wadsworth, M. E., et al. (2016). Poverty and the development of psychopathology. In: M. E. Wadsworth, G. W. Evans, K. Grant, J. S. Carter, & S. Duffy (Eds.), *Development and psychopathology. Volume Four. Risk, resilience, and intervention*, Ch 8 (pp. 215–237). Hoboken: John Wiley & Sons.

Walker, J. S., & Gowen, L. K. (2011). *Community-based approaches for supporting positive development in youth and young adults with serious mental health conditions*. Portland: Research and Training Center for Pathways to Positive Futures, Portland State University.

Watson, A. R. (2000). Non-compliance and transfer from Paediatric to adult transplant unit. *Pediatric Nephrology, 14*, 469–472.

Watson, A. R. (2005). Problems and pitfalls of transition from Paediatric to adult renal care. *Pediatric Nephrology, 20*, 113–117.

Watson, A. R., Harden, P., Ferris, M., Kerr, P. G., Mahan, J., & Ramzy, M. F. (2011). Transition from pediatric to adult renal services: A consensus statement by the international society of nephrology (Isn) and the international pediatric nephrology Association (Ipna). *Pediatric Nephrology, 26*, 1753–1757.

Webster, B. H., Jr., & Bishaw, A. (2006). *U.S. Census Bureau, American Community Survey Reports, ACS-02, Income, Earnings, and Poverty Data From the 2005 American Community Survey*. Washington, DC: U.S. Government Printing Office.

Whitbeck, L., Hoyt, D. R., & Huck, S. M. (1994). Early family relationships, intergenerational solidarity, and support provided to parents by their adult children. *Journal of Gerontology, 49*, S85–S94.

White, S. W., Oswald, D., Ollendick, T., & Scahill, L. (2009). Anxiety in children and adolescents with autism Spectrum disorders. *Clinical Psychology Review, 29*, 216–229.

Yeager, D. S., & Dweck, C. S. (2012). Mindsets that promote resilience: When students believe that personal characteristics can be developed. *Educational Psychologist, 47*(4), 302–314.

Yeung, E., Kay, J., Roosevelt, G. E., Brandon, M., & Yetman, A. T. (2008). Lapse of care as a predictor for morbidity in adults with congenital heart disease. *International Journal of Cardiology, 125*, 62–65.

Permissions

All chapters in this book were first published in HLCHD, by Springer; hereby published with permission under the Creative Commons Attribution License or equivalent. Every chapter published in this book has been scrutinized by our experts. Their significance has been extensively debated. The topics covered herein carry significant findings which will fuel the growth of the discipline. They may even be implemented as practical applications or may be referred to as a beginning point for another development.

The contributors of this book come from diverse backgrounds, making this book a truly international effort. This book will bring forth new frontiers with its revolutionizing research information and detailed analysis of the nascent developments around the world.

We would like to thank all the contributing authors for lending their expertise to make the book truly unique. They have played a crucial role in the development of this book. Without their invaluable contributions this book wouldn't have been possible. They have made vital efforts to compile up to date information on the varied aspects of this subject to make this book a valuable addition to the collection of many professionals and students.

This book was conceptualized with the vision of imparting up-to-date information and advanced data in this field. To ensure the same, a matchless editorial board was set up. Every individual on the board went through rigorous rounds of assessment to prove their worth. After which they invested a large part of their time researching and compiling the most relevant data for our readers.

The editorial board has been involved in producing this book since its inception. They have spent rigorous hours researching and exploring the diverse topics which have resulted in the successful publishing of this book. They have passed on their knowledge of decades through this book. To expedite this challenging task, the publisher supported the team at every step. A small team of assistant editors was also appointed to further simplify the editing procedure and attain best results for the readers.

Apart from the editorial board, the designing team has also invested a significant amount of their time in understanding the subject and creating the most relevant covers. They scrutinized every image to scout for the most suitable representation of the subject and create an appropriate cover for the book.

The publishing team has been an ardent support to the editorial, designing and production team. Their endless efforts to recruit the best for this project, has resulted in the accomplishment of this book. They are a veteran in the field of academics and their pool of knowledge is as vast as their experience in printing. Their expertise and guidance has proved useful at every step. Their uncompromising quality standards have made this book an exceptional effort. Their encouragement from time to time has been an inspiration for everyone.

The publisher and the editorial board hope that this book will prove to be a valuable piece of knowledge for researchers, students, practitioners and scholars across the globe.

List of Contributors

Narayan Sastry, Paula Fomby and Katherine McGonagle
Survey Research Center, Institute for Social Research, University of Michigan, 426 Thompson Street, Ann Arbor, MI 48106, USA

Pamela Salsberry
College of Public Health, Division of Health Behavior, Health Promotion, Institute for Population Health, The Ohio State University, 1841 Neil Avenue, 353 Cunz Hall, Columbus, OH 43210, USA

Rika Tanda
College of Health Science and Professions, Ohio University, Grover Center W133B, Athens, OH 45701, USA

Sarah E. Anderson
The Ohio State University, College of Public Health, 336 Cunz Hall, 1841 Neil Avenue, Columbus, OH 43210, USA

Manmohan K. Kamboj
The Ohio State University, College of Medicine, Endocrinology, Metabolism and Diabetes, Nationwide Children's Hospital, 700 Children's Drive (ED425), Columbus, OH 43205, USA

Todd D. Little
Texas Tech University, Lubbock, TX, USA

Abigail Fraser and Deborah A. Lawlor
Medical Research Council Integrative Epidemiology Unit at the University of Bristol, University of Bristol, Bristol, UK BS8 2BN

Janet M. Catov
Department of Obestetrics and Gynecology, University of Pittsburgh, Pittsburgh, PA 15213, USA
University of Pittsburgh, Department of Epidemiology, Pittsburgh, PA 15261, USA
Magee-Womens Research Institute, Pittsburgh, PA 15213, USA

Janet W. Rich-Edwards
Connors Center for Women's Health and Gender Biology, Brigham and Women's Hospital, Boston, MA 02120, USA
Harvard Medical School, Boston, MA 02115, USA
Harvard School of Public Health, Boston, MA 02120, USA

Stephen L. Buka, Samantha R. Rosenthal and Mary E. Lacy
Department of Epidemiology, Brown University, Providence, RI, USA

Elizabeth C. Cooksey
Center for Human Resource Research, The Ohio State University, Suite 200, 921 Chatham Lane, Columbus, OH 43221, USA

Irene E. Drmic
Hospital for Sick Children, Toronto, ON, Canada

Peter Szatmari
Centre for Addiction and Mental Health, Hospital for Sick Children, University of Toronto, Toronto, ON, Canada

Fred Volkmar
Child Study Center, Yale University School of Medicine, New Haven, CT, USA

Neal Halfon
Department of Pediatrics, David Geffen School of Medicine, UCLA, Los Angeles, CA, USA
Department of Health Policy and Management, Fielding School of Public Health, UCLA, Los Angeles, CA, USA
Department of Public Policy, Luskin School of Public Affairs, UCLA, Los Angeles, CA, USA
Center for Healthier Children, Families and Communities, UCLA, Los Angeles, CA, USA

Christopher B. Forrest
Applied Clinical Research Center, Children's Hospital of Philadelphia, Philadelphia, PA, USA

Richard M. Lerner
Tufts University, Medford, MA, USA

Elaine M. Faustman
Institute for Risk Analysis and Risk Communication, Department of Environmental and Occupational Health Sciences, School of Public Health, University of Washington, Seattle, WA 98105, USA

Ericka Tullis and John Son
Center for Healthier Children, Families and Communities, UCLA, Los Angeles, CA, USA

David Wood
Department of Pediatrics, ETSU College of Medicine, Johnson City, TN 37614, USA

Tara Crapnell, Lynette Lau, Debra Lotstein, Maria Ferris and Alice Kuo
UCLA, Department of Pediatrics, Los Angeles, CA, USA

Ashley Bennett
Department of Pediatrics, USC, Los Angeles, CA, USA

Index

www.ingramcontent.com/pod-product-compliance
Lightning Source LLC
LaVergne TN
LVHW080609210926
848485LV00003B/124